REFERENCE EDITION

Pediatric ESAP™ 2023-2024

Endocrine Society's
Pediatric Endocrine Self-Assessment Program
Questions, Answers, and Discussions

Liuska M. Pesce, MD, Program Chair
Clinical Professor
Pediatric Thyroid Clinic Director
Stead Family Children's Hospital
Division of Pediatric Endocrinology and Diabetes
University of Iowa Carver College of Medicine

Li Chan, MD
Reader in Molecular Endocrinology
and Metabolism
Honorary Consultant in
Paediatric Endocrinology
Centre for Endocrinology
William Harvey Research Institute

Cem S. Demirci, MD
Director, Type 1 Diabetes Program
Connecticut Children's Medical Center

Oscar Escobar, MD
Associate Professor
University of Pittsburgh
School of Medicine
UPMC Children's Hospital of Pittsburgh

Reema L. Habiby, MD
Associate Professor of Pediatrics
Northwestern University
Feinberg School of Medicine
Ann & Robert H. Lurie Children's
Hospital of Chicago

Shana McCormack, MD
Assistant Professor of Pediatrics
Children's Hospital of Philadelphia

Ryan S. Miller, MD
Associate Professor
University of Maryland
School of Medicine

Ron Newfield, MD
Clinical Professor
University of California – San Diego
Rady Children's Hospital San Diego

Siobhan Pittock, MD
Pediatric Endocrinologist
Mayo Clinic

Sripriya Raman, MD
Pediatric Endocrinologist
K S Pediatrics

Christine Trapp, MD
Pediatric Endocrinology, Connecticut
Children's Medical Center
Associate Fellowship Director,
Pediatric Endocrinology
Assistant Professor of Pediatrics,
University of Connecticut
School of Medicine

Halley Wasserman, MD
Assistant Professor
Cincinnati Children's Hospital
Medical Center

Ari Wassner, MD
Medical Director, Thyroid Center
Director, Endocrinology
Fellowship Training Program
Associate Professor of Pediatrics
Boston Children's Hospital
Harvard Medical School

Abbie L. Young, MS, CGC, ELS(D)
Medical Editor

Endocrine Society
2055 L Street NW, Suite 600, Washington, DC 20036
1-888-ENDOCRINE • www.endocrine.org

ENDOCRINE
SOCIETY
Hormone Science to Health

ENDOCRINE
SOCIETY

Hormone Science to Health

The Endocrine Society is the world's largest, oldest, and most active organization working to advance the clinical practice of endocrinology and hormone research. Founded in 1916, the Society now has more than 18,000 global members across a range of disciplines. The Society has earned an international reputation for excellence in the quality of its peer-reviewed journals, educational resources, meetings, and programs that improve public health through the practice and science of endocrinology.

For between-edition updates, visit us at:
endocrine.org/education-and-training/book-updates

Other publications: endocrine.org/publications

ISBN: 978-1-936704-26-2

Library of Congress Control Number: 2022951810

On the Cover: © Shutterstock. Science, Safety, Research, Technology lab tube with a pipette.

OVERVIEW

The Pediatric Endocrine Self-Assessment Program (Pediatric ESAP™) is a self-study curriculum specifically designed for endocrinologists seeking initial certification or recertification in pediatric endocrinology, program directors interested in a training instrument, and clinicians seeking a self-assessment and a broad review of pediatric endocrinology. Pediatric ESAP consists of 100 multiple-choice questions in all areas of pediatric endocrinology, diabetes, growth, and metabolism. There is extensive discussion of each correct answer and references.

Pediatric ESAP is composed of two key components: the online interactive module and the printed book. Upon purchase, learners initially receive access to the online module. To use Pediatric as a true self-assessment tool, learners are strongly encouraged to complete the online interactive self-assessment module first before continuing self-study with the printed book; the online module may be accessed at education.endocrine.org.

LEARNING OBJECTIVES

Pediatric ESAP 2023-2024 allows learners to assess their knowledge of all aspects of pediatric endocrinology. Upon completion of this educational activity, participants will be able to:

- Recognize clinical manifestations of pediatric endocrine, growth, and metabolic disorders and select among current options for diagnosis, management, and therapy.
- Identify risk factors for endocrine and metabolic disorders in pediatric patients and develop strategies for prevention.
- Evaluate pediatric endocrine and metabolic manifestations of systemic disorders.
- Use current, evidence-based clinical guidelines and treatment recommendations to guide diagnosis and treatment of pediatric endocrine and metabolic disorders.

TARGET AUDIENCE

Pediatric ESAP is a self-study curriculum aimed at physicians seeking initial certification or recertification in endocrinology, program directors interested in a testing and training instrument, and clinicians simply wanting a self-assessment and broad review of endocrinology.

STATEMENT OF INDEPENDENCE

The Endocrine Society has a policy of ensuring that the content and quality of this educational activity are balanced, independent, objective, and scientifically rigorous. The scientific content of this activity was developed under the supervision of the Endocrine Society's Pediatric ESAP Faculty Working Group.

DISCLOSURE POLICY

The faculty, committee members, and staff who are in position to control the content of this activity are required to disclose to the Endocrine Society and to learners any relevant financial relationship(s) of the individual or spouse/partner that have occurred within the last 12 months with any commercial interest(s) whose products or services are related to the content. Financial relationships are defined by remuneration in any amount from the commercial interest(s) in the form of grants; research support; consulting fees; salary; ownership interest (eg, stocks, stock options, or ownership interest excluding diversified mutual funds); honoraria or other payments for participation in speakers' bureaus, advisory boards, or boards of directors; or other financial benefits. The intent of this disclosure is not to prevent planners with relevant financial relationships from planning or delivering content, but rather to provide learners with information that allows them to make their own judgments of whether these financial relationships may have influenced the educational activity with regard to exposition or conclusion. The Endocrine Society has reviewed all disclosures and resolved or managed all identified conflicts of interest, as applicable.

The following faculty reported relevant financial relationship(s): **Li Chan, MD,** is an advisory board member of OMass Therapeutics and Great Ormond Street Hospital Children's Charity Research. **Oscar Escobar, MD,** is a board member of the Human Growth Foundation. He is a primary investigator in industry-supported multicentric study for Pfizer, OPKO, and Novo Nordisk. **Shana McCormack, MD,** is an NIH grantee and grant reviewer. She is a grantee of the Doris Duke Charitable Foundation and the Friedreich Ataxia Research Alliance. She is a consultant for Rhythm Pharmaceuticals and Reata Pharmaceuticals. **Ryan S. Miller, MD,** is an NIH grantee. **Ron Newfield, MD,** is a principal investigator for Spruce and Neurocrine for new medications; a consultant for Spruce; a consultant and member of the Independent Safety Committee for Ascendis; a principal investigator for Merck; and a principal investigator for Zealand for dasiglucagon. **Ari Wassner, MD,** is a topic peer reviewer for UpToDate (thyroid).

The following faculty reported no relevant financial relationships: **Cem S. Demirci, MD; Reema L. Habiby, MD; Liuska M. Pesce, MD; Siobhan Pittock, MD; Sripriya Raman, MD; Christine Trapp, MD; and Halley Wasserman, MD.**

The medical editor for this program, **Abbie L. Young, MS, CGC, ELS(D),** reported no relevant financial relationships.

The Endocrine Society staff associated with the development of content for this activity reported no relevant financial relationships.

DISCLAIMERS

The information presented in this activity represents the opinion of the faculty and is not necessarily the official position of the Endocrine Society.

USE OF PROFESSIONAL JUDGMENT:

The educational content in this self-assessment test relates to basic principles of diagnosis and therapy and does not substitute for individual patient assessment based on the health care provider's examination of the patient and consideration of laboratory data and other factors unique to the patient. Standards in medicine change as new data become available.

DRUGS AND DOSAGES:

When prescribing medications, the physician is advised to check the product information sheet accompanying each drug to verify conditions of use and to identify any changes in drug dosage schedule or contraindications.

POLICY ON UNLABELED/OFF-LABEL USE

The Endocrine Society has determined that disclosure of unlabeled/off-label or investigational use of commercial product(s) is informative for audiences and therefore requires this information to be disclosed to the learners at the beginning of the presentation. Uses of specific therapeutic agents, devices, and other products discussed in this educational activity may not be the same as those indicated in product labeling approved by the Food and Drug Administration (FDA). The Endocrine Society requires that any discussions of such "off-label" use be based on scientific research that conforms to generally accepted standards of experimental design, data collection, and data analysis. Before recommending or prescribing any therapeutic agent or device, learners should review the complete prescribing information, including indications, contraindications, warnings, precautions, and adverse events.

ACKNOWLEDGMENT OF COMMERCIAL SUPPORT

This activity is not supported by educational grant(s) or other funds from any commercial supporter.

PUBLICATION DATE: February 2023

Common Abbreviations Used in Pediatric ESAP

ACTH --- corticotropin

ACE inhibitor---------------angiotensin-converting enzyme inhibitor

ALT ---------------------------------------alanine aminotransferase

AST ------------------------------- aspartate aminotransferase

BMI --body mass index

CNS--- central nervous system

CT--- computed tomography

DHEA --dehydroepiandrosterone

DHEA-S-----------------------------dehydroepiandrosterone sulfate

DNA --------------------------------------- deoxyribonucleic acid

DPP-4 inhibitor --------------------- dipeptidyl-peptidase 4 inhibitor

DXA---------------------------- dual-energy x-ray absorptiometry

FDA------------------------------- Food and Drug Administration

FGF-23 --------------------------------- fibroblast growth factor 23

FNA-- fine-needle aspiration

FSH ----------------------------------- follicle-stimulating hormone

GH --- growth hormone

GHRH-------------------------- growth hormone–releasing hormone

GLP-1 receptor agonist-----glucagonlike peptide 1 receptor agonist

GnRH ---------------------------- gonadotropin-releasing hormone

hCG --------------------------------- human chorionic gonadotropin

HDL-- high-density lipoprotein

HIV-----------------------------------human immunodeficiency virus

HMG-CoA reductase inhibitor ---
        3-hydroxy-3-methylglutaryl coenzyme A reductase inhibitor

IGF-1------------------------------------- insulinlike growth factor 1

LDL -- low-density lipoprotein

LH ---luteinizing hormone

MCV ------------------------------------- mean corpuscular volume

MIBG------------------------------------ meta-iodobenzylguanidine

MRI ------------------------------------ magnetic resonance imaging

NPH insulin --------------------- neutral protamine Hagedorn insulin

PCSK9 inhibitor----proprotein convertase subtilisin/kexin 9 inhibitor

PET ---------------------------------- positron emission tomography

PSA -- prostate-specific antigen

PTH --- parathyroid hormone

PTHrP----------------------- parathyroid hormone–related protein

SGLT-2 inhibitor ---------- sodium-glucose cotransporter 2 inhibitor

SHBG -----------------------------sex hormone–binding globulin

T_3 -- triiodothyronine

T_4 --- thyroxine

TPO antibodies --------------------------thyroperoxidase antibodies

TRH------------------------------- thyrotropin-releasing hormone

TRAb --------------------------------------TSH-receptor antibodies

TSH --- thyrotropin

VLDL-------------------------------- very low-density lipoprotein

PEDIATRIC ENDOCRINE SELF-ASSESSMENT PROGRAM 2023-2024

Part I

1 A 10-year-old girl presents for follow-up of Turner syndrome, which was diagnosed by chromosome analysis in infancy. She has since been followed by her pediatric endocrinologist. She has no history of atypical genitalia, developmental delay, or hypothyroidism. Her height gradually drifted down from the 25th percentile to below the 5th percentile at age 7 years, at which point she started GH therapy with good results. Her midparental target height is 64 in (162.5 cm) (~40th percentile).

At today's appointment, her examination findings are notable for Tanner stage 3 breast development. Her height is at the 15th percentile, and her bone age is consistent with chronologic age.

She is doing well in school and has no headaches, vision problems, fatigue, constipation, abdominal pain, or cold intolerance.

Based on her clinical presentation, which of the following is this patient's most likely karyotype?
- A. 45,X monosomy
- B. 45,X/46,XX mosaicism
- C. 45,X/46,XY mosaicism
- D. Ring chromosome X (46,X,r[X])
- E. Xq deletion (46,XX,del[q24])

2 An 8-year-old girl is referred for evaluation of prediabetes. Recent bloodwork documents a fasting plasma glucose concentration of 110 mg/dL (6.1 mmol/L). Her point-of-care hemoglobin A_{1c} value in clinic is 6.0% (42 mmol/mol). Her current height is 47.2 in (120 cm) (9th percentile; Z-score, −1.34), and weight is 198.5 lb (90 kg) (100th percentile; Z-score, 3.9). Review of her previous growth records reveals that she has had progressive rapid weight gain that started during the first year of life. Her parents say that she is "always hungry." Her medical history is notable for vision impairment that was evident by 9 months of age. She has marked photophobia and nystagmus, as well as progressive vision loss. She is in third grade and there are no concerns of intellectual difficulties. Her parents are worried that she is experiencing hearing loss, which is currently being evaluated.

Pertinent physical examination findings include nystagmus, poor visual acuity, moderate acanthosis nigricans on her neck, normal digits, and truncal obesity.

Additional laboratory testing documents a low free T_4 concentration, and levothyroxine is prescribed. Given the suspicion for a monogenic obesity syndrome, genetic testing is discussed with the family.

A pathogenic variant in which of the following genes is most likely to be identified in this patient?
- A. *ALMS1* (ALMS1 centrosome and basal body associated protein)
- B. *BBS1* (Bardet-Biedl syndrome 1)
- C. *LEP* (leptin)
- D. *LEPR* (leptin receptor)
- E. *POMC* (proopiomelanocortin)

3 A 10-year-old boy with autism and sensory processing disorder presents with several months of foot pain and refusal to bear weight. He was previously active in baseball, but over the last several weeks he has been unable to participate because of pain. He has had no known trauma and has no obvious lower-extremity deformity noted on examination. There is no history of easy bruising or bleeding. His mother reports he is a picky eater and does not take a multivitamin. A radiograph is shown (*see image*).

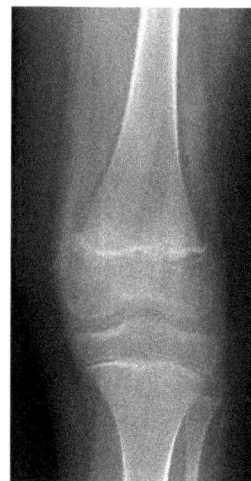

Measurement of which micronutrient or mineral is most likely to reveal the source of this patient's bony abnormalities?
- A. Calcium
- B. Lead
- C. Vitamin C
- D. Vitamin D
- E. Vitamin K

4 A 5-year-old girl has been referred after a recent diagnosis of adrenal insufficiency. She initially presented to her primary care physician with a history of tiredness, reduced appetite, and noticeably hyperpigmented skin.

Laboratory test results:
    Random cortisol = 0.91 μg/dL (4.8-19.5 μg/dL) (SI: 25 nmol/L [133-537 nmol/L])
    ACTH = 1500 pg/mL (<50 pg/mL) (SI: 330 pmol/L [<11 pmol/L])
    Serum urea nitrogen, normal
    Electrolytes, normal
    Serum aldosterone = 5.6 ng/dL (5.4-19.8 ng/dL [supine]) (SI: 155 pmol/L [150-550 pmol/L])
    Renin plasma activity = 1.5 ng/mL per h (0.6-3.8 ng/mL per h)

The patient has an 11-year-old brother diagnosed with attention-deficit/hyperactivity disorder and a 14-year-old brother with essential tremor who is under the care of a neurologist. The parents are consanguineous.

On physical examination, the patient is growing along the 25th percentile for height and weight. She has no dysmorphic features and is hyperpigmented. Her reflexes are very brisk.

Which of the following tests would be most helpful in diagnosing the cause of this patient's adrenal insufficiency?
    A. Barium swallow
    B. Muscle biopsy
    C. Test for tear production (Schirmer test)
    D. Ultrasonography of the adrenal glands
    E. Very long-chain fatty acid measurement

5 A 16-and-9/12-year-old girl with obesity seeks evaluation for elevated LDL cholesterol and total cholesterol. She has limited consumption of eggs, cheese, and red meat. She drinks 2 to 3 cups of 1% milk per week. She eats large amounts of rice and beans and has second helpings several times a week. There are no concerns about fatigue or constipation. Menarche was at age 10 years, and she has regular periods.

She has no clear family history of hypercholesterolemia, except in her paternal grandmother. However, not much is known about her father, as she has lived with her mother for many years. Her mother's height is 62 in (157.5 cm).

On physical examination, her height is 63.8 in (162 cm) (45th percentile for age) and weight is 180.8 lb (82.2 kg) (96th percentile for age) (BMI = 31.3 kg/m² [97th percentile for age]). Her blood pressure is 113/71 mm Hg, and pulse rate is 75 beats/min. She has central adiposity. There is no goiter. She has no acne, hirsutism, acanthosis nigricans, or xanthomas. Breasts and pubic hair are Tanner stage 5. There is no edema. The rest of her examination findings are normal.

Laboratory test results (samples drawn while fasting):
    Total cholesterol = 326 mg/dL (100-169 mg/dL) (SI: 8.44 mmol/L [2.59-4.38 mmol/L])
    LDL cholesterol = 238 mg/dL (0-109 mg/dL) (SI: 6.16 mmol/L [0-2.82 mmol/L])
    HDL cholesterol = 64 mg/dL (>39 mg/dL) (SI: 1.66 mmol/L [>1.01 mmol/L])
    Triglycerides =130 mg/dL (0-89 mg/dL) (SI: 1.47 mmol/L [0-1.01 mmol/L])
    White blood cell count = 7000/μL (3400-10,800/μL) (SI: 7.0 × 10⁹/L [3.4-10.8 × 10⁹/L])
    Hemoglobin = 9.7 g/dL (11.1-15.9 g/dL) (SI: 97 g/L [111-159 g/L])
    Mean corpuscular volume = 89 μm³ (79-97 μm³) (SI: 89 fL [79-97 fL])
    Red cell distribution width = 14.9% (11.7%-15.4%)
    Platelet count = 155 × 10³/μL (150-450 × 10³/μL) (SI: 155 × 10⁹/L [150-450 × 10⁹/L])
    Glucose = 80 mg/dL (70-99 mg/dL) (SI: 4.4 mmol/L [3.9-5.5 mmol/L])
    Sodium = 138 mEq/L (134-144 mEq/L) (SI: 138 mmol/L [134-144 mmol/L])
    Potassium = 4.0 mEq/L (3.5-5.2 mEq/L) (SI: 4.0 mmol/L [3.5-5.2 mmol/L])
    Serum urea nitrogen = 12 mg/dL (5-18 mg/dL) (SI: 4.3 mmol/L [1.8-6.4 mmol/L])

Creatinine = 1.08 mg/dL (0.57-1.00 mg/dL) (SI: 95.5 µmol/L [50.4-88.4 µmol/L])
Albumin = 5.0 g/dL (3.9-5.0 g/dL) (SI: 50 g/L [39-50 g/L])
ALT = 14 U/L (0-24 U/L) (SI: 0.23 µkat/L [0-0.40 µkat/L])

Urinalysis:
    Protein = +1
    Glucose = Negative
    Ketones = Negative
    Leukocytes or red cells = None noted
    Urine specific gravity = 1.027 (1.005-1.030)

Regarding this patient's hypercholesterolemia, which of the following is the best next step?
A. Discuss genetic testing to determine the etiology of her hypercholesterolemia
B. Measure TSH
C. Refer to a dietitian and recommend a diet low in saturated fat
D. Start atorvastatin, 10 mg daily
E. Start ezetimibe, 10 mg daily

6   A 3-and-6/12-year-old girl presents for evaluation of rapid growth. She was born full-term via vaginal delivery after an uncomplicated gestation. Her size was adequate for gestational age, with a birth weight of 7 lb 6 oz (3450 g) (25th percentile; Z-score, –0.65) and birth length of 19.7 in (50 cm) (23rd percentile; Z-score –0.72). She progressed along the 25th percentile for length and weight until age 13 months and then started crossing up percentiles rapidly to well above the 97th percentile. Her parents report a remarkable increase in appetite over the last 1.5 to 2 years. Developmental milestones seem appropriate.

On physical examination, her height is 44.1 in (112 cm) (>97th percentile; Z-score, +3.38) and weight is 55 lb (25 kg) (>97th percentile; Z-score, +3.17). She has no significant dysmorphic features or abnormal skin findings. Breasts and pubic hair are Tanner stage 1. There is no axillary hair, acne, or oiliness of the face or scalp.

Laboratory test results:
    TSH, normal
    Free T₄, normal
    IGF-1 = 950 ng/mL (74-202 ng/mL) (SI: 124.5 nmol/L [9.7-26.5 nmol/L])
    Random GH = 605 ng/mL (0-6 ng/mL) (SI: 605 µg/L [0-6 µg/L])
    Prolactin = 586 ng/mL (3-24 ng/mL) (SI: 26.5 nmol/L [0.1-1.0 nmol/L])

Brain/pituitary MRI demonstrates a pituitary macroadenoma with suprasellar extension.

Which of the following is this patient's most likely diagnosis?
A. McCune-Albright syndrome
B. Neurofibromatosis type 1
C. Sotos syndrome
D. Tatton-Brown-Rahman syndrome
E. X-linked acrogigantism

7   A 16-day-old male newborn with a birth history notable for shoulder dystocia presents to the emergency department with irritability and possible seizures.

On physical examination, he is afebrile. His blood pressure is 88/41 mm Hg, pulse rate is 140 beats/min, weight is 8.8 lb (4 kg) (99th percentile), length is 21.0 in (53.3 cm) (98th percentile), and head circumference is 13.0 in (33 cm) (41st percentile). His mucous membranes are moist. No heart murmur is detected on examination. There is no edema.

Laboratory test results:

    Sodium = 125 mEq/L (136-149 mEq/L) (SI: 125 mmol/L [136-149 mmol/L])

    Potassium = 4.7 mEq/L (4.4-6.6 mEq/L) (SI: 4.7 mmol/L [4.4-6.6 mmol/L])

    Chloride = 96 mEq/L (98-108 mEq/L) (SI: 96 mmol/L [98-108 mmol/L])

    Carbon dioxide = 21 mEq/L (20-27 mEq/L) (SI: 21 mmol/L [20-27 mmol/L])

    Glucose = 76 mg/dL (40-80 mg/dL) (SI: 4.2 mmol/L [2.2-4.4 mmol/L])

    Serum urea nitrogen = 2 mg/dL (5-15 mg/dL) (SI: 0.71 mmol/L [1.79-5.36 mmol/L])

    Creatinine = 0.4 mg/dL (0.25-0.54 mg/dL) (SI: 35.4 µmol/L [22.1-47.7 µmol/L])

    Serum osmolality = 259 mOsm/kg (285-295 mOsm/kg) (SI: 259 mmol/kg [285-295 mmol/kg])

    Urine osmolality = 350 mOsm/kg (50-1400 mOsm/kg) (SI: 350 mmol/kg [50-1400 mmol/kg])

    Spot urinary sodium = 52 mEq/L (SI: 52 mmol/L)

    Arginine vasopressin <1 pg/mL (1.0-13.3 pg/mL)

Which of the following is the most likely cause of this patient's hyponatremia?

    A. Cerebral salt-wasting

    B. Congenital adrenal hyperplasia

    C. Diabetes insipidus

    D. Nephrogenic syndrome of inappropriate antidiuresis

    E. Syndrome of inappropriate antidiuretic hormone secretion

8 A 17-year-old boy presents with 2 weeks of new palpitations, insomnia, and restlessness. He reports no neck swelling or tenderness, eye symptoms, or history of recent viral symptoms. His medical history is notable for depression treated with sertraline, acne treated with minocycline, and asthma treated with as-needed albuterol. He takes no other medications or supplements. He has no family history of thyroid or autoimmune disease.

    Physical examination reveals tachycardia (pulse rate = 120 beats/min) and normal blood pressure. His thyroid gland is normal in size and texture and is nontender. There are no palpable nodules. His eyes are normal.

Laboratory test results:

    TSH = <0.005 mIU/L (0.7-5.7 mIU/L)

    Free T$_4$ = 2.3 ng/dL (0.76-1.46 ng/dL) (SI: 29.6 pmol/L [9.8-18.8 pmol/L])

    Thyroglobulin = 54 ng/mL (<29.4 ng/mL) (SI: 54 µg/L [<29.4 µg/L])

    TPO antibodies = <14.9 IU/mL (<14.9 IU/mL) (SI: <14.9 kIU/L [<14.9 kIU/L])

    Thyroglobulin antibodies = <0.9 IU/mL (<0.9 IU/mL) (SI: <0.9 kIU/L [<0.9 kIU/L])

    Thyroid-stimulating immunoglobulin = 98% (<109%)

    TRAb = <1.75 IU/L (<1.75 IU/L)

In addition to initiating a β-adrenergic blocker for symptomatic relief, which of the following is the most appropriate next step in this patient's management?

    A. Measure erythrocyte sedimentation rate

    B. Measure serum biotin

    C. Question the patient about exogenous thyroid hormone ingestion

    D. Recommend discontinuation of minocycline

    E. Start methimazole treatment

9 Endocrine consultation is requested for an 18-month-old boy who is on a ventilator because of *Staphylococcus aureus* pneumonia. He has underlying adrenal insufficiency that was diagnosed at 2 months of age when he presented with hyperpigmentation.

Laboratory test results at the time of diagnosis:

    Serum sodium = 135 mEq/L (133-146 mEq/L) (SI: 135 mmol/L [133-146 mmol/L])

    Serum potassium = 5.5 mEq/L (3.5-5.3 mEq/L) (SI: 5.5 mmol/L [3.5-5.3 mmol/L])

Serum cortisol = 3.5 μg/dL (7.8-26.2 μg/dL) (SI: 96.6 nmol/L [215.2-722.8 nmol/L])
Plasma ACTH = 550 pg/mL (4.5-48.6 pg/mL) (SI: 121 pmol/L [1.0-10.7 pmol/L])
Serum aldosterone = <0.9 ng/dL (1.4-17.3 ng/dL) (SI: <25 pmol/L [40-480 pmol/L])
Plasma renin activity = 66 ng/mL per h (2.4-37 ng/mL/h [0-11 months])

He is the first child of healthy, nonconsanguineous parents. He was born at 27 weeks' gestation by emergency cesarean delivery for intrauterine growth restriction and suspected fetal distress. Birth weight was 600 g (−4.6 SDS). He had microphallus, hypospadias, and a bifid scrotum. During the neonatal period, he had transient anemia and thrombocytopenia, which were treated with a packed red blood cell transfusion and prophylactic platelet transfusions. Ultrasonography could not identify the adrenal glands. From the age of 7 months, he had multiple episodes of infection, including gastroenteritis, urinary tract infections, respiratory syncytial virus bronchitis, and *Candida albicans* pneumonia requiring multiple hospital admissions. He has developmental delay and is undergoing evaluation for loose stools. He is currently being treated with intravenous hydrocortisone and oral fludrocortisone. He has required both packed red blood cell transfusion and platelet transfusions during this admission.

His intensive care physician inquires about the most likely cause of his adrenal insufficiency.

Which of the following is this patient's most likely diagnosis?
A. Antley-Bixler syndrome
B. Autoimmune polyendocrine syndrome type 1
C. Autoimmune polyendocrine syndrome type 2
D. IMAGe syndrome
E. MIRAGE syndrome

10 A 12-and-3/12-year-old boy with no notable medical history is referred to pediatric endocrinology for evaluation of short stature. His family has moved frequently due to his father's job, and the patient has not had a consistent primary care provider. However, his parents bring a growth chart with compilation of data from different care providers. His height has always been below the 3rd percentile but has progressed parallel to it.

On physical examination, his height is 52.8 in (134 cm) (<3rd percentile; −2.3 SDS) and weight is 64.9 lb (29.5 kg) (<3rd percentile; −2.0 SDS). He has normal body proportions, no dysmorphic features, and Tanner stage 3 pubic hair and genitalia with a testicular volume of 10 mL bilaterally.

Bone age is interpreted to be 13 years. According to the tables of Bayley-Pinneau, he has attained 87.6% of his adult height. This renders a predicted adult height of 60.2 in (152.9 cm) (midparental target height = 68.5 in ± 3.9 in [174 cm ± 10 cm]).

Laboratory testing shows normal IGF-1 concentration for age; normal thyroid function; normal complete blood cell count; negative celiac disease screen; normal inflammatory markers; and normal complete metabolic panel with no evidence of kidney dysfunction, liver dysfunction, or dysglycemia.

Which of the following interventions would be most likely to help improve this patient's final height outcome while minimizing untoward metabolic effects?
A. Aromatase inhibitor
B. Recombinant human GH and a GnRH analogue
C. Recombinant human GH and an aromatase inhibitor
D. Oxandrolone
E. Testosterone cypionate intramuscularly

11 A 3-year-old girl is found to have significant rachitic changes on x-ray done for evaluation of a tibial fracture. Laboratory testing reveals normal serum 25-hydroxyvitamin D and calcium levels but low serum phosphate. Tubular resorption of phosphate is 63%. The FGF-23 concentration is at the high end of normal. Family history is notable for rickets in the father, paternal grandmother, and paternal aunt. The father recalls having a mild bowing deformity that resolved as he got older, whereas his sister and mother did not manifest skeletal issues until late adolescence and young adulthood.

What additional finding is most likely given the child's genetic condition?
   A. Conductive hearing loss
   B. Elevated 1,25-dihydroxyvitamin D_3
   C. Elevated urinary phosphoethanolamine
   D. Low serum alkaline phosphatase
   E. Low serum iron

12 A 13-year-old pubertal boy with obesity (BMI = 30.5 kg/m² [>99th percentile]) presents with polyuria, polydipsia, nocturia, and weight loss. Laboratory testing documents a random blood glucose concentration of 275 mg/dL (15.3 mmol/L) and a hemoglobin A_{1c} level of 10.3% (89 mmol/mol). Urine ketones are negative. His medical history is notable for transient hyperinsulinemic hypoglycemia that required diazoxide treatment until his third birthday and subsequently resolved. He started gaining excess weight in preschool. He has a family history of type 2 diabetes mellitus and obesity.

Which of the following tests would most likely help identify the etiology of this patient's diabetes mellitus?
   A. Genetic testing for *LEP, LEPR, POMC,* and *MC4R* pathogenic variants
   B. Genetic testing for *ABCC8* or *KCNJ11* pathogenic variants
   C. Measurement of antibodies (islet cell, insulin, glutamic acid decarboxylase 65, ZnT8)
   D. Oral glucose tolerance testing and measurement of proinsulin, insulin, and C-peptide
   E. PET and tandem CT of the pancreas

13 A 20-year-old man presents for a follow-up appointment in the pituitary clinic. For the last 10 years, he has been treated for traumatic brain injury–induced central hypothyroidism. He has gained 22 lb (10 kg) in the last year. He states that he can no longer run for an hour a day as he did previously. He has had no changes in his dietary habits. His thyroid hormone, cortisol, gonadotropin, and testosterone concentrations are normal. GH deficiency is suspected.
   The endocrine fellow reports that when she discussed various testing options with the patient, he chose macimorelin (an oral agent) for stimulation testing. The endocrine fellow asks for an explanation of how the agent stimulates GH secretion.

Which of the following describes this agent's mechanism of action when used to test the patient for adult GH deficiency?
   A. Inhibits somatostatin binding to its receptor in pituitary somatotrophs
   B. Stimulates endogenous ghrelin secretion
   C. Stimulates endogenous insulin secretion
   D. Stimulates GH secretagogue receptor 1α in the hypothalamus and pituitary
   E. Stimulates hypoglycemia-induced GH secretion

14 A couple is referred by the genetics clinic for prenatal counseling to discuss a fetal diagnosis of Klinefelter syndrome. Cell-free fetal DNA screening performed due to advanced maternal age revealed an increased risk for 47,XXY. The pregnancy has been unremarkable, and no abnormalities have been identified on fetal ultrasonography. The parents are medically knowledgeable and have questions about treatment with testosterone in infancy.

How should the parents be advised regarding management after delivery?
   A. Initiate testosterone therapy at the time of minipuberty
   B. Measure LH, FSH, and testosterone at 2 months of age to assess the need for testosterone therapy
   C. Perform postnatal chromosome testing on cord blood or peripheral blood to guide decision-making
   D. Plan for follow-up and low-dosage oxandrolone therapy in early childhood
   E. Plan for follow-up at the age of puberty to assess hormonal status and the need for testosterone therapy

15

A 9-year-old girl with obesity is being evaluated for short stature. Records show that her height had been progressing along the 5th percentile, but during the last year, it dropped below the 3rd percentile. Her weight has always been at the 75th percentile (*see image*). The family recently moved from out of state where she had been evaluated by a local endocrinologist.

Laboratory test results:
IGF-1 = 131 ng/mL (SI: 17.2 nmol/L) (–1.3 SDS for age, sex,
    and stage of puberty)
TSH = 6.6 mIU/L (0.7-5.7 mIU/L)
Free T_4 = 1.6 ng/dL (0.78-1.89 ng/dL) (SI: 20.6 pmol/L
    [10.0-24.3 pmol/L])

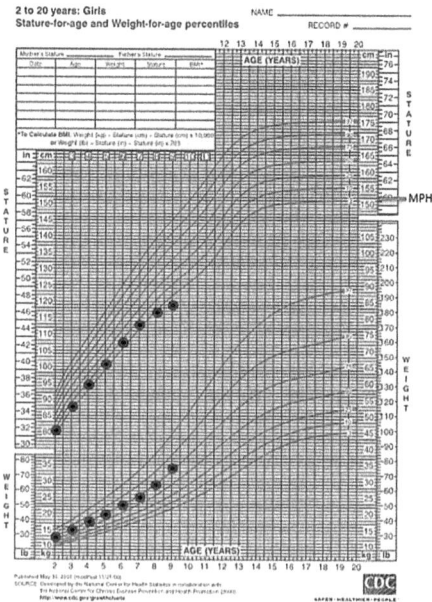

Her former endocrinologist ordered additional testing. Bone age was interpreted to be 8 years and 10 months at a chronologic age of 8 years and 11 months. A GH-stimulation test (arginine-carbidopa/levodopa) documented a peak GH concentration of 7.2 ng/mL (7.2 μg/L).

Her parents were informed that she has GH deficiency and were advised to establish care with an endocrinologist to start GH therapy after their move.

On physical examination, her height is 46.9 in (119 cm) (<3rd percentile; –2.35 SDS), weight is 73 lb (33.2 kg) (75th percentile; +0.69 SDS), and BMI is 23.4 kg/m^2 (97th percentile; +1.92 SDS). No dysmorphic features are observed on examination. She has Tanner stage 2 breast development and stage 1 pubic hair.

Her midparental target height is 59.8 in (152 cm) (5th percentile).

Which of the following is the most appropriate next step in this patient's management?
A. Perform an insulin-tolerance test to exclude GH deficiency before initiating therapy
B. Recommend nutrition consultation and follow-up in 6 months to assess weight, linear growth, and pubertal development
C. Start GH therapy
D. Start GnRH analogue therapy
E. Start levothyroxine replacement therapy

16

A 17-day-old female infant has a mildly elevated TSH concentration. She was born prematurely at 36 weeks' gestation, with a normal birth length and weight. Her mother had gestational diabetes. Findings on intrauterine ultrasonography were abnormal, and she was born with dysmorphic features, including small eyes, blepharophimosis, abnormal ears, bilateral club feet, and knee contractures. She also has bilateral hydronephrosis. After a genetics consultation, whole-genome genetic testing is ordered.

On physical examination, her weight is normal for age at 6.2 lb (2.8 kg). No goiter is present.

Newborn screening at 24 hours of life reported a normal TSH value of 25.99 mIU/L (<29.0 mIU/L).

Laboratory test results:
Day of life 14:
    TSH = 13.74 mIU/L (1.00-10.00 mIU/L)
Day of life 19:
    TSH = 20.50 mIU/L (1.00-10.00 mIU/L)
    Free T_4 = 0.98 ng/dL (0.71-1.85 ng/dL) (SI: 12.6 pmol/L [9.1-23.8 pmol/L])

Neck ultrasonography shows a normal-sized, normally positioned thyroid gland.

While awaiting genetic testing results, which of the following is the best recommendation?
- A. Measure thyroid antibodies; if negative, order congenital hypothyroidism genetic panel
- B. Repeat TSH and free T_4 measurement in 2 weeks before starting levothyroxine
- C. Start levothyroxine, 25 mcg daily
- D. Start levothyroxine, 37.5 mcg daily
- E. Start levothyroxine, 44 mcg daily

17 A 7-year-old girl presents for follow-up. Proopiomelanocortin (POMC) deficiency was diagnosed after she exhibited rapid weight gain and significant hyperphagia in early life. Genetic testing confirmed a pathogenic variant in the *POMC* gene. In clinic today, her height is 48 in (122 cm) (51st percentile; 0.04 SDS), and her weight is 128 lb (58 kg) (99.9th percentile; 3.42 SDS). Her father reports limited success in managing her weight, despite keeping her active in gymnastics and working to limit her dietary intake at home. Over the past 6 months, she has gained 22.1 lb (10 kg). He is very concerned about this continued rapid weight gain, noting that it is starting to limit her physically. He is also worried about the risk for metabolic comorbidities related to severe obesity. He asks whether there is any approved pharmacotherapy that could be considered.

Which of the following medications would be the best recommendation for this patient?
- A. Metformin
- B. Orlistat
- C. Semaglutide
- D. Setmelanotide
- E. Topiramate/phentermine

18 A 14-year-old boy presents for evaluation of tall stature. Review of records from his pediatrician shows that his prenatal course was normal. His birth weight and birth length were appropriate for age. He has hypotonia, speech delay, dyslexia, and autistic spectrum disorder. He is otherwise a healthy child with normal appetite and activity.

On physical examination, he has macrocephaly, large testes (>25 mL), and normal Tanner stage 5 pubic hair distribution. Review of his growth chart documents that his height is 73 in (185.5 cm) (>97th percentile; 2.76 SDS), weight is 130 lb (59 kg) (76th percentile; 0.71 SDS), and BMI is 17.2 kg/m² (18th percentile; –0.65 SDS). His midparental target height is at the 75th percentile.

Laboratory test results:
  IGF-1 = 452 ng/mL (220-574 ng/mL) (SI: 59.2 nmol/L [28.8-75.2 nmol/L])
  TSH = 2.3 mIU/L (0.5-4.8 mIU/L)
  Free T_4 = 1.3 ng/dL (0.90-1.67 ng/dL) (SI: 16.7 pmol/L [11.6-21.5 pmol/L])
  LH = 5.0 mIU/mL (0.4-7.0 mIU/mL) (SI: 5.0 IU/L [0.4-7.0 IU/L])
  FSH = 3.2 mIU/mL (2.6-11.0 mIU/mL) (SI: 3.2 IU/L [2.6-11.0 IU/L])
  Total testosterone = 688 ng/dL (350-970 ng/dL) (SI: 23.9 nmol/L [12.1-33.7 nmol/L])

Which of the following is this patient's most likely diagnosis?
- A. 47,XXY
- B. 47,XYY
- C. Familial tall stature
- D. GH excess
- E. Marfan syndrome

19 A 7-and-7/12-year-old boy with congenital adrenal hyperplasia presents for follow-up. Congenital adrenal hyperplasia (CAH) was diagnosed at age 4-and-6/12 years when he presented with pubic hair and gonadal development. At that time, pubertal assessment revealed Tanner stage 3 genital development and pubic hair. Testicular volumes were 3 mL bilaterally, indicating that he did not have central precocious puberty.

Laboratory test results at diagnosis:
  Androstenedione = 1048.7 ng/dL (<22.9 ng/dL [prepubertal]) (SI: 26.6 nmol/L [<0.8 nmol/L])
  DHEA-S = 214 µg/dL (<185 µg/dL [prepubertal]) (SI: 5.8 µmol/L [<5.0 µmol/L])
  Testosterone = 144 ng/dL (<14 ng/dL [prepubertal]) (SI: 5.0 nmol/L [<0.5 nmol/L])
  17-Hydroxyprogesterone = 5347 ng/dL (<495 ng/dL [prepubertal]) (SI: 162 nmol/L [<15 nmol/L])
  ACTH = 76 pg/mL (<50 pg/mL) (SI: 16.7 pmol/L [<11 pmol/L])
  Aldosterone = 51.3 ng/dL (9.0-34.2 ng/dL [upright]) (SI: 1422 pmol/L [250-950 pmol/L])
  Cosyntropin-stimulation testing (standard):
    Baseline cortisol = 7.6 µg/dL (SI: 209 nmol/L)
    30-minute cortisol = 8.9 µg/dL (SI: 245 nmol/L)
    60-minute cortisol = 8.9 µg/dL (SI: 247 nmol/L)

At the time of diagnosis, the patient's bone age was 12.5 years (chronologic age, 4.5 years).

Genetic testing has confirmed compound heterozygosity for pathogenic variants in the *CYP21A2* gene (c.515T>A and c.293-13C>G). During today's appointment, the patient's mother states that she is 6 weeks pregnant (same father). Following the diagnosis of her first child, she recalls being told that she should inform the endocrinologist immediately if she became pregnant in the future.

After contacting the obstetric team, which of the following is the best recommendation?
  A. Chorionic villus sampling
  B. No intervention until after delivery
  C. Prenatal dexamethasone at a dosage of 10 mcg/kg per day
  D. Prenatal dexamethasone at a dosage of 20 mcg/kg per day
  E. Urgent ultrasonography to determine fetal age

20 A 9-year-old boy sustains a neck injury in a bicycle accident, and neck CT incidentally reveals a thyroid nodule. Thyroid ultrasonography ordered by his pediatrician demonstrates normal background thyroid parenchyma and a 0.8-cm, solid, isoechoic nodule with regular margins in the right thyroid lobe. No calcifications or abnormal lymph nodes are observed. The patient has no symptoms of hypothyroidism or thyrotoxicosis, and his TSH concentration is normal (1.2 mIU/L [reference range, 0.7-5.7 mIU/L]). He has no other notable medical history. His review of systems is positive for an itchy rash on his upper back that has been present since infancy. He lives with his 2 mothers. His biological mother has hypothyroidism, and his paternal family history is unknown.

On physical examination, he has a normal pulse rate and blood pressure. His thyroid gland is normal in size and texture, with no palpable nodules. He has no cervical lymphadenopathy. Skin examination reveals a 2-cm hyperpigmented, lichenified plaque on his left upper back, medial to the scapula. No other skin lesions are present.

Measuring which of the following would be most appropriate as the best next step in this patient's evaluation?
  A. Calcitonin
  B. Radioiodine uptake
  C. Thyroglobulin
  D. TPO antibodies
  E. TRAb

21 A 17-year-old girl presents with recurrent stress fractures of her feet and ankles. She is an avid dancer, often practicing more than 20 hours each week. She regularly sees a sports nutritionist to ensure adequate calcium, vitamin D, and protein in her diet. Her BMI is at the 25th percentile for age. She started puberty approximately 4 years ago but has not yet had menarche. Her linear growth has plateaued over the last 2 years. Her mother did not get her first period until age 16 years. Laboratory testing documents elevated FSH and low serum estradiol.

Which additional finding is most likely to be present?

A. Elevated osteocalcin
B. Elevated total T_4
C. Low bone-specific alkaline phosphatase
D. Low lumbar spine bone density
E. Low total hip bone density

22 A 14-year-old girl felt a small lump in her right neck and she underwent thyroid ultrasonography, which showed a solid, hypoechoic thyroid nodule in the middle of the right lobe, measuring 1.5 cm in greatest dimension, with suggestion of microcalcifications but no extrathyroidal extension. Ultrasonography also revealed a few small lymph nodes in the central neck region, 2 of which on the right side had features suspicious for malignancy. No lateral neck lymphadenopathy was observed on ultrasonography. Her thyroid function was normal, and TPO and thyroglobulin antibodies were not detected. She was referred to pediatric endocrinology.

On physical examination, a firm, right-sided nodule is noted, with no lateral neck lymph nodes palpated. Her weight is 105.8 lb (48 kg), and the rest of the examination findings are unremarkable.

Ultrasound-guided FNA is recommended. Findings are consistent with papillary thyroid cancer (Bethesda VI), and total thyroidectomy with central neck dissection is recommended. The pathology report confirms the diagnosis of papillary thyroid cancer. She has a 1.6-cm right-sided carcinoma with typical psammoma bodies and no extrathyroidal extension. There are 2 foci of papillary thyroid cancer 0.3 cm or smaller in the left lobe. Central neck dissection shows that 8 of 13 small lymph nodes on the right side have metastases (0 of 5 nodes on the left side have metastases).

Her postoperative course is uncomplicated. Levothyroxine, 112 mcg once daily, is initiated, and the dosage is increased 1 month later to 125 mcg daily based on her TSH concentration.

Postoperative laboratory test results:

Analyte	1 Month after surgery (after 1 month of levothyroxine, 112 mcg daily)	2 Months after surgery (after 1 month of levothyroxine, 125 mcg daily)
TSH	1.3 mIU/L	0.35 mIU/L
Free T_4	1.0 ng/dL (SI: 12.87 pmol/L)	1.3 ng/dL (SI: 16.73 pmol/L)
Thyroglobulin antibodies	...	Negative
Unstimulated thyroglobulin	...	<0.1 ng/mL (SI: <0.1 µg/L)

Which of the following is the best next step in this patient's management?

A. Assess the need to order a stimulated thyroglobulin measurement and whole-body ^{123}I scan 6 months postoperatively
B. Increase the levothyroxine dosage to achieve a TSH concentration <0.1 mIU/L
C. Order stimulated thyroglobulin measurement and whole-body ^{123}I scan within 12 weeks postoperatively
D. Order neck CT with contrast now to assess for neck lymphadenopathy
E. Order neck ultrasonography now to assess for neck lymphadenopathy

23   An 11-and-9/12-year-old girl is referred for evaluation of short stature. Her height is 51.2 in (130 cm) (–2.5 SDS), arm span is 48.8 in (124 cm), and midparental target height is–1.8 SDS. Her weight is 72.8 lb (33 kg) (–1.13 SDS), and BMI is 19.5 kg/m^2 (0.53 SDS). She has no other concerns.

On physical examination, she has Tanner stage 3 breast development. Her bone age x-ray is shown (*see image*).

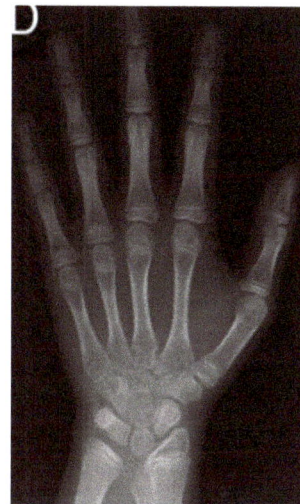

Which of the following would most likely help determine the cause of this patient's short stature?

A.   Basic metabolic panel, complete blood cell count, and erythrocyte sedimentation rate

B.   Forearm x-ray

C.   Free T$_4$ and TSH measurement

D.   GH-stimulation testing

E.   Pituitary MRI

Reprinted from Marchini A et al. *Endocr Rev*, 2016; 37(4). © Endocrine Society.

24   A 17-year-old girl has had type 1 diabetes mellitus for 4 years. She is successfully using glucose sensor technology and is considering insulin infusion pump therapy. Her sensor tracing shows significant swings of glucose readings (*see images*).

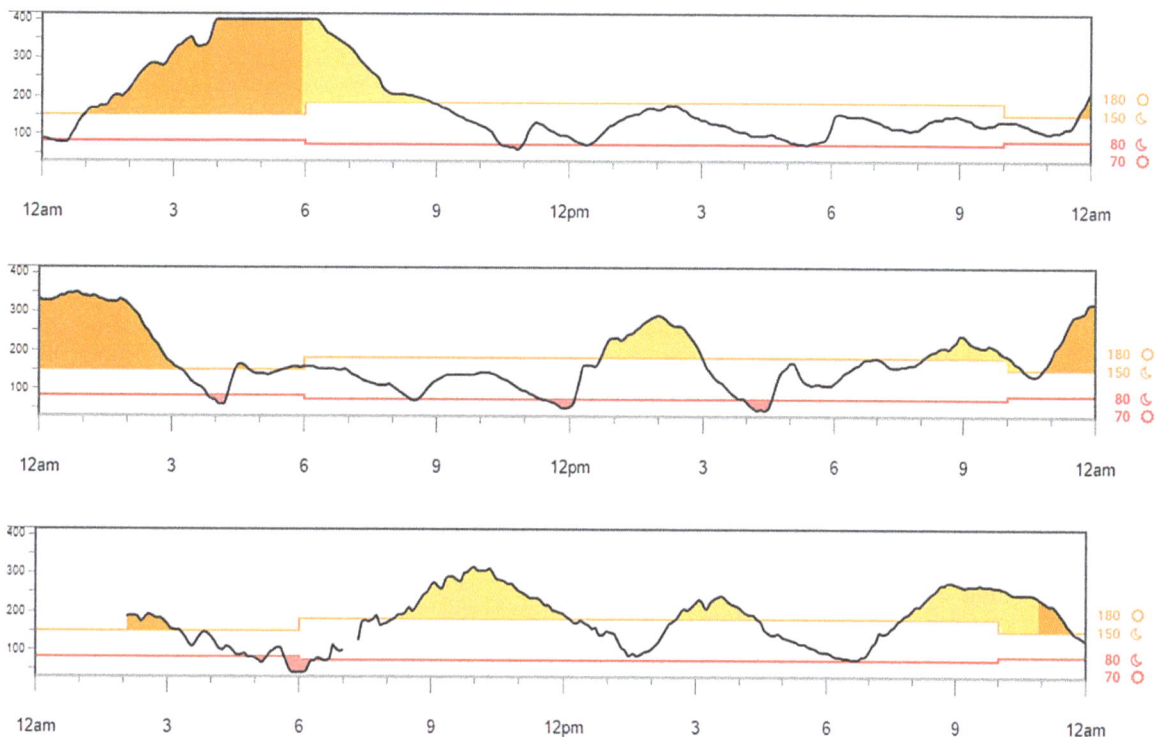

Further questioning indicates that she is "reactive" with insulin administration, waiting to have elevated glucose values on her sensor before administering insulin. This approach leads to frequent episodes of hypoglycemia. She almost never administers a prebolus for any carbohydrates consumed. She is also fearful of overnight hypoglycemia since she had a seizure after "partying" last year. Her most recent hemoglobin A$_{1c}$ value is 8.6% (70 mmol/mol).

Which of the following clinical concerns may delay the transition to pump therapy and require her to attend more education sessions prior to proceeding with pump therapy?
   A. Fear of overnight hypoglycemia
   B. Hemoglobin A_{1c} level greater than 8.5% (>69 mmol/mol)
   C. "Reactive" insulin use for correction of hyperglycemia
   D. The practice of not counting carbohydrates or administering insulin for the carbohydrates consumed
   E. There are no clinical concerns requiring further education before proceeding with pump therapy

25 A 9-year-old girl presents to the endocrinology clinic with concerns of breast discharge. Her family history is notable for multiple endocrine neoplasia type 1 in her father, older sister, and paternal aunt. Review of systems is unremarkable. Review of growth records shows normal linear growth.

On physical examination, her blood pressure is 91/46 mm Hg, pulse rate is 89 beats/min, height is 51.1 in (129.8 cm) (26th percentile), and weight is 68.3 lb (31 kg) (59.8th percentile). There is a small amount of expressible clear discharge from the right breast.

Laboratory test results:
   Prolactin = 217 ng/mL (2-14 ng/mL) (SI: 9.4 nmol/L [0.09-0.61 nmol/L])
   PTH = 73 pg/mL (15-55 pg/mL) (SI: 73 ng/L [15-55 ng/L])
   Ionized calcium = 5.8 mg/dL (4.3-5.4 mg/dL) (SI: 1.44 mmol/L [1.08-1.34 mmol/L])

MRI of the brain shows an 8-mm anterior pituitary mass.

Which of the following should be measured as the best next step in this child's evaluation?
   A. Fasting glucose and insulin
   B. Plasma metanephrines
   C. Serum aldosterone and renin
   D. Serum calcitonin
   E. Serum vasoactive intestinal peptide

26 A 3-year-old boy presents for evaluation of abnormal results on thyroid function tests obtained during an assessment for developmental delay that has been present since infancy. A prior neurologic evaluation revealed that he has severe hypotonia with poor head control, is unable to sit or stand independently, and has intermittent dystonic movements of the limbs. He has cognitive delay and is unable to speak. Brain MRI shows diffusely delayed myelination, decreased white matter volume, and a normal pituitary gland.

On physical examination, his length is –1.4 SD and weight is –3.2 SD for age. Pulse rate and blood pressure are normal. He is not dysmorphic, and his fontanelles are closed. His tongue is normal in size. His thyroid gland is not palpable. His abdomen is scaphoid, with no hepatomegaly or umbilical hernia.

Laboratory test results:
   TSH = 5.2 mIU/L (0.7-5.7 mIU/L)
   Free T_4 = 0.7 ng/dL (0.9-1.9 ng/dL) (SI: 9.0 pmol/L [11.6-24.5 pmol/L])
   Total T_3 = 282 ng/dL (94-241 ng/dL) (SI: 4.3 nmol/L [1.4-3.7 nmol/L])

Genetic testing for pathogenic variants in which of the following genes is most likely to confirm this patient's diagnosis?
   A. *DIO3* (iodothyronine deiodinase 3)
   B. *SECISBP2* (SECIS binding protein 2)
   C. *SLC16A2* (formerly *MCT8*) (solute carrier family 16 member 2)
   D. *THRA* (thyroid hormone receptor alpha)
   E. *THRB* (thyroid hormone receptor beta)

27   A 2-year-old boy is admitted to the hospital with a seizure. He was born at 38 weeks' gestation and had a normal birth weight and birth length. He has always achieved age-appropriate developmental milestones. On physical examination, his height is –2.6 SD and weight is –2.0 SD for age. He has typical prepubertal male genitalia. Laboratory tests ordered in the emergency department show normal electrolytes but a plasma glucose concentration of 36.0 mg/dL (2.0 mmol/L). Brain MRI at an outside facility is shown (*see images*), although the radiology report is not available at this time.

Which of the following is this patient's most likely diagnosis?

   A.   Ectopic posterior pituitary with interrupted pituitary stalk
   B.   Ectopic posterior pituitary within pituitary stalk
   C.   Langerhans-cell histiocytosis
   D.   Normal findings of pituitary gland and stalk
   E.   Pituitary macroadenoma

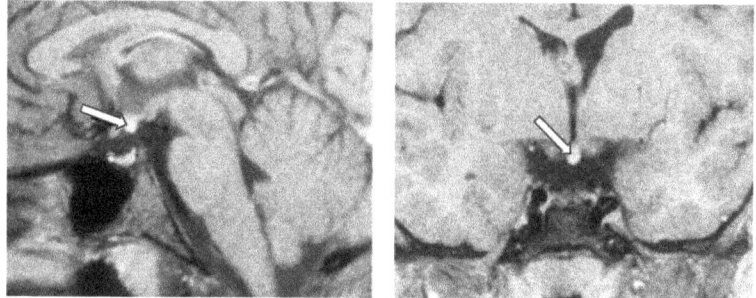

Reprinted from Chen S et al. *J Clin Endocrinol Metab*, 1999; 84(7). © Endocrine Society.

28   A 15-year-old girl was diagnosed with type 2 diabetes mellitus 6 months ago. She has missed several appointments but finally returns for care today. Her BMI is 38 kg/m², and she has moderate to severe acanthosis nigricans on her neck and axillae. Her hemoglobin A_{1c} at the time of diagnosis (initially checked due to concerns about insulin resistance on examination) was 6.8% (51 mmol/mol). Metformin, 1500 mg daily, was prescribed. There is a strong family history of type 2 diabetes in numerous relatives.

At today's appointment, her hemoglobin A_{1c} value is 11.0% (97 mmol/mol) and she has a random glucose measurement of 324 mg/dL (18.0 mmol/L). Urinalysis shows a large amount of glucose and moderate to large ketones. When questioned, the patient reports adherence to her metformin treatment. She has been trying to follow lifestyle modifications and is excited that she has lost 4.4 lb (2 kg) since the last visit. She admits that she has not been routinely checking blood glucose at home.

Which of the following is the most likely finding in her laboratory results that would explain the significant change in her clinical status?

   A.   Elevated C-peptide
   B.   Pancreatic autoantibodies
   C.   Pathogenic variant in the *INS* gene
   D.   Pathogenic variant in the *GCK* gene
   E.   Pathogenic variant in the *KCNJ11* gene

29   A 17-year-old girl has depression and has been brought to the emergency department by her mother after she was missing from home for 4 days. She is hallucinating and is paranoid that people are trying to kill her. She is sexually active and has been on an oral contraceptive pill for a year. She does not take biotin or other supplements. Pediatric endocrinology is consulted due to abnormal thyroid function. Four months ago, she was admitted to the hospital for abdominal pain and vomiting, and she had normal thyroid function at that time.

On physical examination, her temperature is 97.7°F (36.5°C), blood pressure is 136/77 mm Hg, and pulse rate is 115 beats/min. Her height is 61 in (155 cm) (11th percentile), and weight is 145.5 lb (66 kg) (82nd percentile). The following morning, her pulse rate is 92 beats/min. She is alert and in no distress. She is fully pubertal. Findings on eye examination are normal with no exophthalmos. Her thyroid gland is nontender, and there is no goiter or bruit. Her heart has a regular rate and rhythm with no murmur. Her abdomen is soft without hepatosplenomegaly. The rest of the examination findings are unremarkable.

Urine toxicology screen is positive for cannabinoids and methamphetamines.

Additional laboratory test results:

Analyte	Current admission	Prior admission
TSH	0.38 mIU/L	1.29 mIU/L
Total T_4	17.2 µg/dL (SI: 221.4 nmol/L)	...
Free T_4	2.15 ng/dL (SI: 27.7 pmol/L)	1.38 ng/dL (SI: 17.8 pmol/L)
T_3 uptake	25.2%	...
Thyroglobulin antibodies	0.9 IU/mL (SI: 0.9 kIU/L)	...
TPO antibodies	0.13 IU/mL (SI: 0.13 kIU/L)	...
Thyroid-stimulating immunoglobulin	Negative	...

Reference ranges: TSH, 0.35-5.00 mIU/L; total T_4, 4.3-12.5 µg/dL (SI: 55.3-160.9 nmol/L); free T_4, 0.71-1.85 ng/dL (SI: 9.1-23.8 pmol/L); T_3 uptake, 25%-35%; thyroglobulin antibodies, <5.0 IU/mL (SI: <5.0 kIU/L); TPO antibodies, <5.61 IU/mL (SI: <5.61 kIU/L); thyroid-stimulating immunoglobulin, <89%.

This patient's elevated free T_4 and total T_4 are most likely due to which of the following?

A. Graves disease
B. Hashitoxicosis
C. Methamphetamine use
D. Oral contraceptive use
E. Subacute thyroiditis

30 A 9-month-old girl is referred for evaluation of pubic hair development. The mother reports that hair has been present in the pubic area since birth, but that it recently became darker and thicker. She has not noticed the development of axillary hair, adult body odor, breast development, or vaginal discharge. There has been no exposure to exogenous estrogens, tea tree oil, or lavender oil. Perinatal history is uncomplicated; she was born at 40 weeks' gestation, and birth weight was 8 lb (3.6 kg). She has been fed a combination of breast milk, formula, and home-prepared pureed vegetables and fruit. Both parents report normal timing of puberty, and midparental target height is 65 in (165.1 cm). She has a healthy 3-year-old sister who has no signs of puberty.

On physical examination, she has a small amount of fine, light pubic hair, 2 cm of glandular breast tissue bilaterally, and red vaginal mucosa without clitoral enlargement. Length and weight are both at the 85th percentile.

Laboratory test results (sample drawn at 8 AM):
  LH = 0.853 mIU/mL (<0.3 mIU/mL) (SI: 0.853 IU/L [<0.3 IU/L])
  Estradiol (sensitive) = 2.6 pg/mL (<16 pg/mL) (SI: 9.5 pmol/L [<58.7 pmol/L])
  17-Hydroxyprogesterone = 84 ng/dL (0-82 ng/dL) (SI: 2.55 nmol/L [0-2.48 nmol/L])
  TSH, normal
  Free T_4, normal

Which of the following is the best step in this patient's initial management?

A. Brain MRI and initiation of a GnRH agonist to treat central precocious puberty
B. Continued monitoring for pubertal progression
C. Cosyntropin-stimulation testing to assess for congenital adrenal hyperplasia
D. FSH measurement to distinguish minipuberty from central precocious puberty
E. GnRH-stimulation testing to assess for central precocious puberty

31

Two years ago, a 16-year-old girl underwent total thyroidectomy and bilateral cervical lymph node dissection for papillary thyroid carcinoma. The postoperative stimulated thyroglobulin concentration was 245 ng/mL (245 μg/L), and whole-body scintigraphy after radioactive iodine therapy (^{131}I 150 mCi) showed multiple foci of iodine uptake in the lungs. Chest CT demonstrated bilateral pulmonary nodules (0.8-1.2 cm) consistent with metastases. One year later, the stimulated thyroglobulin concentration was 230 ng/mL (230 μg/L), and chest CT showed that some lung nodules had decreased in size and others remained stable. Another dose of radioactive iodine (^{131}I 200 mCi) was administered, and posttreatment whole-body scintigraphy showed no significant pulmonary uptake.

Now, 2 years after initial treatment, the stimulated thyroglobulin concentration is 358 ng/mL (358 μg/L). Chest CT demonstrates that many of the pulmonary nodules have increased in size. Pulmonary function is normal, and the patient is asymptomatic.

Which of the following is the optimal next step in this patient's evaluation and management?
A. Cytotoxic chemotherapy with doxorubicin and cisplatin
B. External beam radiation to bilateral lung fields
C. Genetic testing of resected tumor tissue for a molecularly targetable driver variant
D. Radioactive iodine (^{131}I) therapy, 250 mCi
E. Radioactive iodine (^{131}I) therapy, maximum tolerated dose as determined by dosimetry

32

An 18-year-old man with a history of primitive neuroectodermal tumor of the pineal gland diagnosed at age 6 years presents to the endocrine clinic with generalized fatigue, which has worsened over the past year.

His tumor was treated with gross total resection and chemotherapy with cisplatin, cyclophosphamide, and vincristine. He received craniospinal irradiation (36 Gy) with boost to the third ventricle. The estimated dose to the pituitary was 40.5 Gy with minimal thyroid exposure. As a child, he was treated with a GnRH agonist for central precocious puberty and with GH for GH deficiency. He discontinued GH therapy at age 16 years, as he had reached his final adult height and no longer wanted to take GH injections.

On physical examination, his height is 64 in (162.5 cm) and weight is 143 lb (65 kg). His blood pressure is 90/50 mm Hg, and pulse rate is 100 beats/min. He has long legs, a short-appearing trunk, and increased abdominal adiposity. His skin is normal. Pubic hair and genitalia are Tanner stage 5, and testicular volume is 12 mL bilaterally.

Laboratory test results:
Hemoglobin = 12.3 g/dL (12-16 g/dL) (SI: 123 g/L [120-160 g/L])
Hematocrit = 36% (36-46%) (SI: 0.36 [0.36-0.46])
Sodium = 141 mEq/L (136-149 mEq/L) (SI: 141 mmol/L [136-149 mmol/L])
Potassium = 4.0 mEq/L (3.9-5.7 mEq/L) (SI: 4.0 mmol/L [3.9-5.7 mmol/L])
Free T$_4$ = 1.4 ng/dL (0.98-1.63 ng/dL) (SI: 18.0 pmol/L [12.6-21.0 pmol/L])

Which of the following is the most important diagnostic test to order now?
A. Cosyntropin-stimulation test
B. Gonadotropin (LH, FSH) measurement
C. Prolactin measurement
D. Serum IGF-1 measurement
E. TSH measurement

33

A 15-year-old girl with a history of polycystic ovary syndrome and prediabetes presents for follow-up in clinic. At her last visit several months ago, pharmacologic treatment of obesity was discussed because of continued weight gain despite lifestyle changes. After an extensive discussion of the risks and benefits associated with different pharmacologic options for weight management in adolescents, she opted to start liraglutide, given subcutaneously once daily.

Which of the following best describes the mechanism of action for liraglutide in this setting?

A. Activates melanocortin 4 receptors in areas of the hypothalamus associated with appetite regulation, as well as increases resting energy expenditure

B. Decreases gastric emptying and has effects on hypothalamic nuclei involved in the regulation of appetite

C. Decreases hepatic glucose production, reduces intestinal glucose absorption, and increases insulin sensitivity

D. Inhibits gastric and pancreatic lipases, leading to decreased absorption of dietary fat

E. Stimulates the release of norepinephrine in the hypothalamus, leading to appetite suppression

34 A previously healthy 13-year-old boy was involved in a severe motor vehicle crash resulting in traumatic brain injury and quadriplegia. Sequelae of his injuries include diabetes insipidus, central hypothyroidism, and adrenal insufficiency. In addition, he now receives all his nutrition via a gastric tube. Before the accident, he was reported to have normal growth and pubertal development. Approximately 4 months into his prolonged hospitalization, he was noted to have hypercalcemia with hypercalciuria. There have been no changes in his neurologic status or feeding tolerance.

Laboratory test results:
  Calcium = 14.3 mg/dL (8.5-10.0 mg/dL) (SI: 3.58 mmol/L [2.1-2.5 mmol/L])
  Phosphate = 4.3 mg/dL (2.8-5.1 mg/dL) (SI: 1.39 mmol/L [0.9-1.6 mmol/L])
  Alkaline phosphatase = 93 U/L (141-460 U/L) (SI: 1.55 μkat/L [2.35-7.68 μkat/L])
  PTH = 4 pg/mL (15-87 pg/mL) (SI: 4 ng/L [15-87 ng/L])
  25-Hydroxyvitamin D = 33.3 ng/mL (20.0-60.0 ng/mL) (SI: 83.1 nmol/L [49.9-149.8 nmol/L])
  Urinary calcium-to-creatinine ratio = 0.47 (<0.2)

He is currently on hydrocortisone replacement (11 mg/m^2 per day) and levothyroxine, 88 mcg daily (with normal free T$_4$ levels), and subcutaneous desmopressin to maintain normal urine output. Hyperhydration is attempted, but due to concerns about sodium balance and edema, this is discontinued. A trial of calcitonin is also attempted, without significant response.

Which of the following interventions is the best next step to safely reduce this patient's serum calcium concentration?

A. Initiate stress-dose steroids

B. Start cinacalcet

C. Start denosumab

D. Start pamidronate

E. Switch to enteral feeds with lower calcium content

35 A 15-year-old girl felt some lumps in her neck when she tried on a new necklace. Her pediatrician ordered ultrasonography of her thyroid and neck, which revealed 2 moderate-sized nodules in her right thyroid lobe (largest 2.6 cm), a smaller nodule in the left lobe, and suspicious lymph nodes in the right lateral neck. FNA biopsy of the nodules and 1 of the lymph nodes confirmed that she has papillary thyroid cancer. She undergoes total thyroidectomy with bilateral central neck dissection and right lateral neck dissection.

Her PTH concentration 1 hour postoperatively is 20.0 pg/mL (8.5-72.5 pg/mL) (SI: 20.0 ng/L [8.5-72.5 ng/L]), and her calcium concentration at 6 PM (4 hours after surgery) is 8.8 mg/dL (8.5-10.5 mg/dL) (SI: 2.2 mmol/L [2.1-2.6 mmol/L]).

Which of the following is the best next step in this patient's management?

A. Discharge the patient home the next day

B. Repeat calcium and PTH measurement at midnight

C. Repeat calcium measurement the next morning

D. Start oral calcitriol

E. Start oral calcium and remeasure calcium 4 hours later

36 A 6-year-old boy is referred for evaluation of short stature. He was born full-term via normal vaginal delivery after an uncomplicated pregnancy with minimal prenatal care. Birth length was 21.7 in (55 cm) (97th percentile), and birth weight was 9 lb 11 oz (4400 g) (97th percentile). The growth chart from the primary care provider shows that his length/height progressively dropped from the 97th percentile at birth to the 25th percentile by age 4 years and to below the 3rd percentile by age 6 years. His weight shows a similar pattern.

On physical examination, his height is 40.9 in (104 cm) (<3rd percentile; height SDS, –2.25), weight is 35.2 lb (16 kg) (<3rd percentile; weight SDS, –2.13), and head circumference is 21.3 in (54 cm) (98th percentile). He has dysmorphic features, which include posteriorly rotated ears, slight ocular hypertelorism, left-sided palpebral ptosis, pectus excavatum, and widely spaced nipples. There are no abnormal skin findings. He has a systolic murmur in the second intercostal space to the left of the sternum.

The patient has 5 siblings. His 9-year-old brother was also large for gestational age, and his current height now plots below the 3rd percentile. He has facial features that are similar to those of the patient's. The other siblings are unaffected. His father's height is 68.9 in (175 cm), and his mother's height is 65.8 in (167 cm). The parents are first-degree cousins, have normal intellect, and have no dysmorphic features.

Based on the clinical assessment, Noonan syndrome is suspected.

Among the genes associated with Noonan syndrome, pathogenic variant(s) in which of the following most likely explains this patient's history and clinical findings?
   A. *CBL* (Cbl proto-oncogene)
   B. *LZTR1* (leucine zipper like transcription regulator 1)
   C. *NF1* (neurofibromin 1)
   D. *PTPN11* (protein tyrosine phosphatase nonreceptor type 11)
   E. *SOS1* (SOS Ras/Rac guanine nucleotide exchange factor 1)

37 A 17-year-old girl with known cystic fibrosis (homozygous Delta 508 pathogenic variant) undergoes yearly oral glucose tolerance testing. She is asymptomatic and specifically has no polyuria, polydipsia, or nocturia. Her BMI is 20.3 kg/m² (Z-score, –0.06). She follows the diet recommended by her pulmonology clinic dietitian. Her hemoglobin A_{1c} value is 5.8% (40 mmol/mol).

Oral glucose tolerance test results (after standard 75-g glucose solution):

Time	Glucose
0 min	88 mg/dL (SI: 4.9 mmol/L)
60 min	185 mg/dL (SI: 10.3 mmol/L)
120 min	128 mg/dL (SI: 7.1 mmol/L)

Which of the following diabetes treatment options would be best suited for this patient?
   A. Basal and bolus regimen with insulins glargine and lispro
   B. Basal insulin with long-acting glargine
   C. Meal bolus insulin with rapid-acting lispro
   D. No treatment but monitor blood glucose with either a glucose meter (fasting and 1 hour postprandial) or glucose sensor
   E. Oral glycemic agent repaglinide before each meal

38 A 10-year-old boy had abnormal findings on thyroid function testing ordered in the primary care setting for evaluation of obesity. His BMI is 25.5 kg/m² (98th percentile), and it has been slowly increasing over the past 5 years. His linear growth has been normal. He is otherwise healthy, has no developmental or academic problems, and takes no medications or supplements. He reports no symptoms of hypothyroidism or thyrotoxicosis.

On physical examination, his height is at the 79th percentile and weight is at the 98th percentile. Heart rate and blood pressure are normal. His thyroid gland is normal in size and texture, with no nodules. Aside from obesity, the rest of his examination findings are normal.

Laboratory test results:
    TSH = 3.4 mIU/L (0.7-5.7 mIU/L)
    Total T_4 = 15.3 µg/dL (4.7-12.4 µg/dL) (SI: 200 nmol/L [60-160 nmol/L])

Which of the following is the most likely molecular mechanism underlying this patient's findings?
    A. Duplication of the thyroxine-binding globulin gene (*SERPINA7*)
    B. Increased binding affinity of albumin for T_4
    C. Increased binding affinity of prealbumin (transthyretin) for T_4
    D. Increased binding affinity of thyroxine-binding globulin for T_4
    E. Pathogenic variant in the thyroid hormone receptor β gene (*THRB*)

39 A 9-year-old girl is followed in the endocrinology clinic for premature breast development and intermittent vaginal bleeding that first began at 18 months of age. During a recent episode of bleeding, laboratory tests were ordered and pelvic ultrasonography was performed.

Laboratory test results:
    LH = 0.1 mIU/mL (0.02-12.0 mIU/mL) (SI: 0.1 IU/L [0.02-12.0 IU/L])
    FSH = 0.1 mIU/mL (1.0-6.0 mIU/mL) (SI: 0.1 IU/L [1.0-6.0 IU/L])
    Estradiol = 247 pg/mL (<16 pg/mL) (SI: 906.7 pmol/L [<58.7 pmol/L])

Pelvic ultrasonography shows that the right ovary is enlarged for age and contains a simple cystic lesion with peripheral daughter cysts/follicles. A 2.3 × 1.5-cm, irregular, echogenic, mass-like area is adjacent to the inferior aspect of the ovary with some associated cysts. A 1.7-cm left paraovarian simple cystic lesion is observed.

Which of the following signal transduction pathways accounts for her clinical presentation?
    A. Activation of a JAK-STAT pathway
    B. Activation of adenylate cyclase
    C. Activation of tyrosine kinases
    D. Smad phosphorylation
    E. Stimulation of gene transcription through hormone response elements

40 A 7-year-old boy presents for a follow-up visit in the weight management clinic. He has a history of rapid weight gain since he was very young. Despite the lifestyle modifications that his family has tried very hard to implement, he has continued to gain weight (13.2 lb [6 kg] in the past 6 months). His current height is 47.2 in (120 cm) (35th percentile; –0.38 SDS), and weight is 114.6 lb (52 kg) (99th percentile; 3.47 SDS). The family is frustrated and expresses concern that regardless of what they do, he just seems to gain weight. They are convinced that his metabolism is "slow" and want to know if there is a way to better assess this, so they can work with a dietician to tailor an improved plan.

Which of the following is the best way to assess this patient's resting energy expenditure?
    A. Accelerometry
    B. Direct calorimetry
    C. Indirect calorimetry
    D. Measurement of basal metabolic rate
    E. Owen equation for resting energy expenditure

41 A 6-year-old girl presents for evaluation of a several-month history of axillary hair, pubic hair, and breast development. She has no history of seizures, headaches, or vision problems and developmental history is normal. Her parents confirm there has been no exposure to exogenous sources of estrogen. A bone age x-ray at the chronologic age of 6 years 4 months is equivalent to 8 years 10 months. Review of her growth chart shows that she has been gaining in height percentiles.

On physical examination, her height is at the 93rd percentile, weight is at the 96th percentile, and BMI is at the 93rd percentile. She has Tanner stage 3 pubic hair and stage 3 breast development (6-7 cm bilaterally). Findings on neurologic examination are normal.

Laboratory results (drawn at 8 AM):
    LH = 0.88 mIU/mL (<0.3 mIU/mL) (SI: 0.88 IU/L [<0.3 IU/L])
    Estradiol (sensitive) = 21.0 pg/mL (<16 pg/mL) (SI: 77.1 pmol/L [<58.7 pmol/L])

Which of the following is the best next step in this patient's management?
    A. Order genetic testing for causes of central precocious puberty
    B. Perform GnRH-stimulation testing to confirm the diagnosis
    C. Perform pelvic ultrasonography
    D. Perform thyroid function testing to rule out primary hypothyroidism
    E. Provide counseling on the risk of type 2 diabetes mellitus

42 A 15-year-old girl has classic salt-wasting congenital adrenal hyperplasia that was diagnosed at birth. Her current treatment regimen is hydrocortisone, 7.5 mg 3 times daily (13 mg/m² per day), and 9α-fludrocortisone, 100 mcg once daily. Over the last month, she has been experiencing intermittent headaches and dizziness during the course of the day (no consistency in timing of symptoms).

Laboratory test results:
    Serum sodium = 137 mEq/L (133-146 mEq/L) (SI: 137 mmol/L [133-146 mmol/L])
    Potassium = 4.9 mEq/L (3.5-5.3 mEq/L) (SI: 4.9 mmol/L [3.5-5.3 mmol/L])
    Serum urea nitrogen = 10.6 mg/dL (7.0-21.8 mg/dL) (SI: 3.8 mmol/L [2.5-7.8 mmol/L])
    Creatinine = 0.7 mg/dL (0.5-1.0 mg/dL) (SI: 62 μmol/L [45-84 μmol/L])
    Plasma renin activity = 3.8 ng/mL per h (0.6-3.8 ng/mL per h)
    17-Hydroxyprogesterone = 336.6 ng/dL (SI: 10.2 nmol/L)
    Serum testosterone = 17.3 ng/dL (8.6-49.0 ng/dL) (SI: 0.6 nmol/L [0.3-1.7 nmol/L])
    DHEA-S = 14.8 μg/dL (59.0-287.8 μg/dL) (SI: 0.4 μmol/L [1.6-7.8 μmol/L])
    Androstenedione = 106.0 ng/dL (57.3-154.7 ng/dL) (SI: 3.7 nmol/L [2.0-5.4 nmol/L])
    Cortisol = 15.9 μg/dL (SI: 440 nmol/L)

Which of the following is the best next step in this patient's management?
    A. Increase the 9α-fludrocortisone dosage
    B. Increase the hydrocortisone dosage
    C. Measure blood pressure while the patient is laying down and standing
    D. Order a complete blood cell count
    E. Perform head MRI

43 A 7-year-old girl is seen for multiple pituitary hormone deficiencies secondary to craniopharyngioma diagnosed and resected at age 4 years. She is treated with GH, levothyroxine, hydrocortisone, and desmopressin. Her family has recently moved, and they seek to establish care. Review of her medical records indicates that she has missed several follow-up appointments, and her last clinic visit was 1 year ago. She has had 2 visits to the emergency department for vomiting and diarrhea, and "adrenal crisis" was diagnosed. She was sent home after receiving intravenous hydrocortisone and hydration. Her family was educated about the management of her condition. Her growth velocity is 2 cm/y.

On physical examination, her height is 41.3 in (105 cm) (<1st percentile), weight is 48.5 lb (22 kg) (42nd percentile), and BMI is 20 kg/m² (96th percentile). Her body surface area is 0.78 m².

Current daily medications are GH, 1 mg subcutaneous injection daily; levothyroxine, 62.5 mcg daily; and hydrocortisone, 12.5 mg daily (5 mg morning, 5 mg afternoon, and 2.5 mg evening).

Laboratory test results (sample drawn the morning of the clinic visit):
IGF-1 = 60 ng/mL (49-267 ng/mL) (SI: 7.9 nmol/L [6.4-35.0 nmol/L])
TSH, not ordered
Free T₄ = 0.7 ng/dL (0.90-1.67 ng/dL) (SI: 9.0 pmol/L [11.6-21.5 pmol/L])
Basic metabolic panel, normal

Which of the following is the best next step in this patient's management?
A. Increase GH dosage to 1.1 mg daily
B. Increase hydrocortisone dosage to 15 mg daily (5 mg morning, 5 mg afternoon, 5 mg evening)
C. Increase levothyroxine dosage to 75 mcg daily and repeat laboratory tests in 4 weeks
D. Report the family to the local child protection services
E. Screen for social determinants of health

44 A 16-year-old boy presents with a 4-week history of fatigue and excess thirst. He has felt dizzy, lightheaded, and cold for the last 2 days and has also noticed diminished urine output. His appetite has been reduced and he has lost weight. His only medication is risperidone, which was started 2 months ago. He has had no sick contacts.

On physical examination, he appears anxious and ill. His blood pressure is 112/68 mm Hg, pulse rate is 135 beats/min, respiratory rate is 32 breaths/min, temperature is 100.2°F (37.9°C), and BMI is 41.5 kg/m². His lungs are clear to auscultation. His abdomen is difficult to palpate, but there is no tenderness or detected mass. His extremities are cold, and capillary refill is longer than 3 seconds.

In the office, his point-of-care glucose value is greater than 600 mg/dL (>33.3 mmol/L).

Laboratory test results:
Plasma glucose = 852 mg/dL (70-99 mg/dL) (SI: 47.3 mmol/L [3.9-5.5 mmol/L])
Serum sodium = 148 mEq/L (136-142 mEq/L) (SI: 148 mmol/L [136-142 mmol/L])
Serum bicarbonate = 16 mEq/L (21-28 mEq/L) (SI: 16 mmol/L [21-28 mmol/L])
Serum β-hydroxybutyrate = 2.1 mg/dL (<3.0 mg/dL) (SI: 201.7 μmol/L [<288.2 μmol/L])
Serum potassium = 5.8 mEq/L (3.5-5.0 mEq/L) (SI: 5.8 mmol/L [3.5-5.0 mmol/L])
pH = 7.29 (7.35-7.45)

Which of the following options would be the best initial management for this patient?
A. Long-acting insulin subcutaneous bolus: 0.5 unit/kg
B. Normal saline intravenous bolus: 10 mL/kg
C. Normal saline intravenous bolus: 20 mL/kg
D. Regular insulin intravenous bolus: 0.1 unit/kg
E. Regular insulin intravenous drip: 0.1 unit/kg

45 An 8-year-old boy presents with recurrent spells concerning for seizure activity. His mother reports that he has episodes at school and at home where his hands flex in and he falls to the floor. These episodes, which occur more than 10 times per day, seem to happen more often when he is active, but they are not associated with altered mental status. Since early childhood, he has grown at the 50th percentile for both height and weight. He does not have any obvious dysmorphic features. He is an average student. Review of his medical history shows that he had a normal serum calcium concentration in the first month of life.

An evaluation is done, and the pertinent laboratory test results are shown:

Calcium = <5.0 mg/dL (8.5-10.1 mg/dL) (SI: 1.3 mmol/L [2.1-2.5 mmol/L])
Phosphate = 10.2 mg/dL (3.7-6.5 mg/dL) (SI: 3.3 mmol/L [1.2-2.1 mmol/L])
Magnesium = 1.9 mg/dL (1.7-2.4 mg/dL) (SI: 0.78 mmol/L [0.70-0.99 mmol/L])
Albumin = 3.5 g/dL (3.5-4.7 g/dL) (SI: 35 g/L [35-47 g/L])
PTH = 1000 pg/mL (15-87 pg/mL) (SI: 1000 ng/L [15-87 ng/L])
25-Hydroxyvitamin D = 27.2 ng/mL (20.0-60.0 ng/mL) (SI: 67.9 nmol/L [49.9-149.8 nmol/L])
1,25-Dihydroxyvitamin D = 47.4 pg/mL (19.9-79.3 pg/mL) (SI: 123.2 pmol/L [51.7-206.2 pmol/L])

He is started on calcium and calcitriol with resultant improvement in bone metabolites.

Which of the following is most likely to be discovered on additional evaluation?

A. Advanced bone age
B. Ectopic ossification on skeletal survey
C. Elevated GH
D. Elevated TSH
E. Low intelligence quotient scores

46 An 11-year-old boy is referred for evaluation of short stature. He was born full term with a birth weight of 7 lb (3.2 kg) and has been healthy. However, his parents have been concerned about his growth for the last 5 years. His father's height is 69 in (175.3 cm), and his mother's height is 65 in (165.1 cm). He eats a balanced diet and feels well, except for a history of frequent mouth sores. He does not take any medications.

On physical examination, pubic hair and genitalia are Tanner stage 1. Testicles are descended bilaterally. He has inguinal lymphadenopathy. BMI is 15.83 kg/m² (Z-score, 0.92 [18th percentile]). The rest of the examination findings are normal.

At a chronologic age of 11 years, bone age is interpreted to be 8 years with a predicted adult height of 65.5 in (166.4 cm).

Laboratory test results:

White blood cell count = 9100/μL (4500-13,000/μL)
(SI: 9.1 × 10⁹/L [4.5-13.0 × 10⁹/L])
Hemoglobin = 12 g/dL (12.7-17.0 g/dL) (SI: 120 g/L
[127-170 g/L])
Tissue transglutaminase IgA and quantitative IgA,
normal
TSH = 3.5 mIU/L (0.3-4.2 mIU/L)
Free T₄ = 1.3 ng/dL (0.9-1.7 ng/dL) (SI: 17.11 pmol/L
[11.58-21.88 pmol/L])
IGF-1 = 117 ng/mL (52-391 ng/mL) (SI: 15.3 nmol/L
[6.8-51.2 nmol/L])
Erythrocyte sedimentation rate = 14 mm/h
(0-15 mm/h)
Liver enzymes, normal
Electrolytes, normal

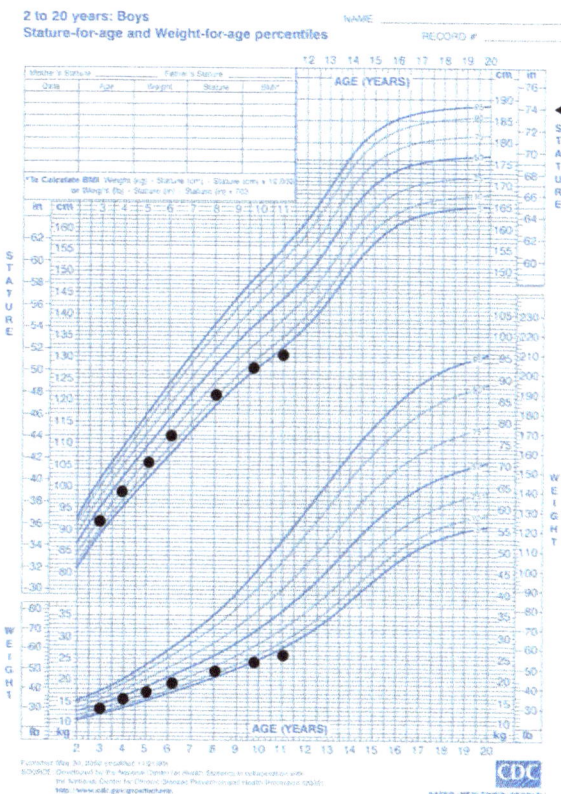

Findings on ultrasonography of the abdomen, scrotum, and testicles are normal except for inguinal lymphadenopathy.

Which of the following is the best next step in evaluating this patient?
- A. Arginine and insulin-stimulation test
- B. Chromosome microarray analysis
- C. Fecal calprotectin measurement
- D. FSH measurement
- E. IGFBP-3 measurement

47 A 12-year-old boy with a genetic diagnosis of triple-A syndrome and attention-deficit/hyperactivity disorder presents for follow-up. His sister (the family's index case) presented with primary adrenal insufficiency at age 5 years. The patient is under the care of the general pediatric team. Last year, he underwent a standard cosyntropin-stimulation test that demonstrated a peak cortisol value of 20.2 μg/dL (557 nmol/L) at 60 minutes. He has been growing well, and his body surface area is 1.25 m². Results of a repeated short cosyntropin-stimulation test (250 mcg) are shown (*see table*).

Time	Cortisol
0 min	7.1 μg/dL (SI: 196 nmol/L)
30 min	11.6 μg/dL (SI: 320 nmol/L)
60 min	13.6 μg/dL (SI: 375 nmol/L)

Laboratory test results:
Plasma ACTH = 19 pg/mL (<50 pg/mL) (SI: 4.2 pmol/L [<11.0 pmol/L])
Plasma renin activity = 1.0 ng/mL per h (0.5-3.5 ng/mL per h)
Aldosterone = 12.6 ng/dL (9.0-34.2 ng/dL) [upright]) (SI: 350 pmol/L [250-950 pmol/L])
Urea and electrolytes normal

Which of the following is the best next step in this patient's management?
- A. Contact a biochemist to review his results
- B. Contact a geneticist to review his diagnosis
- C. Start emergency hydrocortisone only
- D. Start hydrocortisone treatment, 10 mg daily (5 mg, 2.5 mg, 2.5 mg)
- E. Start hydrocortisone treatment, 15 mg daily (5 mg, 5 mg, 5 mg)

48 A 12-year-old boy presents to the emergency department with a 1-month history of polyuria and polydipsia, drinking 10 to 15 L of water per day. His medical history and family history are unremarkable. On physical examination, his blood pressure is 127/67 mm Hg and pulse rate is 96 beats/min. His height is 57.7 in (146.5 cm), and weight is 120.5 lb (54.8 kg) (BMI = 25.4 kg/m²). He has very mild right esotropia with normal extraocular function. Genitalia and pubic hair are Tanner stage 3, and testicular volume is 4 to 5 mL bilaterally. The rest of his examination findings are normal. After 4 hours of nothing-by-mouth status in preparation for head MRI, his serum sodium concentration is 155 mEq/L (155 mmol/L).

MRI shows a heterogeneous, T1-hypointense, T2-isointense, enhancing mass involving the sella and suprasellar region, measuring approximately 1.7 × 1.1 × 1.7 cm (superior-inferior × anteroposterior × transverse) (*see image, arrows*). The pituitary gland and infundibulum cannot be separately identified from the mass. There is mass effect/involvement of the hypothalamus, inferior third ventricle, and optic chiasm.

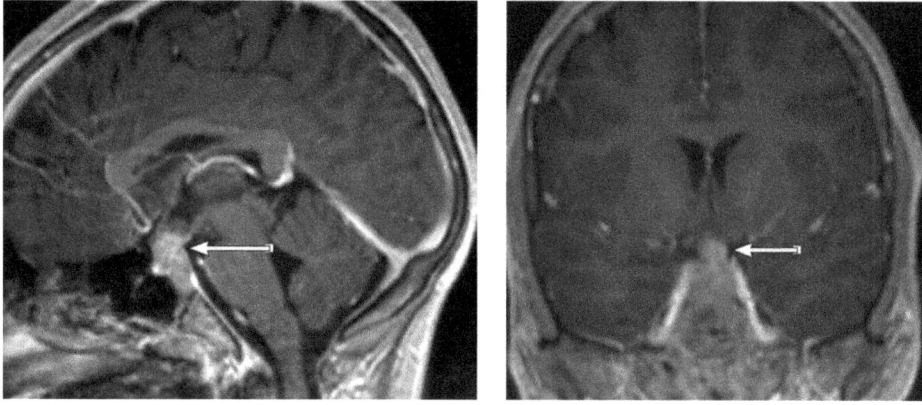

Which of the following is this patient's most likely diagnosis?
A. Craniopharyngioma
B. Chiasmatic glioma
C. Germ-cell tumor
D. Langerhans-cell histiocytosis
E. Rathke cleft cyst

49 A 14-year-old Hispanic girl is referred for evaluation of irregular menses. She underwent menarche at age 11 years and reports that menstrual periods have always been irregular, typically occurring every 6 to 10 weeks. She has no concerns about hair growth on her face or chest, but she does have hair growth on her lower abdomen. She has mild acne that is well controlled with topical treatment and a history of complex migraine headaches. Her growth chart reveals that her height has followed along higher percentiles, while her weight has been increasing in percentiles since approximately age 7 years. There is a family history of irregular menses in her mother and type 2 diabetes in both parents and maternal grandparents.

On physical examination, her blood pressure is 130/70 mm Hg. Her height is 65.6 in (166.6 cm) (Z score = 0.97), weight is 236 lb (107 kg) (Z score = 2.77), and BMI is 38.6 kg/m² (Z score = 2.5). Pubertal development is adult. Findings are notable for dark, thickened skin on her neck.

Laboratory test results:
FSH = 7.3 mIU/mL (0.64-10.98 mIU/mL) (SI: 7.3 IU/L [0.64-10.98 IU/L])
LH = 21.8 mIU/mL (0.04-10.80 mIU/mL) (SI: 21.8 IU/L [0.04-10.80 IU/L])
Prolactin = 17.6 ng/mL (3.2-20.0 ng/mL) (SI: 0.77 nmol/L [0.14-0.87 nmol/L])
TSH = 3.73 mIU/L (0.4-4.5 mIU/L)
Total testosterone = 50 ng/dL (<40 ng/dL) (SI: 1.74 nmol/L [1.39 nmol/L])
Free testosterone = 9.2 ng/dL (0.1-7.4 ng/dL) (SI: 0.32 nmol/L [0.003-0.26 nmol/L])
Total cholesterol = 141 mg/dL (<170 mg/dL) (SI: 3.65 mmol/L [<4.40 mmol/L])
HDL cholesterol = 46 mg/dL (>45 mg/dL) (SI: 1.19 mmol/L [>1.17 mmol/L])
LDL cholesterol = 87 mg/dL (<110 mg/dL) (SI: 2.25 mmol/L [<2.85 mmol/L])
Triglycerides = 39 mg/dL (<90 mg/dL) (SI: 0.44 mmol/L [<1.02 mmol/L])
Hemoglobin A$_{1c}$ = 6.3% (<5.7%) (45 mmol/mol [<39 mmol/mol])

In addition to counseling on lifestyle modification, which of the following is the most appropriate management option for this patient?
A. Hormonal contraceptive
B. Hormonal contraceptive and metformin
C. Metformin
D. Metformin and spironolactone
E. Ultrasonography to assess for polycystic ovaries

50   A 12-year-old girl with obesity and end-stage kidney disease secondary to autosomal dominant polycystic kidney disease receives a kidney transplant from a living donor. Her hemoglobin A_{1c} level before kidney transplant was 5.8% (40 mmol/mol) with a fasting glucose concentration of 96 mg/dL (5.3 mmol/L). She develops hyperglycemia immediately after kidney transplant while on high-dosage corticosteroid therapy and requires insulin initiation as part of postoperative care in the hospital. Four weeks after kidney transplant, her steroid dosage is reduced. The family is asked to monitor blood glucose with the provided glucose meter, and insulin is discontinued.

Twelve weeks after kidney transplant, the patient's daily medications include the following:
    Mycophenolate, 500 mg twice daily
    Tacrolimus, 3 mg twice daily
    Prednisone, 5 mg once daily (body surface area, 1.62 m²)

At today's appointment, her hemoglobin A_{1c} level is 6.8% (51 mmol/mol).

The download from the glucose meter (average 5.2 measurements daily) shows the following:
    14-day average glucose: 221 mg/dL (12.3 mmol/L)
    30-day average glucose: 202 mg/dL (11.2 mmol/L)

Which of the following treatment options would best help this patient achieve better glycemic control?

    A. Initiate GLP-1 receptor agonist therapy
    B. Initiate metformin therapy
    C. Initiate sulfonylurea therapy
    D. Monitor blood glucose without any medical intervention
    E. Restart insulin therapy

---

51   A 3-year-old boy is referred for abnormal findings on thyroid ultrasonography. At an annual well-child visit, bilateral cervical lymphadenopathy was noted, and it had been present for several weeks. He is otherwise healthy, was born at term, and is fully immunized. He has no prior hospitalizations or surgeries. His family history is remarkable for hypothyroidism in his maternal grandmother, and there is no family history of thyroid cancer or other endocrine disorders.

Neck ultrasonography shows prominent bilateral cervical lymph nodes with normal morphology. Also noted is a 7-mm hypoechoic focus in the right thyroid lobe with multiple areas of hyperechogenicity. A lesion with decreased echogenicity that contains multiple areas of hyperechogenicity is located inferior to the thyroid (*see images*).

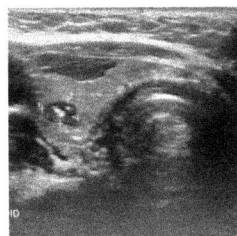

Right thyroid.

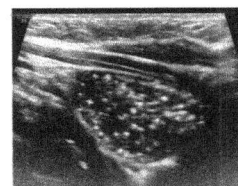

Inferior to right thyroid on the right side.

Which of the following is the best next step in this patient's management?

    A. Measure calcium, phosphate, and PTH
    B. Measure serum calcitonin
    C. Perform CT of the neck and chest
    D. Perform FNA biopsy of the thyroid nodule under ultrasound guidance
    E. Reassure the family that no intervention is needed

---

52   A 16-year-old girl is found to have parathyroid adenomas involving 2 of 4 glands after evaluation for kidney stones revealed hypercalcemia and hypercalciuria. Her family history is notable for her mother having hyperparathyroidism as a teenager, which was treated with subtotal parathyroidectomy, and a pituitary tumor in her 20s. A paternal uncle had thyroid carcinoma as a teenager. Her maternal grandmother also has a history of kidney stones and severe gastric ulcers.

This patient is most likely to have a pathogenic variant in which of the following genes?
- A. *CASR*
- B. *CDC73*
- C. *CDKN1B*
- D. *MEN1*
- E. *RET*

53 A 7-and-4/12-year-old boy presents with failure to thrive and hyperpigmentation.

Laboratory test results:
Cortisol (9 AM) = 4.5 µg/dL (>7.2 µg/dL) (SI: 125 nmol/L [>200 nmol/L])
ACTH = 280 pg/mL (9-52 pg/mL) (SI: 61.6 pmol/L [2.0-11.4 pmol/L])
Peak cortisol after standard short cosyntropin-stimulation test (250 mcg) = 12.3 µg/dL (>19.9 µg/dL) (SI: 340 nmol/L [>550 nmol/L])
Renin = 1.0 ng/mL per h (0.5-3.5 ng/mL per h)
Aldosterone = 4.3 ng/dL (3.6-30.6 ng/dL) (SI: 120 pmol/L [100-850 pmol/L])
IGF-1 = 404.5 ng/mL (152.7-648.9 ng/mL) (SI: 53 nmol/L [20-85 nmol/L])
Urea and electrolytes, normal

On physical examination, he is prepubertal and examination findings are unremarkable except for hyperpigmentation.
He has 2 siblings. His parents are Irish Travellers and second cousins. The patient was born at term, and birth weight was –2.5 SDS. His current height is –2.7 SDS. Bone age is normal.

This patient's condition is most likely explained by pathogenic variants in which of the following genes?
- A. *AIRE* (autoimmune regulator)
- B. *CDKN1C* (cyclin dependent kinase inhibitor 1C)
- C. *MCM4* (minichromosome maintenance complex component 4)
- D. *SAMD9* (sterile α motif domain–containing protein 9)
- E. *SGPL1* (sphingosine-1-phosphate lyase 1)

54 A 6-year-old girl is referred by her pediatrician for possible management of short stature. Her height is 39.6 in (100.6 cm) (SDS, –4.28), and her weight is 41.8 lb (19.0 kg) (SDS, –0.44).
Physical examination findings are remarkable for the presence of significant disproportion with short limbs and an upper-to-lower segment ratio of 1.8 (normal for age = 1.1), genu varum, short fingers, trident configuration of the hands, marked lumbar lordosis, macrocephaly, prominent forehead, midface hypoplasia, and depressed nasal bridge.
Her mother has similar characteristics.

A medication with which of the following mechanisms of action would be most appropriate for managing this child's short stature?
- A. Activation of FGFR3
- B. Activation of natriuretic peptide receptor 2
- C. Enhancement of production of IGF-1
- D. Neutralization of FGF-23
- E. Suppression of somatostatin

55 A 17-year-old boy with obesity and no relevant medical history presents with 3 to 4 days of abdominal pain, nausea, and vomiting. In the emergency department, he is determined to be hyperglycemic and acidotic. Findings on abdominal CT are nonspecific. The treatment protocol for diabetic ketoacidosis is initiated after the initial laboratory results return (*see table*). Twenty-four hours later, his clinical status improves.

Laboratory test	Initial presentation	24 Hours later	Reference range
Blood glucose	528 mg/dL (SI: 29.3 mmol/L)	230 mg/dL (SI: 12.8 mmol/L)	65-99 mg/dL (fasting); 65-139 (nonfasting) (SI: 3.6-5.5 mmol/L [fasting]; 3.6-7.7 mmol/L [nonfasting])
Sodium	128 mEq/L (SI: 128 mmol/L)	145 mEq/L (SI: 145 mmol/L)	135-146 mEq/L (SI: 135-146 mmol/L)
Potassium	4.3 mEq/L (SI: 4.3 mmol/L)	3.2 mEq/L (SI: 3.2 mmol/L)	3.8-5.1 mEq/L (SI: 3.8-5.1 mmol/L)
Bicarbonate	5 mEq/L (SI: 5 mmol/L)	18 mEq/L (SI: 18 mmol/L)	23-29 mEq/L (SI: 23-29 mmol/L)
Venous blood gas pH	7.0	7.30	7.31-7.41
β-Hydroxybutyrate	52.1 mg/dL (SI: >5 mmol/L)	Not measured	<2.81 mg/dL (SI: <0.4-0.5 mmol/L)
Lactic acid	36.0 mg/dL (SI: 4.0 mmol/L)	Not measured	4.5-19.8 mg/dL (SI: 0.5-2.2 mmol/L)
Urine ketones	Large	Large	Small: <20 mg/dL (SI: <1.0 mmol/L) Moderate: 30-40 mg/dL (SI: 1.0-3.0 mmol/L) Large: >80 mg/dL (SI: >3.0 mmol/L)

His regimen is switched to subcutaneous insulin, and he is tolerating an oral diet. Within few hours, he reports recurrence of abdominal pain and nausea. His abdomen is firm and diffusely tender. Laboratory workup documents recurrence of lactic acidosis. His pain intensifies, and the on-call resident orders abdominal x-ray, which shows multiple dilated and fluid-filled loops.

Which of the following is the most appropriate next step to manage this patient's recurring abdominal pain and nausea?
A. Initiate a liquid diet
B. Initiate intravenous proton-pump inhibitor therapy
C. Perform abdominal MRI
D. Restart the insulin drip and intravenous fluids
E. Seek urgent surgical consultation

56 A 19-month-old boy presents to the emergency department with acute dehydration after 1 day of vomiting and diarrhea in addition to a history of thirst, high urine output, and difficulty gaining weight despite supplementation for 6 months. Prior to this illness, his mother reports that he drank 1.0 to 1.2 L per day and would try to drink from any source he could find (eg, bathtub, flowerpots, puddles, toilets). His pediatrician had recommended liquid caloric supplementation because he had difficulty gaining weight. Over the 24 hours, he developed vomiting and diarrhea without fever.

At age 4 years, his mother was diagnosed with central diabetes insipidus and was treated with twice-daily oral desmopressin with good effect. She found she needed somewhat more desmopressin during each of her pregnancies. The patient's 5-year-old sister is healthy and has neither excess thirst nor excess urination.

On physical examination, he appears moderately dehydrated and has mild tachycardia. Length is 31.9 in (81 cm) (22nd percentile), weight is 22 lb (10 kg) (5th percentile), and weight-for-length is at the 11th percentile.

Laboratory test results:
Serum sodium = 152 mEq/L (136-142 mEq/L) (SI: 152 mmol/L [136-142 mmol/L])
Urine osmolality = 118 mOsm/kg (150-1150 mOsm/kg) (SI: 118 mmol/kg [150-1150 mmol/kg])
Serum glucose = 92 mg/dL (70-99 mg/dL) (SI: 5.1 mmol/L [3.9-5.5 mmol/L])

He is admitted to the hospital for fluid resuscitation and initiation of desmopressin, to which he responds well, with decreases in urine output and thirst.

Which of the following best explains the likely molecular pathogenesis of this patient's underlying condition?

    A. Impaired action of vasopressin at its distal nephron receptor encoded by the *AVPR2* gene

    B. Impaired posttranslational processing of the preprovasopressin precursor peptide

    C. Inadequate transcription of the *AVP* gene encoding vasopressin

    D. Inadequate translation of vasopressin from *AVP* mRNA

    E. Increased clearance of circulating vasopressin

57 A 5-and-6/12-year-old boy is referred for poor growth. Review of his growth chart documents a height of 41.4 in (105.2 cm) (7th percentile; –1.49 SDS), weight of 44.8 lb (20.3 kg) (58th percentile; 0.23 SDS), and BMI of 18.4 kg/m^2 (95th percentile; 1.67 SDS). Midparental target height is at 50th percentile. Review of records from his pediatrician shows that he was born at 37 weeks' gestation to a G7P3 mother. His birth weight and length were appropriate for gestational age. No developmental delays are present. He has polyuria but no enuresis.

    On physical examination, he has genu valgum.

Laboratory test results:

    Complete blood cell count, normal

    Bicarbonate = 22 mEq/L (24-34 mEq/L) (SI: 22 mmol/L [24-34 mmol/L])

    Calcium = 9.3 mg/dL (8.4-10.5 mg/dL) (SI: 2.3 mmol/L [2.1-2.6 mmol/L])

    Magnesium = 2.0 mg/dL (1.7-2.5 mg/dL) (SI: 0.8 mmol/L [0.7-1.0 mmol/L])

    Phosphate = 3.1 mg/dL (3.7-4.7 mg/dL) (SI: 1.0 mmol/L [1.2-1.5 mmol/L])

    Alkaline phosphatase = 723 U/L (38-405 U/L) (SI: 12.1 μkat/L [0.6-6.8 μkat/L])

    1,25-Dihydroxyvitamin D = 57 pg/mL (31-87 pg/mL) (SI: 148.2 pmol/L [80.6-226.2 pmol/L])

    25-Hydroxyvitamin D = 18 ng/mL (30-100 ng/mL) (SI: 44.9 nmol/L [74.9-249.6 nmol/L])

    PTH = 56 pg/mL (8-72 pg/mL) (SI: 56 ng/L [8-72 ng/L])

    Urinary calcium-to-creatinine ratio = 0.6 mg/mg (<0.28 for children aged 19 months to 6 years)

Which of the following is this patient's most likely diagnosis?

    A. Fanconi syndrome

    B. Hereditary hypophosphatemic rickets with hypercalciuria

    C. Vitamin D deficiency rickets

    D. Vitamin D–resistant rickets type 1

    E. Vitamin D–resistant rickets type 2

58 A 4-year-old nonHispanic Black boy presents for a new-patient visit. His grandmother reports that he began gaining weight rapidly during infancy, and she is worried that he continues to gain weight. His current height is 41.7 in (106 cm) (77.5th percentile), weight is 50.7 lb (23 kg) (>99th percentile), and BMI is 20.5 kg/m^2 (>99th percentile for age). She notes that multiple relatives struggle with overweight/obesity, and she would like to address these concerns now, so her grandchild can avoid future metabolic complications.

Compared with this patient, which of the following children is at the highest risk for pediatric obesity?

    A. American Indian male

    B. Asian female

    C. Asian male

    D. Hispanic male

    E. NonHispanic White female

59 A 4-and-2/12-year-old boy is referred for evaluation of short stature. Results of a GH-stimulation test (arginine-insulin tolerance test) show a peak GH concentration of 1.6 ng/mL (1.6 µg/L), consistent with GH deficiency. His height SDS is –3.02, and his height has been drifting further below the third percentile in the past 2 years.

MRI of the brain and pituitary gland is performed (*see image*).

Based on the image, which combination of MRI and clinical findings is most likely in this patient?

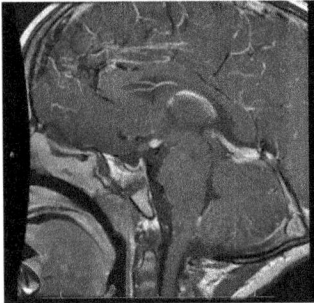

Answer	MRI findings	Clinical findings
A.	Normal hypothalamic-pituitary axis	Isolated idiopathic GH deficiency
B.	Craniopharyngioma	Multiple pituitary hormone deficiencies
C.	Hypoplastic adenohypophysis + ectopic posterior pituitary + interrupted pituitary stalk	GH deficiency and neurogenic diabetes insipidus
D.	Rathke cleft cyst	Isolated GH deficiency
E.	Hypoplastic adenohypophysis + ectopic posterior pituitary + interrupted pituitary stalk	Multiple anterior pituitary hormone deficiencies

60 A 17-year-old boy presents for evaluation of pubertal delay. He was referred by his pediatrician for evaluation of small testes. He reports first noticing signs of puberty at age 13 years. He states he has normal sense of smell and has no headaches or vision problems. He has completed the 11th grade and reports doing well in school. He has a twin sister and a 14-year-old sister; both have undergone menarche. His father states that he was very delayed in completion of his own pubertal development; thus, he has not been concerned about his son's development. Midparental target height is 67 in (170.2 cm) (24th percentile).

At today's appointment, examination findings are notable for prepubertal-appearing genitalia. Stretched penile length is 5 cm, and testicular volume is 2 mL bilaterally. Pubic hair is Tanner stage 4. His height is 66.4 in (168.7 cm) (15th percentile), and BMI is normal.

Laboratory test results:
LH = <0.3 mIU/mL (1.7-8.6 mIU/mL) (SI: <0.3 IU/L [1.7-8.6 IU/L])
FSH = 1.6 mIU/mL (1.5-12.4 mIU/mL) (SI: 1.6 IU/L [1.5-12.4 IU/L])
Total testosterone = 8.6 ng/dL (150-785 ng/dL) (SI: 0.3 nmol/L [5.2-27.2 nmol/L])

Which of the following is the most likely cause of this patient's presentation?
A. 47,XXY karyotype
B. Variant in the *ANOS1* (*KAL1*) gene
C. Variant in the *NR0B1* (*DAX1*) gene
D. Variant in the *SRY* gene
E. Variant in the *TACR3* gene

61 A 3-and-8/12-year-old girl presents to the bone clinic for evaluation of recurrent fractures. She had been limping and was found to have a fracture of her right proximal tibia and fibula last week. The month prior, she fractured her left radius after falling out of bed.

On physical examination, her right foot is casted. She is pale and mildly tachycardic. She has lost 2.2 lb (1 kg) over the last 3 months. She refuses to walk, instead wanting to be carried by her parents.

Dietary intake includes 24 to 32 oz of fortified cow's milk daily. Her parents report that she has abdominal pain and constipation. There is no hematochezia. Abdominal x-ray reveals vertebral compression deformities of T9 through T11. No other radiographic abnormalities are noted.

Which of the following is most likely to diagnose her underlying condition?
A. *COL1A1* genetic testing
B. Complete blood cell count
C. DXA scan
D. 25-Hydroxyvitamin D measurement
E. Tissue transglutaminase antibody measurement

62 A 17-year-old boy with type 1 diabetes mellitus presents for follow-up. Diabetes was diagnosed at 18 months of age. He is a senior in high school and reports adequate skills of diabetes self-management. He is physically active and captain of the swim team. He has been accepted to a 4-year college. He has no vision problems, headaches, imbalance, erectile dysfunction, polyuria, or nocturia.

His hemoglobin A_{1c} values have varied over the past 15 years. He is on a multiple daily insulin injection regimen and seldom uses glucose sensor technology. On review of available blood vs sensor glucose values, there is variation with a standard deviation of 80 mg/dL (4.4 mmol/L). He reports hypoglycemia unawareness.

On physical examination, his blood pressure is 108/65 mm Hg, and pulse rate is 55 beats/min. His height, weight, and BMI are at the 50th percentile. He has mild to moderate lipohypertrophy at insulin injection sites. Nondilated funduscopic examination reveals no change in vessel structure.

He was examined by an ophthalmologist within the past year, and a retinal image captured by a digital camera appears normal. Results from recent laboratory tests are within the reference range. Urine analysis shows glycosuria but is negative for ketones or protein.

Which of the following is the best next step to identify this patient's potential risk for diabetes mellitus–related complications?
A. Diabetic neuropathy screening
B. Dilated retinal examination
C. Fasting lipid profile
D. 24-Hour blood pressure monitoring
E. 24-Hour urine collection to determine albumin-to-creatinine ratio

63 A 7-year-old girl with a history of high-risk neuroblastoma diagnosed at 28 months of age is referred for growth evaluation. Her treatment included radiotherapy to the right orbit (1800 cGy) because her vision was threatened, surgery (status post right adrenalectomy), multiagent chemotherapy, 2 stem-cell transplant procedures, right flank radiation (2160 cGy), immunotherapy, and cis-retinoic acid. She is the shortest child in her first-grade class and is upset that she is shorter than her younger brother.

Review of her growth chart shows that her height had been at the 50th percentile until age 4 years when height deceleration began. Her current height is at less than the third percentile despite adequate weight gain. Her most recent annualized growth velocity was 3.5 cm/y.

On physical examination, she is alert and appears well. Breast and pubic hair are Tanner stage 1.

Laboratory test results:
   Complete blood cell count, normal
   Metabolic profile, normal
   Thyroid function, normal
   Celiac disease screening, negative

Results of provocative testing are indicative of GH deficiency.

Which of the following is the most likely etiology of GH deficiency in this child?
- A. Cis-retinoic acid
- B. Multiagent chemotherapy
- C. Right flank radiotherapy
- D. Right orbit radiotherapy
- E. Stem-cell transplant (without total-body irradiation)

64 A 7-and-1/12-year-old boy is evaluated for poor growth. His height and weight growth charts are shown (*see images*). His BMI is normal. At age 6 years, he underwent assessment for short stature and was found to have low IGF-1 and IGFBP-3 concentrations and delayed bone age. The family did not follow-up with endocrinology after that visit, as they were worried about the adverse effects of agents used in GH-stimulation testing and GH therapy. Now, the family reestablishes care because his little sister (3 years younger) is already taller than he is. His growth velocity is 1.5 in (3.8 cm) per year. His birth weight and length are appropriate for gestational age. He is otherwise healthy. He has no developmental delays.

On physical examination, he is prepubertal with male genitalia that appear small for his age. Stretched penile length is 3 cm.

His bone age is delayed by 2 years.

Laboratory test results:
- Complete blood cell count, normal
- IGF-1 = 24 ng/mL (81-255 ng/mL) (SI: 3.1 nmol/L [10.6-33.4 nmol/L])
- IGFBP-3 = 1.3 mg/L (1.4-5.2 mg/L)
- Free T$_4$ = 0.7 ng/dL (0.7-1.5 ng/dL) (SI: 9.0 pmol/L [9.0-19.3 pmol/L])
- TSH = 2.51 mIU/L (0.70-4.17 mIU/L)

Which of the following is the most appropriate next step in this patient's management?
- A. Order arginine-clonidine GH provocative testing
- B. Perform pituitary-directed MRI
- C. Reassure the family that he has constitutional delay of growth and puberty
- D. Refer to a nutritionist to improve caloric intake and promote weight gain
- E. Start GH therapy

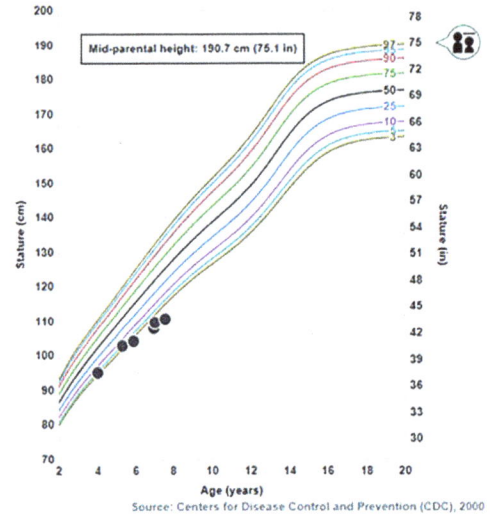

Mid-parental height: 190.7 cm (75.1 in)

Source: Centers for Disease Control and Prevention (CDC), 2000

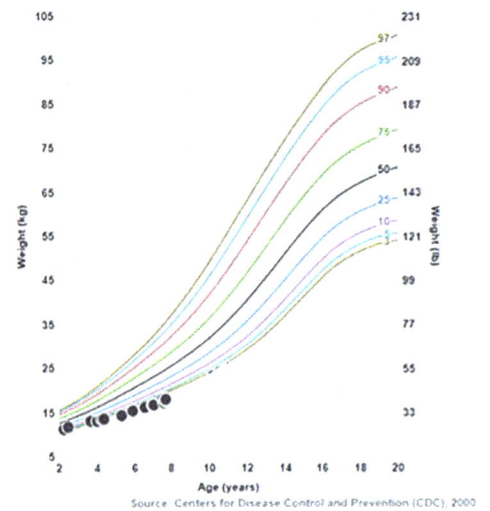

Source: Centers for Disease Control and Prevention (CDC), 2000

65 A 9-month-old boy presents for follow-up of congenital hypothyroidism. His serum TSH concentration at diagnosis was 354 mIU/L, and he began treatment with levothyroxine at 9 days of age. Four weeks ago, his levothyroxine dosage was increased from 50 mcg to 56 mcg daily, based on his thyroid function tests at that time. His parents administer his levothyroxine consistently each day by crushing the tablet, suspending the powder in 5 mL of cow milk–based formula, and administering it orally by syringe.

On physical examination, he has a normal pulse rate and blood pressure, and he appears alert. His growth and weight gain have been normal. His thyroid gland is not palpable. He has normal muscle tone.

Laboratory test results:

Measurement	4 Weeks ago	This visit	Reference range
TSH	7.4 mIU/L	3.7 mIU/L	0.7-5.7 mIU/L
Free T$_4$	1.3 ng/dL (SI: 16.7 pmol/L)	2.0 ng/dL (SI: 25.7 pmol/L)	0.8-1.8 ng/dL (SI: 10.3-23.2 pmol/L)

Which of the following is the most appropriate next step in this patient's management?
  A. Continue the current levothyroxine dosage
  B. Increase the levothyroxine dosage to achieve a target TSH value of 0.5 to 2.0 mIU/L
  C. Measure free T$_4$ by a dialysis method
  D. Recommend administering levothyroxine in soy-based formula instead of cow milk–based formula
  E. Reduce the levothyroxine dosage to avoid elevation of free T$_4$

66 A 25-day-old male baby presents to the emergency department with poor weight gain and poor feeding. He is apyrexial, hypotensive, and tachycardic.

Laboratory test results:
  Plasma sodium = 125 mEq/L (135-145 mEq/L) (SI: 125 mmol/L [135-145 mmol/L])
  Plasma potassium = 6.8 mEq/L (3.5-5.0 mEq/L) (SI: 6.8 mmol/L [3.5-5.0 mmol/L])
  Plasma bicarbonate = 18.0 mEq/L (17.0-25.0 mEq/L) (SI: 18.0 mmol/L [17.0-25.0 mmol/L])
  pH = 7.27 (7.35-7.45)
  Creatinine = 0.68 mg/dL (0.42-1.01 mg/dL) (SI: 60 µmol/L [37-89 µmol/L])
  Urinary potassium = 20 mEq/L (<20 mEq/L) (SI: 20 mmol/L [<20 mmol/L])
  Urinary sodium = 16 mEq/L (<20 mEq/L) (SI: 16 mmol/L [<20 mmol/L])
  Serum aldosterone = 1406 ng/dL (14-108 ng/dL) (SI: 39,000 pmol/L [400-3000 pmol/L])
  Plasma renin activity = 250 nmol/L per h (1.9-29.0 nmol/L per h)
  Plasma glucose, normal

He was born at term to nonconsanguineous parents. His birth weight was 8 lb 10 oz (3900 g). He had an uncomplicated delivery and was discharged home 2 days after birth.

Which of the following is this patient's most likely diagnosis?
  A. Congenital adrenal hyperplasia
  B. Congenital adrenal hypoplasia
  C. Pseudohypoaldosteronism type 1
  D. Pseudohypoaldosteronism type 2
  E. Pyelonephritis

67 A 6-year-old boy is seen for follow-up for a suspected disorder of sexual development. His prenatal course was unremarkable, and he was born at full term. At birth he was noted to have hypospadias, chordee, and nonpalpable testes. Laboratory testing in the neonatal period was notable for a 46,XY karyotype and presence of the *SRY* gene. Pelvic ultrasonography showed small structures in the inguinal canals most likely representing testes. Laparoscopic orchidopexy demonstrated normal left testicular tissue and atrophic testicular tissue from the right gonad without evidence of ovarian tissue.

Physical examination findings are notable for a normal-sized phallus, single left testis, and distal hypospadias. His height is at the 39th percentile.

Laboratory test results (obtained at 5 weeks of age):

    Total testosterone = 146 ng/dL (60-400 ng/dL) (SI: 5.1 nmol/L [2.1-13.9 nmol/L])

    LH = 8.3 mIU/mL (0.2-7.8 mIU/mL) (SI: 8.3 IU/L [0.2-7.8 IU/L])

    FSH = 10.0 mIU/mL (0.2-22.2 mIU/mL) (SI: 10.0 IU/L [0.2-22.2 IU/L])

    Antimullerian hormone = 12.4 ng/mL (32.8-262.7 ng/mL) (SI: 88.6 pmol/L [234.3-1876.4 pmol/L])

Which of the following is this patient's most likely diagnosis?

A. 3β-Hydroxysteroid dehydrogenase deficiency (congenital adrenal hyperplasia)

B. 46,XY ovotesticular disorder

C. 5α-Reductase deficiency

D. Partial androgen insensitivity syndrome

E. Partial gonadal dysgenesis

68 A 7-year-old girl presents for follow-up regarding weight concerns. On physical examination, her height is 47.2 in (120 cm), weight is 55 lb (24.9 kg), and BMI is 17.4 kg/m² (83rd percentile for age). She has a history of asthma. Since her last follow-up visit 6 months ago, she has gained 8.8 lb (4 kg). When talking with the family about her lifestyle habits, her mother reports that she participates in a dance class for 30 minutes twice weekly. She also has a 60-minute physical education class once weekly at school. At home, she occasionally goes outside to ride her bike or play basketball with her brother, but she is more interested in spending time on the computer. Her mother inquires whether she is active enough for her age.

Which of the following is the best recommendation to give this family regarding her physical activity level?

A. Engage in 30 minutes of moderate-to-vigorous intensity physical activity 5 days of the week

B. Engage in 60 minutes of moderate-to-vigorous intensity physical activity 7 days of the week

C. Engage in physical activity throughout the day (no specific time recommendations)

D. Enroll her in longer dance classes so that she engages in 60 minutes of moderate-to-vigorous intensity physical activity at least 3 days of the week

E. Family does not need to make any changes to her physical activity level since she has a normal BMI for age

69 A 12-and-2/12-year-old girl who has been followed for tall stature for 9 years presents for a follow-up appointment. She was born full term via cesarean delivery, and her birth weight and length were adequate for gestational age. Her father's height is 76 in (193 cm), and her mother's height is 73.5 in (186.7 cm). Her father recently died at age 42 years of a heart attack.

On physical examination, the patient's height is 72.7 in (184.7 cm) (>99th percentile; height SDS: +4.54), weight is 213.2 lb (96.7 kg) (>99 percentile; weight SDS: +2.97), and BMI is 28.4 kg/m² (>97th percentile). Her arm span is 77.5 in (196.8 cm), and her upper-to-lower segment ratio is 0.865. She has dolichocephaly, enophthalmos, retrognathia, pectus carinatum, kyphosis, protruding heels, and high-arched feet. Pubic hair is Tanner stage 1, and breasts are early Tanner stage 2. She has no axillary hair.

Genetic test results:

    Karyotype = 46,XX

    Microarray interpretation = normal female

    MC4R genetic testing = negative

    Macrocephaly/overgrowth disorders gene panel (11 genes) = no abnormalities

    Congenital disorders of glycosylation panel = normal

Measurement	Age 10 years, 11 months	Age 12 years, 2 months
TSH	Normal	...
Free T$_4$	Normal	...
IGF-1	262 ng/mL (SI: 34.3 nmol/L)	...
Prolactin	6.4 ng/mL (SI: 0.28 nmol/L)	...
Estradiol	...	27 pg/mL (SI: 99.1 pmol/L)
FSH (ultrasensitive)	...	2.59 mIU/mL (SI: 2.59 IU/L)
LH	...	1.27 mIU/mL (SI: 1.27 IU/L)

IGF-1 reference range: 125-541 ng/mL (SI: 16.4-70.9 nmol/L)

Bone age is interpreted to be 12 years 6 months. Predicted adult height according to Bayley-Pinneau is 77.2 in (196.2 cm).

Which of the following is the best next step in this patient's management?
- A. Echocardiography
- B. Genetic testing for variants in the estrogen receptor gene
- C. Genetic testing for variants in the *FBN1* gene
- D. Oral glucose tolerance test
- E. Reassuring the family

70 A 14-year-old boy presents for evaluation of new-onset thyrotoxicosis with a 1-month history of severe anxiety, difficulty focusing, heat intolerance, diarrhea, and 10-lb (4.5-kg) weight loss. He has a history of long QT syndrome due to an *SCN5A* pathogenic variant. He had severe and prolonged arrhythmia at age 7 years resulting in cardiac arrest and severe cardiac dysfunction. He has had a cardiac denervation procedure and has both a pacemaker and an implantable cardioverter-defibrillator. His arrhythmias are currently well controlled on a combination of flecainide and amiodarone (stable dosages for the past 2 years). His thyroid function has been followed regularly; over the past year, results have documented mildly elevated free T$_4$, normal TSH, and normal T$_3$.

His mother has ulcerative colitis, and there is no other autoimmune disease in the family.

On physical examination, his height is 61.1 in (155.1 cm) and weight is 111.6 lb (50.6 kg) (BMI = 21.03 kg/m^2). His blood pressure is 103/68 mm Hg, and pulse rate is 78 beats/min.

He appears anxious and has a mild tremor. Examination of the neck reveals no goiter and no bruit over the thyroid gland. Eye appearance is normal without proptosis. He has lid lag, but eye movements are normal.

Laboratory test results:
    TSH = <0.01 mIU/L (0.5-4.3 mIU/L)
    Free T$_4$ = 5.6 ng/dL (1.0-1.6 ng/dL) (SI: 72.08 pmol/L [12.87-20.59 pmol/L])
    Total T$_3$ = 279 ng/dL (91-218 ng/dL) (SI: 4.30 nmol/L [1.40-3.36 nmol/L])
    TRAb = <1.10 IU/L (0-1.75 IU/L)

Thyroid ultrasonography shows normal echogenicity, normal vascularity, and no masses.

Which of the following is the best next step in this child's management?
- A. Arrange for urgent subtotal thyroidectomy
- B. Perform a radioactive uptake scan with ^{123}I
- C. Perform a ^{99m}Tc pertechnetate uptake scan
- D. Start propranolol
- E. Stop amiodarone

71 An 11-and-5/12-year-old boy who is 6 months status post endoscopic endonasal near-total resection of craniopharyngioma presents for ongoing endocrine care. No additional treatment for craniopharyngioma has been recommended by his neurooncology team. He initially presented with headaches and increased intracranial pressure. He has multiple pituitary hormone deficiencies (central diabetes insipidus, central hypothyroidism, and adrenal insufficiency).

On physical examination, his height percentile has decreased from the 12th percentile at diagnosis (Z-score, −1.17) to the 5th percentile (Z-score, −1.63), and his annualized growth velocity is 3.1 cm/y despite adequate thyroid hormone replacement. His midparental height is at the 75th percentile. He has also developed hypothalamic obesity, with his BMI increasing from the 73rd percentile at diagnosis (Z-score, 0.62) to the 98th percentile now (Z-score, 2.21).

On physical examination, genitalia and pubic hair are Tanner stage 1.

His IGF-1 Z-score is −3.1 for Tanner stage. His bone age is delayed by 2 years. Surveillance MRI performed the morning of the clinic visit demonstrates expected postsurgical changes and radiologically stable disease. The neurooncologist recommends another surveillance MRI in 6 months.

His short stature is causing him distress, particularly at school, and he is concerned that his younger sibling is already taller than he is.

In addition to engaging the clinical social worker to provide support to the child and family, which of the following is the best management plan?
- A. Counsel the family that GH therapy is contraindicated
- B. Observe for another 12 months, then offer GH therapy if there is no tumor recurrence
- C. Offer GH therapy and perform MRI sooner, 3 months after GH initiation
- D. Offer GH therapy with no changes to planned MRI surveillance
- E. Recommend provocative testing to establish the diagnosis of GH deficiency

72 A 17-year-old boy has a 10-year history of suboptimally controlled type 1 diabetes mellitus. He was lost to follow-up for 7 months and now returns to endocrinology after a recent emergency department visit for dizziness. In the emergency department, he was hyperglycemic but was not in diabetic ketoacidosis. His urine toxicology screen was negative except for cannabis. Thyroid function was also normal.

For the past 8 weeks, he has had daily symptoms of fatigue, headache, postural dizziness, palpitations, loss of appetite, and intermittent nausea. He has also been experiencing "burning" pain in both feet that is worse at night. He initially attributed the pain to playing basketball. He has no joint pain or rash and no vision changes. He is a high school senior, and his grades are poor. He vapes nicotine daily and describes moderate marijuana use. He states he does not use other illicit drugs or alcohol.

He is currently on a multiple daily insulin injection regimen. His basal insulin dosage is 0.6 units/kg per day, which he misses once or twice per week. He is nonadherent to rapid-acting insulin and takes a correction bolus only when he "feels" his blood glucose is "high." He often senses that his blood glucose is low when he is physically active, triggering consumption of glucose-containing beverages.

On physical examination, his blood pressure is 133/85 mm Hg, pulse rate is 57 beats/min, and respiratory rate is 26 breaths/min. His height is at the 75th percentile, and weight is at the 25th percentile. Interim weight loss is 6.6 lb (3 kg). In general, he appears anxious, irritable, and thin. He has no goiter or exophthalmos. Respiratory examination findings are normal with good air entry and no added sounds. Muscle tone and power are normal, but his reflexes are diminished in the bilateral lower extremities. The dorsalis pedis arteries are palpable bilaterally.

Neurologic evaluation shows bilateral, symmetric distal impaired light touch sensation up to the ankles. He has cold hands and feet.

His last point-of-care hemoglobin A_{1c} value was 11.1% (98 mmol/mol). Today's measurement is 11.5% (102 mmol/mol). There are no results from a glucose meter to review.

Urine analysis is positive for glucose and small ketones but no protein.

Which of the following is the best next step in this patient's management?
- A. Another urine toxicology screen
- B. Celiac disease screening
- C. Electrocardiography and cardiac evaluation
- D. 24-Hour urine collection for proteinuria
- E. MRI of the brain

73 A 7-and-10/12-year-old girl is referred for evaluation of short stature. She was born small-for-gestational-age at 40 weeks' gestation via normal vaginal delivery. Birth weight was 5 lb 1.5 oz (2310 g) (−2.06 SDS), birth length was 17.5 in (44.5 cm) (−2.18 SDS), and head circumference was 11.9 in (30.2 cm) (−3.1 SDS). She met developmental milestones appropriately. She has an individualized educational plan at school due to mild learning disability. Her medical history is otherwise unremarkable. No previous growth records are available but, per parental report, she did not display catch-up growth.

Her father was born small-for-gestational-age with a birth weight of 4 lb 13.6 oz (2200 g) (−2.08 SDS) and birth length of 17.3 in (44 cm) (−2.22 SDS). He received GH therapy and reached an adult height of 64.9 in (165 cm). Her mother's height is 64.5 in (164 cm).

On physical examination, the patient's height is 44.6 in (113.4 cm) (−2.42 SDS), weight is 37.0 lb (16.8 kg) (−3.03 SDS), and BMI is 13 kg/m² (−2.1 SDS). Her head circumference is 19.1 in (48.5 cm) (−2.5 SDS). Pubic hair and breasts are Tanner stage 1. There are no dysmorphic features. Body proportions are normal.

Laboratory test results:
IGF-1 = 350 ng/mL (112-276 ng/mL)
(SI: 45.9 nmol/L [14.7-36.1 nmol/L])
Thyroid function, normal
Erythrocyte sedimentation rate, normal
C-reactive protein, normal
Celiac screen, negative

Bone age is 6 years and 10 months.

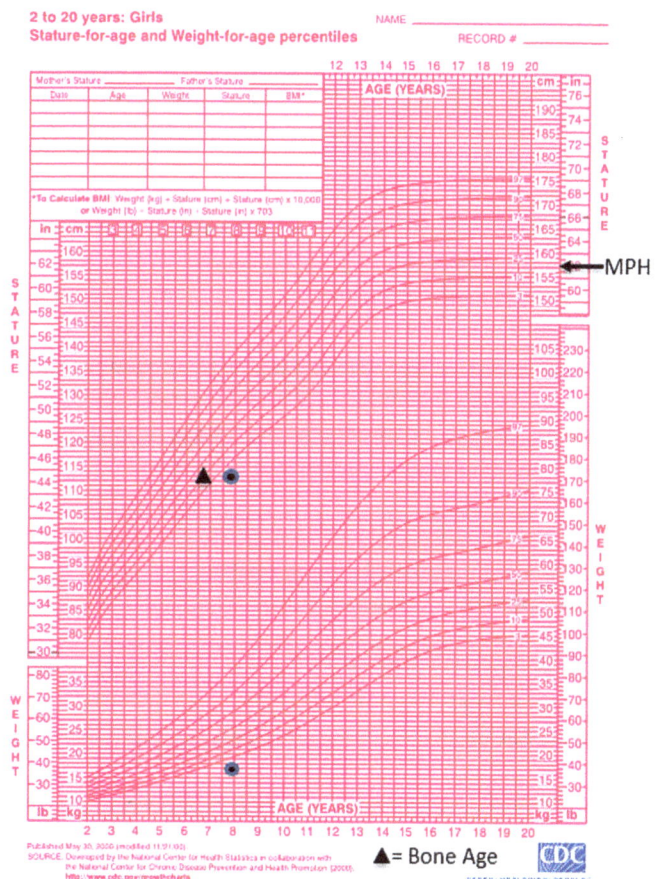

A pathogenic variant in which of the following genes most likely explains the etiology of this child's short stature?
- A. *PAPPA2*
- B. *GHR*
- C. *IGF1*
- D. *IGF1R*
- E. *STAT5B*

74 A 15-year-old girl presents for evaluation of abnormal laboratory studies, which were ordered by her primary care physician to investigate 6 weeks of increasing fatigue and low energy. For the past 2 days, the patient has been extremely tired, hardly able to get out of bed. She describes weight loss of 8 lb (3.6 kg) over the past month due to reduced appetite. She has occasional nausea but no vomiting, diarrhea, or constipation. Over the past 3 to 4 months, she has noticed diffuse thinning of her hair and unusually heavy menstrual periods. She reports no neck swelling, dysphagia, or voice changes. Her mother has celiac disease, and a maternal aunt has autoimmune thyroiditis.

On physical examination, her blood pressure is 94/52 mm Hg and pulse rate is 96 beats/min. She appears tired. Her eyes are normal. Mucous membranes are slightly dry. Her thyroid gland is symmetrically enlarged to twice normal size and is firm and bosselated in texture, with no palpable nodules. Findings on abdominal examination are normal. Her skin is cool and dry.

Laboratory test results:
TSH = 63.0 mIU/L (0.7-5.7 mIU/L)
Free T$_4$ = 0.65 ng/dL (0.8-1.8 ng/dL) (SI: 8.37 pmol/L [10.3-23.2 pmol/L])
TPO antibodies = >1000 IU/mL (<14.9 IU/mL)
Sodium = 131 mEq/L (135-145 mEq/L) (SI: 131 mmol/L [135-145 mmol/L])
Potassium = 5.4 mEq/L (3.5-5.0 mEq/L) (SI: 5.4 mmol/L [3.5-5.0 mmol/L])
Chloride = 102 mEq/L (99-111 mEq/L) (SI: 102 mmol/L [99-111 mmol/L])
Bicarbonate = 20 mEq/L (22-30 mEq/L) (SI: 20 mmol/L [22-30 mmol/L])
Blood urea nitrogen = 40 mg/dL (5-18 mg/dL) (SI: 14.3 mmol/L [1.8-6.4 mmol/L])
Creatinine = 0.9 mg/dL (0.3-1.0 mg/dL) (SI: 79.6 μmol/L [26.5-88.4 μmol/L])
Glucose = 64 mg/dL (60-99 mg/dL) (SI: 3.6 mmol/L [3.3-5.5 mmol/L])

Which of the following is the most appropriate next step in this patient's management?
A. Initiate levothyroxine at full replacement dosage
B. Initiate levothyroxine at half the replacement dosage for 2 weeks, then increase to full replacement dosage
C. Measure 8-AM serum cortisol and ACTH
D. Measure serum tissue transglutaminase IgA and total IgA
E. Perform thyroid ultrasonography

75 A 6-year-old boy has hypoparathyroidism secondary to a calcium-sensing receptor pathogenic variant. He is currently managed with calcium carbonate and calcitriol. He is prescribed calcium carbonate, 60 mg/kg elemental calcium daily (divided in twice daily dosing, taken with meals), and calcitriol, 0.25 mcg once daily. He was previously on sevelamer, 3 packets daily. However, this medication was discontinued because of intolerance.

Laboratory test results:
Calcium = 7.4 mg/dL (8.0-10.5 mg/dL) (SI: 1.85 mmol/L [2.0-2.63 mmol/L])
Ionized calcium = 3.96 mg/dL (3.40-5.80 mg/dL) (SI: 0.99 mmol/L [0.85-1.45 mmol/L])
Phosphate = 7.8 mg/dL (2.8-6.9 mg/dL) (SI: 2.5 mmol/L [0.90-2.23 mmol/L])
Magnesium = 1.9 mg/dL (1.7-2.4 mg/dL) (SI: 0.78 mmol/L [0.70-0.98 mmol/L])
Albumin = 3.6 g/dL (2.6-4.7 g/dL) (SI: 36 g/L [26-47 g/L])
Urinary calcium-to-creatinine ratio = 0.35 (<0.20)

Kidney ultrasonography shows no nephrocalcinosis.

Which of the following changes is the best next step in managing this patient's calcium-phosphate balance?
A. Increase dosage of calcium carbonate to 90 mg/kg elemental calcium divided 3 times daily
B. Increase dosage of calcitriol to twice daily
C. Resume sevelamer
D. Start a low-phosphate diet
E. Start recombinant human PTH injections

76 A 17-year-old young man underwent a sleeve gastrectomy 7 months ago. His preoperative weight was 309 lb (140 kg) (BMI = 45.5 kg/m²). He was lost to follow-up after his initial postoperative visit and now presents with a current weight of 247 lb (112 kg) (BMI = 36.3 kg/m²). He has not been consistently taking his prescribed postoperative supplementation. He has frequent nausea and vomiting that has worsened in recent weeks. His mother reports noticing that he seems clumsier, and he reports feeling like his balance is "off." He also has blurry vision, and his mother has noticed that his eyes do not seem to be in sync at times.

Which of the following nutritional deficiencies is most likely producing these symptoms in this patient?
  A. Ferritin
  B. Vitamin A
  C. Vitamin B_1
  D. Vitamin B_{12}
  E. Vitamin D

77 A 13-day-old male infant is hospitalized for seizures, and endocrinology is consulted for evaluation of abnormal thyroid function test results. The infant was born at 38 weeks' gestation after an uncomplicated pregnancy. The mother was treated with levothyroxine for hypothyroidism during pregnancy. At 7 days of life, the infant developed generalized seizures that have been refractory to initial management. He is currently treated with phenobarbital, levetiracetam, pyridoxine, biotin, and midazolam.

On physical examination, the infant's weight, length, and weight-for-length are normal. His temperature is 98.4°F (38.9°C), pulse rate is 140 beats/min, and blood pressure is 92/52 mm Hg. The infant is calm and has decreased appendicular muscle tone. The cranial fontanelles are open and of normal size. His eyes are normal, and the thyroid gland is not palpable. Findings on cardiac, pulmonary, and abdominal examination are normal. His skin is warm and dry.

Laboratory test results:
  TSH = <0.005 mIU/L (1.7-9.1 mIU/L)
  Free T_4 = >7.77 ng/dL (1.6-3.8 ng/dL) (SI: 100.0 pmol/L [10.3-23.2 pmol/L])

Measurement of which of the following is most likely to be normal in this infant?
  A. Free T_3
  B. Thyroid-stimulating immunoglobulin
  C. Total T_3
  D. Total T_4
  E. TRAb

78 A 4-year-old girl is referred for evaluation of poor growth. Her mother did not receive prenatal care, and she was delivered at home. She was placed in foster care when she was 5 months old, and she was subsequently adopted when she was 18 months old. She was at less than the 1st percentile for height and weight at the time of adoption. Her weight improved with supplemental enteral feeds via a gastrostomy tube. She has had 3 hospital admissions for pneumonia since infancy. She has large, loose, and foul-smelling stools. There are no developmental delays. Her weight is at the 3rd percentile, but height is still less than the 1st percentile. Her BMI is at the 10th percentile. Midparental height is at the 65th percentile.

Laboratory test results:
  IGF-1 = 35 ng/mL (21-157 ng/mL) (SI: 4.6 nmol/L [2.8-20.6 nmol/L])
  IGFBP-3 = 4.2 mg/L (1.71-4.93 mg/L)
  Free T_4 = 0.9 ng/dL (0.7-1.5 ng/dL) (SI: 11.6 pmol/L [9.0-19.3 pmol/L])
  TSH = 2.51 mIU/L (0.70-4.17 mIU/L)

Which of the following is the most appropriate next step in this patient's management?
- A. Perform GH provocative testing
- B. Order karyotype analysis
- C. Refer back to dietician to improve caloric intake and weight gain
- D. Refer to pulmonology
- E. Screen for celiac disease

79 A 5-year-old boy presents for evaluation of signs of puberty. His parents noticed he had adult body odor at 2 to 3 years of age, and he recently started developing pubic hair. He has no acne or axillary hair growth. He has had some behavioral concerns over the past year that his parents have attributed to distance learning. They also note that he is much taller than his peers even though they themselves are not tall.

His mother's height is 66 in (167.6 cm), and she underwent menarche at age 11 years. His father's height is 68 in (172.7 cm), and he underwent puberty a little earlier than average.

On physical examination at today's appointment, the patient's vital signs are normal. Findings are notable for a stretched penile length of 9 cm, testicular volume of 2 mL bilaterally, and Tanner stage 2 pubic hair. His height is 51.6 in (131 cm) (>99th percentile), and BMI is normal.

His bone age is 12 years at a chronological age of 5 years.

Laboratory test results:
Total testosterone (liquid chromatography/tandem mass spectrometry) = 113.7 ng/dL (2.5-10.0 ng/dL) (SI: 3.95 nmol/L [0.87-0.35 nmol/L])
LH = 0.04 mIU/mL (0.02-0.30 mIU/mL) (SI: 0.04 IU/L [0.02-0.30 IU/L])
Androstenedione = 766 ng/dL (0-22 ng/dL) (SI: 26.7 nmol/L [0-0.77 nmol/L])
17-Hydroxyprogesterone = 306 ng/dL (0-90 ng/dL) (SI: 9.27 nmol/L [0-2.73 nmol/L])

Which of the following is the best next step in this patient's care?
- A. Perform adrenal MRI
- B. Perform brain MRI
- C. Perform cosyntropin-stimulation testing
- D. Prescribe an antiandrogen and an aromatase inhibitor
- E. Prescribe hydrocortisone

80 A 13-and-10/12-year-old boy (family-reported Black race) presents for evaluation of growth deceleration. In addition to decreased growth (average annualized growth velocity was 2.6 cm/y over past 3 years), he has had accelerated weight gain and central adiposity.

On physical examination, his genitalia are Tanner stage 2. Bone age is concordant with chronologic age.

Routine screening laboratory studies for impaired growth do not disclose an etiology.

Additional laboratory studies are performed. After nighttime administration of 1 mg dexamethasone, he has nonsuppressed 8-AM cortisol (15 μg/dL [413.8 nmol/L]) and elevated ACTH (89.1 pg/mL [19.6 pmol/L]) with an appropriate dexamethasone concentration. The midnight salivary cortisol value is elevated in one specimen and high-normal in the other. There is 89% suppression of cortisol after administration of 8 mg dexamethasone (15 μg/dL [413.8 nmol/L] → 1.7 μg/dL [46.9 nmol/L]).

Relative to nonminority patients, this patient is more likely to have which of the following based on what is known about racial/ethnic disparities in this condition?
- A. Diagnosis at a younger age
- B. Diagnostic uncertainty after initial testing
- C. Disease recurrence after initial therapy
- D. Predisposing genetic variant
- E. Treatment nonresponse in clinical trials

81 A 16-year-old girl was diagnosed with type 1 diabetes mellitus 3 months ago. She initially presented in diabetic ketoacidosis and was admitted to the intensive care unit. Her current treatment regimen consists of multiple daily insulin injections. She monitors blood glucose with a glucose meter and does not wish to wear a continuous glucose monitoring device. Her hemoglobin A_{1c} value at today's clinic visit is 7.4% (57 mmol/mol), improved from 11.5% (102 mmol/mol) at the time of diagnosis. Her family is supportive, yet hints that insulin injections are becoming contentious and anxiety provoking. She often "mentally disengages" from her parents and prefers to be left alone regarding diabetes-related tasks. She seems to complete all steps of her diabetes care, and her family is happy to report that she quite independent in this regard. She admits searching the internet for possible diabetes cures and wishes that it would resolve. She is also active in social media and claims that venting reduces her stress; she has gained many followers. At the end of the clinic visit, she asks about an app that she uploaded to her smart phone to help calculate insulin doses and would like help to confirm settings for accuracy.

Which of her coping mechanisms will most likely yield the best metabolic outcomes and improved quality of life?
- A. Avoiding her parents to maximize her independence
- B. Mental disengagement to reduce stress
- C. Searching for a cure and wishful thinking that diabetes will resolve
- D. Use of the phone app
- E. Use of venting/social media for relaxation

82 A 3-day-old premature baby boy is referred for abnormal thyroid function test results. His mother did not receive prenatal care and went into premature labor at 29 weeks and 2 days' gestation. The mother's most recent laboratory tests document undetectable TSH and a free T_4 concentration of 4.2 ng/dL (54.06 pmol/L). The infant is intubated and ventilated.

On physical examination, his length is 14.8 in (37.6 cm) (29th percentile), weight is 2.29 lb (1.04 kg) (12th percentile), pulse rate is 147 beats/min, respiratory rate is 37 breaths/min, and blood pressure is 84/52 mm Hg. He has no dysmorphic features. Examination findings are unremarkable. The thyroid gland is not enlarged. His phallus is normal, and testes are undescended bilaterally.

Laboratory test results:
Newborn screen for congenital hypothyroidism (TSH) (age-dependent), normal
TSH = 0.02 mIU/L (0.7-15.2 mIU/L)
Free T_4 = 0.4 ng/dL (0.9-2.5 ng/dL) (SI: 5.15 pmol/L [11.58-32.18 pmol/L])
Total T_3 = 22 ng/dL (73-288 ng/dL) (SI: 0.34 nmol/L [1.12-4.44 nmol/L])
TRAb = 2.15 IU/L (0-1.75 IU/L)

These laboratory findings are most likely due to which of the following?
- A. *FOXE1* pathogenic variant
- B. Prematurity
- C. *PROP1* pathogenic variant
- D. *TBL1X* pathogenic variant
- E. Untreated maternal hyperthyroidism

83 A 6-year-old girl is referred to pediatric endocrinology because of pubic and axillary hair growth that began 1 year ago. She was born at term to nonconsanguineous parents. There is no family history of early puberty. Her mother has obesity, oligomenorrhea, and hirsutism.

On physical examination, the patient's breasts are Tanner stage 1 and pubic hair is Tanner stage 3. She also has axillary hair.

Bone age is advanced (interpreted to be 8.5 years).

Laboratory test results:

DHEA-S = <14.8 µg/dL (22.1-169.7 µg/dL) (SI: <0.4 µmol/L [0.6-4.6 µmol/L])

DHEA = 5.19 ng/mL (1.15-5.19 ng/mL) (SI: 18 nmol/L [1.3-18.0 nmol/L])

Androstenedione = 117.5 ng/dL (4.0-68.8 ng/dL) (SI: 4.10 nmol/L [0.14-2.40 nmol/L])

Testosterone = 17.3 ng/dL (0.86-18.7 ng/dL) (SI: 0.6 nmol/L [0.03-0.65 nmol/L])

LH = <0.2 mIU/mL (0.2-1.3 mIU/mL) (SI: <0.2 IU/L [0.2-1.3 IU/L])

FSH = 2.0 mIU/mL (0.2-3.7 mIU/mL) (SI: 2.0 IU/L [0.2-3.7 IU/L])

Estradiol = 4.9 pg/mL (4.9-14.2 pg/mL) (SI: <18 pmol/L [18-52 pmol/L])

17-Hydroxyprogesterone = 42.9 ng/dL (6.6-191.4 ng/dL) (SI: 1.30 nmol/L [0.20-5.80 nmol/L])

Cortisol = 5.1 µg/dL (3.6-18.1 µg/dL) (SI: 140 nmol/L [100-500 nmol/L])

Pathogenic variants in which of the following genes are the most likely cause of this patient's condition?

    A. *CYP11B1*

    B. *CYP17A1*

    C. *CYP21A2*

    D. *MKRN3*

    E. *PAPSS2*

84 A 15-year-old girl presents for evaluation of irregular menses and fatigue. She reports that she started showing signs of puberty at age 9 years and had her first period 2 years later. Her menstrual cycles have never been regular, occurring once every 3 to 4 months. She has significant acne that she treats with over-the-counter topical medications and has excess hair on her abdomen. She gets tired with regular activity and feels dizzy if she stands up too fast. She reports no concern for weight loss or excessive weight gain. Her medical history is notable only for tympanostomy tube placement and adenotonsillectomy.

On physical examination, she has dark, coarse hair on her abdomen and sides of her face and cystic acne on her back. She has no hyperpigmentation or acanthosis nigricans. Her height is 64.1 in (162.9 cm), and weight is 116.5 lb (52.8 kg) (BMI = 19.9 kg/m² [45th percentile]). Her blood pressure is 104/71 mm Hg.

Laboratory test results:

Hemoglobin A_{1c} = 5.6% (4.8%-5.6%) (SI: 38 mmol/mol [29-38 mmol/mol])

TSH = 0.57 mIU/L (0.45-4.50 mIU/L)

Total testosterone (liquid chromatography/tandem mass spectrometry) = 53 ng/dL (20.0-38.0 ng/dL) (SI: 1.8 nmol/L [0.69-1.32 nmol/L])

Prolactin = 29.3 ng/mL (4.8-23.3 ng/mL) (SI: 1.27 nmol/L [0.21-1.01 nmol/L])

LH = 17.8 mIU/mL (0.5-41.7 mIU/mL) (SI: 17.8 IU/L [0.5-41.7 IU/L])

FSH = 6.0 mIU/mL (1.6-17.0 mIU/mL) (SI: 6.0 IU/L [1.6-17.0 IU/L])

Cortisol = 11.8 µg/dL (6.2-19.4 µg/dL) (SI: 325.5 nmol/L [171.1-535.2 nmol/L])

Androstenedione = 120 ng/dL (41-262 ng/dL) (SI: 0.42 nmol/L [1.43-9.14 nmol/L])

DHEA-S = 346 µg/dL (110.0-433.2 µg/dL) (SI: 9.38 µmol/L [2.98-11.7 µmol/L])

17-Hydroxyprogesterone = 200 ng/dL (20-265 ng/dL) (SI: 6.06 nmol/L [0.61-8.03 nmol/L])

Which of the following interventions is most likely to be helpful?

    A. Cabergoline, 0.25 mg twice weekly

    B. Combined oral contraceptive once daily

    C. Hydrocortisone, 8-10 mg/m² per day divided 3 times daily

    D. Metformin, 1000 mg twice daily

    E. Spironolactone, 40 mg once daily

85 A 10-year-old boy has a medical history of obesity, asthma, attention-deficit/hyperactivity disorder, and aggression. His mother shares that his behaviors have been escalating in recent months. He has been followed by a psychiatrist who prescribed risperidone 3 months ago. His mother is alarmed because he seems to be gaining weight more easily than in the past, and she reports that he has gained 8 lb (3.6 kg) in the past 2 months. Because of these concerns, she has been speaking to his psychiatrist about switching medications, but she also wants to know how other psychiatric medications compare with his current therapy regarding weight effects.

It is most accurate to tell her that he is likely to have more severe weight gain if his current medication is switched to which of the following?
- A. Bupropion
- B. Duloxetine
- C. Fluoxetine
- D. Haloperidol
- E. Olanzapine

86 A 7-year-old girl presents for follow-up of primary congenital hypothyroidism that was present on newborn screening. The patient was born at 36 weeks' gestation and was small for gestational age (length Z-score, –2.71; weight Z-score, –2.45). Her initial diagnosis was delayed because of poor follow-up in primary care. At 9 weeks of age, her serum TSH concentration was 15.6 mIU/L (1.7-9.1 mIU/L) and total T_4 concentration was 5.6 µg/dL (6.2-17.0 µg/dL) (SI: 72.1 nmol/L [79.8-218.8 nmol/L]). She was treated with levothyroxine until age 3 years, at which time she was euthyroid on a levothyroxine dosage of 37.5 mcg daily. She was subsequently lost to follow-up.

She returns to clinic because her 2-week-old maternal half-brother was just diagnosed with primary congenital hypothyroidism on newborn screening. The patient's mother stopped administering her levothyroxine 4 years ago, after her last visit. She has no symptoms.

She has a learning disorder and speech delay. Her mother is healthy and has no history of thyroid disease. The patient's midparental height is 62 in (157.5 cm).

On physical examination, her height is at the 0.3 percentile (Z-score, –2.73), weight is at the 18th percentile, and BMI is at the 80th percentile. Arm span and upper-to-lower segment ratio are normal. Her blood pressure is 88/68 mm Hg, and pulse rate is 106 beats/min. She is not dysmorphic and has no frontal bossing. Her thyroid gland is normal. She has short 4th and 5th metacarpals. The rest of her examination findings are normal.

Laboratory test results:
TSH = 12.9 mIU/L (0.34-5.0 mIU/L)
Free T_4 = 0.9 ng/dL (0.9-1.9 ng/dL) (SI: 11.6 pmol/L [10.3-23.2 pmol/L])
TPO antibodies = <10 IU/mL (0-14.9 IU/mL)
Thyroglobulin antibodies = <20 IU/mL (0-24.9 IU/mL)
IGF-1= 92 ng/mL (80-233 ng/mL) (SI: 12.1 nmol/L [10.5-30.5 nmol/L])
Karyotype = 46,XX

Which of the following is the most appropriate next step in this patient's evaluation?
- A. Measure serum calcium and PTH
- B. Measure serum TRAb
- C. Perform genetic testing for SHOX deficiency
- D. Perform GH-stimulation testing
- E. Perform ^{123}I thyroid scintigraphy

87 A 16-and-5/12-year-old boy with GH deficiency returns for follow-up. He has been receiving recombinant human GH (rhGH) since age 6 years when GH deficiency was diagnosed via an arginine-insulin tolerance test, which showed a peak GH value of 6.2 ng/mL (6.2 µg/L) 30 minutes after insulin administration. Cortisol response to insulin-induced hypoglycemia was normal.

He initially presented at age 5 years and 5 months for evaluation of short stature and a noticeable decline in growth velocity over the preceding 2 years. At that time, his height was below the 3rd percentile (−2.5 SDS). Tests performed during his initial evaluation showed a low IGF-1 concentration of 26 ng/mL (3.4 nmol/L) (IGF-1 Z-score, −2.16) with low IGFBP-3. Thyroid function, kidney function, liver function, and electrolytes were normal. Screening for celiac disease was negative. His bone age was 1 year behind his chronologic age. Brain MRI performed after the arginine-insulin tolerance test showed a small anterior pituitary gland. The posterior pituitary bright spot was in the normal location, and the pituitary stalk was normal.

His current height is 66.1 in (168 cm) (19th percentile; height SDS, −0.85) and is within his midparental height range. At a visit 6 months earlier, his height was 65.8 in (167.2 cm), rendering a height velocity of 1.6 cm/y. Pubic hair and genitalia are Tanner stage 5, and testicular volume is 20 mL.

His current GH dosage represents 0.23 mg/kg weekly.

Current laboratory test results:
IGF-1 = 360 ng/mL (180-501 ng/mL) (SI: 47.2 nmol/L [23.6-65.6 nmol/L])
TSH = 3.7 mIU/L (0.5-4.8 mIU/L)
Free T$_4$ = 1.2 ng/dL (0.93-1.60 ng/dL) (SI: 15.4 pmol/L [12.0-20.6 pmol/L])

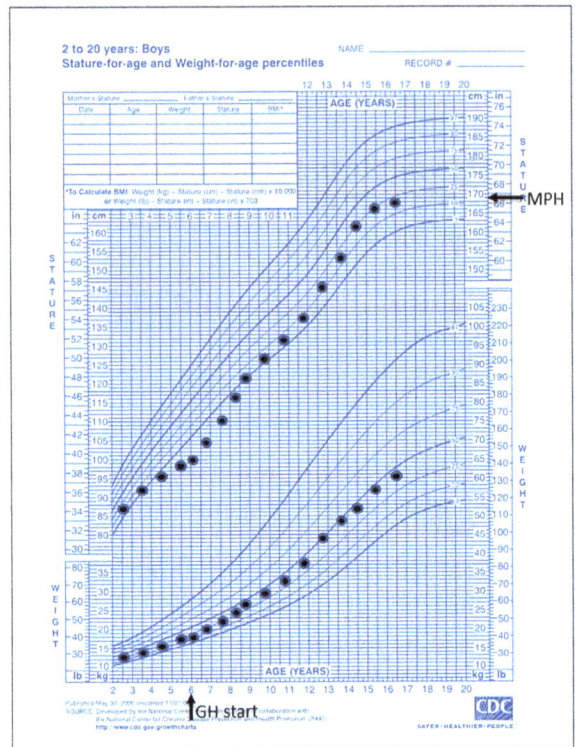

Which of the following is the most appropriate next step in this patient's management?
A. Decrease the GH dosage to the adult replacement dosage starting at 0.04 mg/kg weekly
B. Discontinue GH and measure IGF-1 in 1 to 2 months
C. Discontinue GH and reassure the patient and family
D. Optimize the GH dosage to the pubertal dosage of 0.4 mg/kg weekly
E. Perform an insulin tolerance test

88 A 15-year-old girl presents for evaluation of a recently diagnosed thyroid nodule. She self-identified a lump in her neck several years ago and raised the concern at a recent sports physical. She does not think the lump has changed recently; it is not painful or tender and she has no difficulty swallowing. Her voice is normal. There is no family history of thyroid disease. She has no history of radiation exposure. She is otherwise healthy.

On physical examination, her height is 63.9 in (162.5 cm), and weight is 123.5 lb (56 kg) (BMI = 21.3 kg/m^2). Her blood pressure is 111/72 mm Hg, and pulse rate is 74 beats/min. Her neck is asymmetric. She has a palpable, firm nodule in the left lobe of the thyroid gland. She has bilateral cervical lymphadenopathy with multiple small (<1 cm), firm, mobile, nontender lymph nodes.

Neck ultrasonography reveals a 2.6-cm hypoechoic nodule in the left thyroid lobe with irregular margins and several tiny areas of hyperechogenicity with acoustic shadowing. Blood flow to the nodule is similar to that of the surrounding tissue. The remaining thyroid gland appears inhomogeneous in echogenicity with normal blood flow. She has multiple enlarged lymph nodes in the anterior neck bilaterally with nodes maintaining normal architecture.

Ultrasound-guided biopsy of the left-sided nodule reveals Bethesda IV cytology (suspicious for follicular neoplasm). Molecular genetic testing of the cytology sample reveals the presence of a *DICER1* pathogenic variant.

Which of the following is the best next step in this patient's management?

   A. Evaluate for cystic nephroma and ovarian malignancy

   B. Perform left thyroid lobectomy

   C. Perform total thyroidectomy

   D. Perform total thyroidectomy and central compartment lymph node dissection

   E. Recommend closely monitoring with ultrasonography

89

A medical student is seeing patients in clinic. The next patient is an 8-year-old Black girl, and her growth chart is being reviewed ahead of the visit. Her height is 50 in (127 cm), and weight is 64.2 lb (29.1 kg). The medical student calculates the child's BMI to be 18 kg/m², which is at the 82nd percentile for age. The student asks how well the patient's BMI correlates with her actual adiposity.

Which of the following most accurately describes this patient's BMI and how to interpret her BMI and its ability to detect adiposity?

Answer	BMI	Interpretation
A.	Normal for age and sex	No excess adiposity
B.	Overweight for age and sex	BMI has high sensitivity for detecting excess adiposity
C.	Normal for age and sex	BMI has low sensitivity for detecting excess adiposity
D.	Overweight for age and sex	BMI has low specificity for detecting excess adiposity
E.	Normal for age and sex	BMI has low specificity for detecting excess adiposity

90

An 11-month-old girl with congenital heart disease presents with failure to thrive. She has been having trouble tolerating her feeds and appears dehydrated on examination. In addition, physical examination findings are notable for a broad forehead, flat nasal bridge, upturned nasal tip, wide mouth, and micrognathia. She has a 2/6 systolic ejection murmur.

Laboratory test results:
   Calcium = 14.4 mg/dL (8.2-11.2 mg/dL) (SI: 3.6 mmol/L [2.1-2.8 mmol/L])
   Phosphate = 4.8 mg/dL (4.3-7.4 mg/dL) (SI: 1.6 mmol/L [1.39-2.39 mmol/L])
   Magnesium = 2.6 mg/dL (1.6-2.6 mg/dL) (SI: 1.07 mmol/L [0.66-1.07 mmol/L])
   Albumin = 4.8 g/dL (2.6-4.7 g/dL) (SI: 48 g/L [26-47 g/L])
   Alkaline phosphatase = 105 U/L (73-300 U/L) (SI: 1.75 μkat/L [1.22-5.00 μkat/L])
   PTH = <3 pg/mL (15-87 pg/mL) (SI: <3 ng/L [15-87 ng/L])
   25-Hydroxyvitamin D = 24.0 ng/mL (20.0-60.0 ng/mL) (SI: 59.9 nmol/L [50.0-150.0 nmol/L])
   1,25-Dihydroxyvitamin = <5.0 pg/mL (47.1-151.0 pg/mL) (SI: <13.0 pmol/L [122.0-393.0 pmol/L])

She receives a single dose of pamidronate, and serum calcium normalizes over the next 48 hours. She returns for follow-up in 4 months and has gained weight well. Her serum calcium concentration is 11.0 mg/dL (2.8 mmol/L).

Which of the following is recommended regarding calcium management for this patient?

   A. Furosemide

   B. Low-calcium diet

   C. Monitoring serum calcium every 4 to 6 months until age 2 and then every 2 years thereafter

   D. Second dose of pamidronate

   E. Vitamin D supplementation

91 A 4-year-old girl presents for evaluation of precocious puberty. Her parents report that she started exhibiting breast and pubic hair development, adult body odor, and acne approximately 4 to 5 months ago, and she has recently been growing faster. Her parents also express some concern regarding her vision. Her midparental target height is 66 in (167.6 cm). Her mother underwent menarche at age 12 years, and her dad reports normal timing of pubertal development.

Physical examination findings are notable for Tanner stage 3 breast and pubic hair development and many small, scattered hyperpigmented macules. Her height is 41.3 in (105 cm), and weight is 44 lb (20 kg) (BMI = 18.1 kg/m²).

Bone age is 6 years, 10 months.

Laboratory test results:
LH = 2.2 mIU/mL (0-0.5 mIU/mL) (SI: 2.2 IU/L [0-0.5 IU/L])
FSH = 6.3 mIU/mL (0.2-11.1 mIU/mL) (SI: 6.3 IU/L [0.2-11.1 IU/L])
Estradiol = 18.2 pg/mL (<16 pg/mL) (SI: 66.8 pmol/L [<58.7 pmol/L])
Thyroid function, normal

Which of the following conditions is most consistent with this patient's presentation?
A. Craniopharyngioma
B. Hypothalamic hamartoma
C. Langerhans cell histiocytosis
D. Neurofibromatosis type 1
E. Peutz-Jeghers syndrome

92 A 6-and-6/12-year-old girl presents for assessment of adrenal insufficiency. She was born at term weighing 8 lb 3 oz (3700 g). Her postnatal course was unremarkable. Since age 1 and a half years, she has been overweight and has had overt hyperphagia. She has had several hospital admissions for respiratory tract infections, diarrhea, and vomiting.

Her BMI is +4 SDS. Her mother's BMI is 27.5 kg/m² and her father's BMI is 21 kg/m². Her parents are first cousins of Pakistani origin. Like her parents, she has dark hair and normal skin pigmentation.

Laboratory test results:
Serum sodium = 133 mEq/L (130-142 mEq/L) (SI: 133 mmol/L [130-142 mmol/L])
Potassium = 4.5 mEq/L (3.6-6.2 mEq/L) (SI: 4.5 mmol/L [3.6-6.2 mmol/L])
Serum cortisol (random) = 2.1 µg/dL (6.7-22.6 µg/dL) (SI: 57 nmol/L [185-624 nmol/L])
Plasma ACTH = 2081 pg/mL (9.1-50.0 pg/mL) (SI: 458 pmol/L [2-11 pmol/L])

Which of the following genetic diagnoses best explains this patient's phenotype?
A. Deletion of the paternally inherited 15q11.2-q13 region
B. Maternal uniparental disomy (chromosome 15)
C. Pathogenic variant in the *BBS* genes
D. Pathogenic variants in the *MC4R* gene
E. Pathogenic variants in the *POMC* gene

93 A 9-month-old girl is referred for concerns of failure to thrive. She was born via spontaneous normal vaginal delivery at 38 weeks' gestation. She had normal prenatal and postnatal courses. Results of newborn screening were normal. She has no developmental delays. She was exclusively breastfed until age 6 months. She continues to breastfeed now and eats some solid food.

Findings on physical examination are normal. Her pediatrician is concerned because her weight-for-length is at the lower end of the growth chart (*see images*).

CDC Length-for-Age Growth Chart
Birth to 36 months: girls
Length-for-age and weight-for-age percentiles

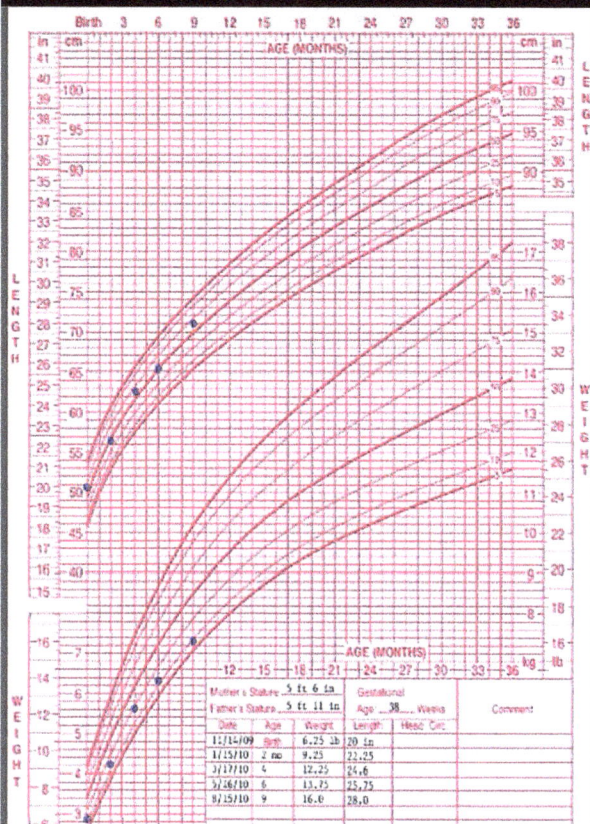

CDC Weight-for-Length Growth Chart
Birth to 36 months: girls
Head circumference-for-age and weight-for-length percentiles

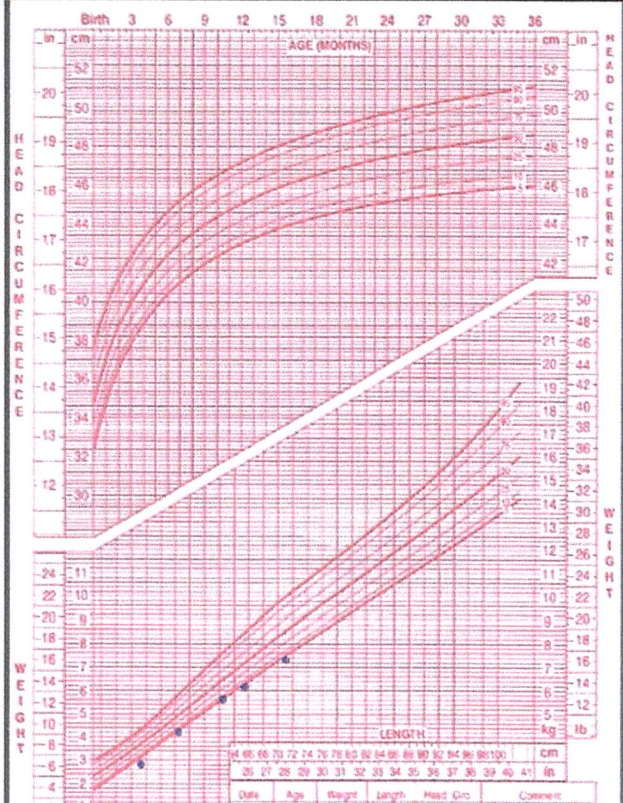

Date	Age	Weight	Length	Head Circ	Comment
11/14/09	Birth	6.25 lb	20 in		
1/15/10	2 mo	9.25	22.25		
3/17/10	4	12.25	24.6		
5/26/10	6	13.75	25.75		
8/15/10	9	16.0	28.0		

Mother's Stature 5 ft 6 in   Father's Stature 5 ft 11 in   Gestational Age 38 Weeks

Modified from *Growth Chart Training: Using the WHO Growth Charts*. Centers for Disease Control and Prevention, U.S. Department of Health and Human Services. https://www.cdc.gov/nccdphp/dnpao/growthcharts/who/examples/example1.htm

Which of the following is the most appropriate next step in this patient's management?

A. Measure free T_4 and TSH
B. Reassure the family that her growth and weight gain are normal
C. Refer for nutritional consultation
D. Screen for celiac disease
E. Supplement feedings with infant formula

94 A 12-year-old girl with autism is referred for evaluation of multiple thyroid nodules. The nodules were noticed incidentally when head CT was performed after a head injury. She has significant developmental delay and is nonverbal, but as far as her parents are aware, her neck does not seem to bother her. She has no symptoms suggestive of hypothyroidism or hyperthyroidism, and her parents have not noticed any lumps in her neck. She is adopted and her parents do not have any information about her family history.

On physical examination, her height is 59.5 in (151.2 cm) and weight is 119 lb (54 kg) (BMI = 23.6 kg/m²). Her blood pressure is 106/68 mm Hg. There are no palpable nodules in the thyroid gland, and she has bilateral shotty anterior cervical chain lymphadenopathy.

Neck ultrasonography, which she tolerates well, reveals heterogeneous echotexture throughout the thyroid gland with multiple small (subcentimeter), isoechoic nodules bilaterally that have smooth margins, no internal calcifications, and normal internal blood flow.

Laboratory test results:
TSH = 2.3 mIU/L (0.5-4.3 mIU/L)
Free T$_4$ = 1.3 ng/dL (1.0-1.6 ng/dL) (SI: 16.73 pmol/L [12.87-20.59 pmol/L])

Which of the following is the best next step in this child's management?
A. Arrange follow-up ultrasonography in 3 months
B. Measure TPO antibodies
C. Proceed with ultrasound-guided FNA biopsy of the largest nodule on each side of the gland
D. Recommend total thyroidectomy
E. Refer to medical genetics

95 An 18-year-old Asian American woman with acquired hypothyroidism secondary to Hashimoto thyroiditis is referred to endocrinology with the concern of episodic hypoglycemia. For the past month, she has had frequent episodes of headache, sweating, tremors, palpitations, and acute hunger that resolves with food consumption. She reports adherence to her levothyroxine regimen (75 mcg daily). She also takes alpha-lipoic acid, 200 mg 3 times daily, as a dietary supplement for weight loss, which was prescribed by her naturopathic practitioner. Her family history is notable for 3 generations of Hashimoto thyroiditis on her maternal side. She has no access to insulin or any other diabetes medication.

On physical examination, she appears anxious. Her vital signs are normal. BMI is 31 kg/m^2. Palpation of her thyroid gland reveals normal size, no asymmetry, and no nodules. She has no skin lesions.

Laboratory test results (sample drawn while fasting):
Glucose = 48 mg/dL (65-99 mg/dL [fasting]; 65-139 [nonfasting]) (SI: 2.7 mmol/L [3.6-5.5 mmol/L (fasting); [3.6-7.7 mmol/L (nonfasting)])
Insulin = 55.0 μIU/mL (<19.6 μIU/mL) (SI: 382.0 pmol/L [<136.1 pmol/L])
Free T$_4$ = 1.3 ng/dL (0.8-1.4 ng/dL) (SI: 16.7 pmol/L [10.3-18.0 pmol/L])
TSH = 2.3 mIU/L (0.5-4.5 mIU/L)

Which of the following assessments would best help establish the diagnosis?
A. *ABCC8* gene sequencing
B. Alpha-lipoic acid measurement with urine toxicology screening
C. *HNF1A* gene sequencing
D. Insulin autoantibody titers
E. Oral glucose tolerance test with measurement of insulin and C-peptide

96 A 14-year-old boy with renal cell carcinoma has been treated with ipilimumab (anticytotoxic lymphocyte-associated protein 4 [CTLA4] antibody) for the last 12 weeks. He has developed severe headaches, vision changes, polydipsia, polyuria, and fatigue. His blood pressure and blood glucose concentration are normal.

MRI of the brain and pituitary demonstrates diffuse pituitary enlargement and homogenous enhancement following contrast.

Laboratory test results are consistent with central diabetes insipidus, ACTH deficiency, and central hypothyroidism.

He is managed with desmopressin, supraphysiologic steroids, and thyroid hormone replacement. After 2 weeks, headache and vision changes resolve, as does pituitary enlargement, but pituitary hormone deficits persist. Supraphysiologic steroid dosages are tapered to physiologic dosages over 1 month.

Which of the following best explains this patient's presentation?
A. Autoimmune hypophysitis
B. Direct CNS toxicity of ipilimumab
C. Pituitary apoplexy
D. Pseudotumor cerebri syndrome
E. Renal cell carcinoma metastatic to the hypothalamus/pituitary

97 A 2-week-old male newborn is referred because of poor weight gain. His 6-year-old brother has simple virilizing congenital adrenal hyperplasia (CAH). His parents are first cousins. He was born at 37 weeks' gestation with a birth weight of 5 lb 15 oz (2700 g). His mother had high blood pressure during the pregnancy and takes a nasal spray for hay fever. Newborn screening on day 4 of life documented a 17-hydroxyprogesterone concentration of 363 ng/dL (11 nmol/L) (reference range for full-term babies <825 ng/dL [<25 nmol/L]).

On physical examination, he has typical male genitalia with bilateral descended testes and some scrotal hyperpigmentation.

His 17-hydroxyprogesterone concentration is 4950 ng/dL (<231 ng/dL) (SI: 150 nmol/L [<7 nmol/L]). Hydrocortisone is started and genetic testing is ordered.

Which of the following is the most likely cause of this baby's newborn screening result?
  A. Low birth weight
  B. Male sex
  C. Maternal preeclampsia
  D. Maternal use of nasal spray
  E. Newborn screening performed outside the typical testing window

98 A 10-year-old girl who started GH therapy 6 months ago for idiopathic short stature has had headaches in the last 2 weeks that sometimes wake her from sleep. She occasionally has blurry vision and vomiting with these headaches, and she missed the last 2 days of school. Her mother took her to the emergency department yesterday where she had normal findings on physical examination. Laboratory workup done in the emergency department showed normal results from a metabolic panel, complete blood cell count, liver function tests, and thyroid function tests. Findings on head CT were interpreted as normal. She was sent home on ibuprofen, which has helped her headaches some. Her current GH dosage is 0.3 mg/kg weekly.

Which of the following is the most appropriate next step in this patient's management?
  A. Continue ibuprofen as needed for headaches and reassure the family
  B. Decrease the GH dosage to 0.15 mg/kg weekly and follow-up in 1 week
  C. Refer her to neurology for migraine headaches
  D. Start acetazolamide therapy, 10 mg/kg daily (once daily)
  E. Stop GH therapy and urgently refer her to ophthalmology

99 A 14-year-old boy presents to the emergency department after a high-velocity motor vehicle accident. Imaging was notable for a tibia fracture, but the radiologist also commented that all the long bones appeared dense with thick cortices and narrow medullary cavities. He has no fracture history, height is 63.0 in (160 cm), dentition is normal for age, and he has no dysmorphic facial features other than mild hypertelorism. Puberty has started. His only medication is a multivitamin.

Which of the following best explains this patient's presentation?
  A. Excessive fluoride consumption
  B. Gain-of-function variant in *LRP5* (low-density lipoprotein receptor-related protein 5)
  C. Gain-of-function variant in *SOST* (sclerostin)
  D. Loss-of-function variant in *CLCN7* (chloride channel)
  E. Loss-of-function variant in *CTSK* (cathepsin K)

100 A 6-year-old boy presents for evaluation of abnormal thyroid function test results. He was initially evaluated by a neurologist because of inattention, hyperactivity, and impulsive behavior that have caused significant difficulty in school. Neuropsychological evaluation revealed low-normal cognitive function. In response to his parents reporting staring spells, the neurologist ordered electroencephalography and brain MRI, which both had normal findings. Attention-deficit/hyperactivity disorder was diagnosed. Prior to initiating treatment with methylphenidate, the neurologist performed a laboratory evaluation that revealed abnormal thyroid function.

The patient was adopted at age 2 years; his prenatal, birth, and family histories are unknown. He has no significant medical history since adoption. His mother reports that he always seems to feel warm. He is gaining weight normally. He has frequent bowel movements but no diarrhea. He has no vomiting, difficulty swallowing, headaches, vision changes, palpitations, shortness of breath, or syncope.

On physical examination, his height is 48 in (121.8 cm) (87th percentile) and weight is 47.2 lb (21.4 kg) (56th percentile) (BMI = 14.4 kg/m² [17th percentile]). His blood pressure is 102/63 mm Hg, and pulse rate is 77 beats/min. He appears well, and his eyes are normal. His skin and hair are normal in appearance and texture. His thyroid gland is firm and diffusely enlarged to 2.5-fold normal size, with no nodules. No cervical lymphadenopathy is present. Findings on cardiac, respiratory, and abdominal examination are normal.

Laboratory test results:
  TSH = 3.61 mIU/L (0.7-5.7 mIU/L)
  Total T_4 = 19.4 µg/dL (6.0-14.2 µg/dL) (SI: 249.7 nmol/L [77.2-182.8 nmol/L])
  Free T_4 = 4.92 ng/dL (1.0-2.1 ng/dL) (SI: 63.3 pmol/L [12.9-27.0 pmol/L])
  Total T_3 = 328 ng/dL (94-241 ng/dL) (SI: 5.1 nmol/L [1.4-3.7 nmol/L])
  TPO antibodies = <10.0 IU/mL (0-14.9 IU/mL)
  Thyroglobulin antibodies = <20 IU/mL (0-24.9 IU/mL)
  TRAb = 7% (<10%)

Which of the following is the most appropriate next step in this patient's management?

A. Initiate methimazole
B. Measure free T_4 by a dialysis method
C. Perform ^{123}I thyroid uptake and scan
D. Recommend proceeding with treatment of attention-deficit/hyperactivity disorder
E. Refer for near-total thyroidectomy

PEDIATRIC ENDOCRINE SELF-ASSESSMENT PROGRAM 2023-2024

Part II

1

ANSWER: B) 45,X/46,XX mosaicism

Turner syndrome is defined as a chromosomal disorder that affects phenotypic females who have 1 intact X chromosome and complete or partial absence of the second sex chromosome with 1 or more clinical feature(s). While the karyotype does not always predict the phenotype, some generalizations can be made that allow more individualized counseling on expected manifestations.

Primary hypogonadism is one of the most common features of Turner syndrome; most affected females have no breast development and have primary amenorrhea. However, up to 30% of females with Turner syndrome have a milder phenotype, which can manifest as breast development followed by pubertal arrest, adult breast development with amenorrhea, or normal pubertal progression followed by menarche. Girls with mosaicism (Answer B) are significantly more likely to undergo puberty and have spontaneous pregnancies than those with 45,X monosomy (Answer A). However, it is important to be aware that a small proportion of girls with a 45,X karyotype can undergo spontaneous puberty and menarche and even achieve spontaneous pregnancy. As this patient has breast development but no evidence of virilization or other unusual features, she most likely has mosaic Turner syndrome.

Other X chromosome anomalies seen in Turner syndrome are often associated with characteristic features. Girls with a ring X chromosome (Answer D) are more likely to have intellectual disability and other findings not typically associated with Turner syndrome, such as atypical facial features and syndactyly. Individuals with deletions of the short arm of chromosome X involving the *SHOX* gene (short stature homeobox) can be expected to have short stature and other skeletal anomalies associated with Turner syndrome. However, girls with deletions distal to Xq24 (Answer E) may have primary or secondary amenorrhea without short stature or any other features of Turner syndrome; thus, they may be identified as having premature ovarian insufficiency, not Turner syndrome.

Individuals with 45,X/46,XY mixed gonadal dysgenesis may have phenotypic features of Turner syndrome with normal female appearance or may have mild to severe virilization. However, normal isosexual development without virilization would not be expected, thus 45,X/46,XY mosaicism (Answer C) is incorrect. Laparoscopic gonadectomy of streak gonads is recommended for female patients with Y-chromosome mosaicism because gonadoblastomas have a high risk of malignant transformation.

Educational Objective
Identify genotype-phenotype relationships in Turner syndrome.

Reference(s)

Gravholt CH, Andersen NH, Conway GS, et al; International Turner Syndrome Consensus Group. Clinical practice guidelines for the care of girls and women with Turner syndrome: proceedings from the 2016 Cincinnati International Turner Syndrome Meeting. *Eur J Endocrinol.* 2017;177(3):G1-G70. PMID: 28705803

2

ANSWER: A) *ALMS1* (ALMS1 centrosome and basal body associated protein)

The child in this vignette has a clinical history that is most suspicious for Alström syndrome, which is a ciliopathy. Alström syndrome is a very rare autosomal recessive form of monogenic obesity. The prevalence is 1 to 10 in 1,000,000 persons. Alström syndrome is characterized by progressive cone-rod dystrophy that develops within the first year of life. By the second decade of life, most patients are blind. In addition to early-onset obesity and hyperphagia, progressive sensorineural hearing loss can affect up to 70% of patients, as can cardiomyopathy and hepatic and kidney dysfunction. Patients may have developmental delay, but intelligence is usually unaffected. Patients with Alström syndrome are also at high risk for endocrine dysfunction, including type 2 diabetes mellitus, hypothyroidism, short stature, and hypogonadism. The disorder is caused by pathogenic variants in the *ALMS1* gene (Answer A), which is located on chromosome 2p13.

Bardet-Biedel syndrome is defined as a ciliopathy, similar to Alström syndrome. It is a very heterogeneous disorder, but in addition to severe, early-onset obesity, affected patients will develop night blindness by late childhood and continued progressive cone-rod dystrophy into adolescence, postaxial polydactyly or syndactyly, hypogonadism, intellectual impairment, and kidney disease. While more than 20 different genes have been implicated in Bardet-Biedel syndrome, pathogenic variants in *BBS1* (Answer B) and *BBS10* are most common in European and White populations, accounting for 20% to 30% of those with Bardet-Biedel syndrome.

Congenital leptin deficiency leads to severe, early-onset obesity starting soon after birth. It is caused by pathogenic variants in the *LEP* gene (Answer C). It is extremely uncommon, with fewer than 30 cases reported in the literature. Pathogenic variants in the *LEPR* gene (Answer D) result in leptin receptor deficiency. *LEPR* pathogenic variants are found in 2% to 3% of patients who present with severe early-onset obesity. In addition to early-onset obesity, patients with congenital leptin deficiency and leptin receptor deficiency demonstrate marked hyperphagia and hypogonadotropic hypogonadism. They may also be at risk for immune dysfunction.

Pathogenic variants in the *POMC* gene (Answer E) result in proopiomelanocortin (POMC) deficiency. Patients with POMC deficiency exhibit early-onset obesity and hyperphagia. Additionally, they are at risk for central adrenal insufficiency due to ACTH deficiency and central hypothyroidism. Some affected patients will also be diagnosed with GH deficiency and/or gonadotropin deficiency. While not true for all patients with POMC deficiency, red hair and pale skin have been described as a result of deficient production of melanocyte-stimulating hormone.

Educational Objective
Identify the phenotypic features seen in patients with Alström syndrome.

Reference(s)
Tahani N, Maffei P, Dollfus H, et al. Consensus clinical management guidelines for Alström syndrome. *Orphanet J Rare Dis.* 2020;15(1):253. PMID: 32958032

Han JC, Reyes-Capo DP, Liu CY, et al. Comprehensive endocrine-metabolic evaluation of patients with Alström syndrome compared with BMI-matched controls. *J Clin Endocrinol Metab.* 2018;103(7):2707-2719. PMID: 29718281

3 ANSWER: C) Vitamin C

Vitamin C deficiency (Answer C), or scurvy, is a rare cause of metabolic bone disease, but it has been reported in several recent case series, often involving children with autism spectrum disorder and severely restricted diets. This patient's vitamin C concentration was undetectable at less than 5 μmol/L. Vitamin C is an important cofactor for collagen hydroxylation and cross-linking. During periods of rapid growth, vitamin C deficiency results in abnormal production of the bony matrix. Without the collagen framework, bones are osteopenic with thin cortices, especially within the epiphyses. However, if vitamin D and calcium intake are adequate, mineralization occurs normally. Vitamin C is a water-soluble vitamin, and deficient intake for as few as 1 to 3 months can result in these skeletal changes. The recommended daily allotment of vitamin C is highest during adolescence at 75 mg, or the equivalent of 1 cup of oranges, strawberries, or broccoli. Considering vitamin C deficiency is important in patients who have restricted diets.

In contrast, rickets due to deficiency of vitamin D (Answer D), calcium (Answer A), or phosphorus results in excessive osteoid formation that is unmineralized. The growth plate is widened with fraying at the metaphyses—features not seen in this child's x-ray.

The figures contrast the radiographic appearance of vitamin C deficiency (*figure A*) and vitamin D deficiency (*figure B*). Both patients represented in the figures had nutritional deficiencies due to restricted eating behaviors as part of autism spectrum disorder.

In Figure A, the bones of the child presented in this vignette appear osteoporotic. The dashed white lines show dense sclerotic bands at the zone of provisional calcification (Frankel lines) as mineralization occurs normally, but collagen formation is decreased. Peripheral extension of this zone of calcification results in "beaking" (*noted by the asterisk*). The cortices are thin, especially at the epiphyses (*dashed black lines*). This

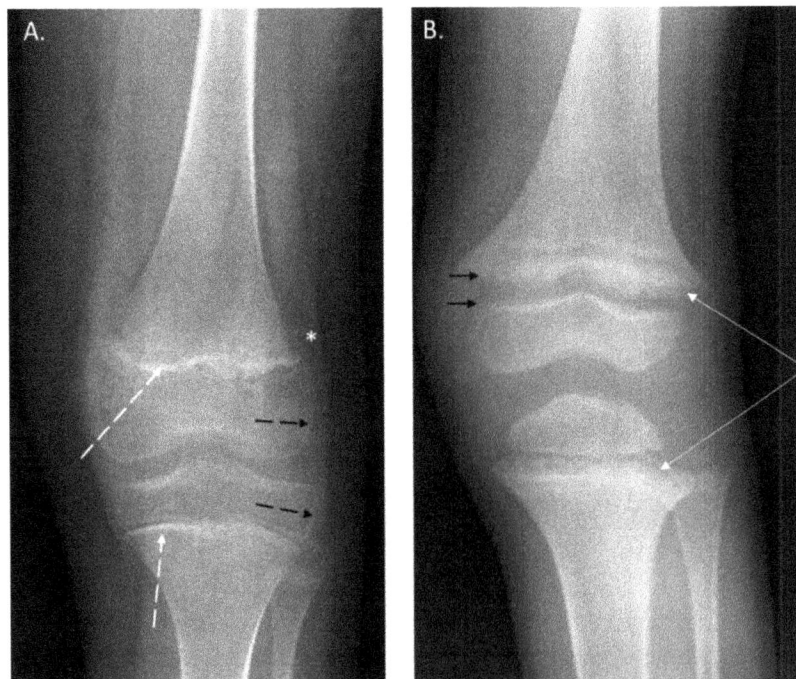

image does not clearly show subperiosteal hemorrhage nor the Trummerfeld zone, which represents hemorrhage directly adjacent to the Frankel line. In some cases, this is an area where fractures occur. Figure B is an x-ray of a 6-year-old boy. The solid white lines show fraying of the metaphysis with irregular borders. Metaphyses are significantly wider than adjacent epiphyses. The solid black lines show widening of the growth plate where normal chondrocyte proliferation continues.

Lead poisoning (Answer B) can be a cause of dense metaphyseal lines, but findings of thin cortices of the epiphyses and periosteal reaction would not be expected. Skeletal changes of lead poisoning also reflect chronic exposure, whereas this child's symptoms are more acute.

Vitamin K (Answer E) is involved in the carboxylation of many bone proteins and the regulation of bone resorption. Vitamin K deficiency been associated with reduced bone density and fracture in adults on anticoagulant therapy. There are no classic radiographic features of vitamin K deficiency.

Educational Objective
Distinguish radiographic findings of vitamin C deficiency from those of vitamin D deficiency.

Reference(s)

Perkins A, Sontheimer C, Otjen JP, Shenoi S. Scurvy masquerading as juvenile idiopathic arthritis or vasculitis with elevated inflammatory markers: a case series. *J Pediatr.* 2020;218:234-237.e2. PMID: 31843213

Chang CY, Rosenthal DI, Mitchell DM, Handa A, Kattapuram SV, Huang AJ. Imaging findings of metabolic bone disease. *Radiographics.* 2016;36(6):1871-1887. PMID: 27726750

4 **ANSWER: C) Test for tear production (Schirmer test)**

This child has triple-A syndrome with a combination of adrenal insufficiency and hyperreflexia. Triple-A syndrome (AAAS) is a rare autosomal recessive disorder characterized by the triad of **a**lacrima (an inability to produce tears), **a**chalasia of the esophageal cardia, and **a**drenal failure. Pathogenic variants in the *AAAS* gene, which encodes the nuclear pore protein ALADIN, cause triple-A syndrome. Alacrima is the earliest and most consistent manifestation of triple-A syndrome, and it is often present from birth (93%-100%). Alacrima is diagnosed by performing the Schirmer test (Answer C) to determine deficiency in tear production. Small lacrimal ducts have been observed on MRI in affected patients, and autonomic dysfunction of the lacrimal glands has been suggested as a mechanism. Alacrima can be overlooked unless specifically inquired about or investigated. A barium swallow (Answer A) would be helpful in diagnosing achalasia, although this is a less frequent or consistent feature in triple-A syndrome (overall frequency of 57%-86%) than alacrima, and has an average age of onset of 6.4 to 8.19 years. Symptoms and severity of achalasia can be progressive.

More than 200 cases of triple-A syndrome have been described worldwide. This condition is very heterogeneous clinically, with wide variability in age of onset, presence of features, and symptom severity. Most recent reports suggest that the 3 cardinal features (alacrima, achalasia, and adrenal insufficiency) are present in 58% to 70% of affected patients.

In individuals with triple-A syndrome, adrenal insufficiency most commonly presents in mid-childhood, with a median age of onset of 4 years, but its onset can vary from birth to 35 years. Histologic examination the adrenal glands in deceased individuals reveals atrophy of the adrenal cortical zona fasciculata and zona reticularis. The proportion of patients with triple-A syndrome who have adrenal insufficiency with mineralocorticoid deficiency is variable and depends on the cohort studied (ranging from 10% to 50%). The pathophysiology of mineralocorticoid deficiency is unknown and may be due to progressive degeneration of zona glomerulosa and/or autonomic dysfunction.

A wide range of neurologic and autonomic features have been associated with triple-A syndrome and, in fact, these can be the only presenting features. Autonomic dysfunction is reported in one-third of affected patients. Approximately 70% of affected patients have progressive neurodegenerative features that can be very disabling (*see box*). The median age of onset is 12 years, with a range of 1.1 to 40 years. Because of variable neurologic abnormalities, individuals with triple-A syndrome may be incorrectly diagnosed with juvenile amyotrophic lateral sclerosis, Charcot-Marie-Tooth disease, or other neurologic disorders. Skin changes such as palmoplantar hyperkeratosis can also be present. There is no genotype-phenotype correlation. Clinical heterogeneity exists in patients who have the same *AAAS* pathogenic variants, as well as among affected individuals within the same family.

Box. Features Associated With Triple-A Syndrome

System	Features
Endocrine	• Adrenal insufficiency (78%-79%) (mineralocorticoid deficiency reported in 10%-50%) • Osteoporosis • Short stature (70%) • Delayed puberty (28% especially in males) • Amenorrhea (hypogonadotropic hypogonadism, 4%) • Low DHEA-S (100%)
Ophthalmologic	• Alacrima/hypolacrima (earliest, most consistent manifestation, within the first year of life, 93%-100%) • Optic atrophy • Anisocoria/abnormal pupillary responses
Gastrointestinal	• Achalasia (57%-86%) • Dysphagia (26%) • Regurgitation • Weight loss/failure to thrive • Chronic cough
Autonomic	• Postural hypotension • Bladder dysfunction • Anisocoria/abnormal pupillary responses • Increased/decreased sweating • Heart arrhythmias/abnormal heart responses • Sexual dysfunction (13%)
Neurologic (72%)	• Decreased muscle tone/muscle atrophy/muscle weakness • Hyperreflexia (57%) • Extensor plantar responses • Ataxia/clumsiness • Pes cavus • Gait disturbances • Dysarthria/nasal speech • Parkinsonism/extrapyramidal symptoms • Sensory impairment • Sensorineural deafness • Microcephaly • Intellectual disability (can progress) • Dementia • Epilepsy • Polyneuropathy • Upper and lower motor neuron signs
Dermatologic (71%)	• Hyperpigmentation (43%) • Palmoplantar and punctate hyperkeratosis • Cutis anserine • Incomplete dermatoglyphics
Oral	• Xerostomia • Fissured tongue • Dental caries • Edentulism • Fungal infections
Dysmorphism	• Narrow face • Long philtrum • Down-turned mouth
Respiratory	• Chronic respiratory symptoms/recurrent infections

Adapted from the following references (note that the frequency of these findings varies significantly depending on cohort studies and inclusion criteria):

Flokas ME, Tomani M, Agdere L, Brown B. Triple A syndrome (Allgrove syndrome): improving outcomes with a multidisciplinary approach. *Pediatric Health Med Ther*. 2019;10:99-106.

Polat R, Ustyol A, Tuncez E, Gurna T. A broad range of symptoms in Allgrove syndrome: single center experience in Southeast Anatolia. *J Endocrinol Invest*. 2020;43(2):185-196.

Patt H, Koehler K, Lodha S, et al. Phenotype-genotype spectrum of AAA syndrome from Western India and systematic review of literature. *Endocr Connect*. 2017;6(8):901-913.

Prasad R, Metherell LA, Clark AJ, Storr HL. Deficiency of ALADIN impairs redox homeostasis in human adrenal cells and inhibits steroidogenesis. *Endocrinology*. 2013;154(9):3209-3218.

Muscle biopsy (Answer B) would be beneficial in diagnosing Duchenne muscular dystrophy in a child with adrenal insufficiency. This combination can be seen in patients with a contiguous deletion in which deletion of the *NR0B1* gene in males leads to adrenal hypoplasia congenita together with Duchenne muscular dystrophy and/or glycerol kinase deficiency. In this case, one would see reduced reflexes. Also, the patient in this vignette is female, so a muscle biopsy is not necessary.

Very long-chain fatty acid measurement (Answer E) is an important part of evaluating boys presenting with adrenal insufficiency to exclude adrenoleukodystrophy due to pathogenic variants in the *ABCD1* gene. In adrenoleukodystrophy, increased tendon reflexes can be associated with adrenal insufficiency. Because this patient is female, measuring very long-chain fatty acids is incorrect. However, there are emerging data on women with *ABCD1* gene variants who develop myelopathy at a later age than affected men.

Ultrasonography of the adrenal glands (Answer D) is rarely helpful in diagnosing the cause of adrenal insufficiency unless it is due to infection, hemorrhage, or infarction, and its usefulness is operator dependent.

Educational Objective
Diagnose triple-A syndrome in a child with adrenal insufficiency and hyperreflexia.

Reference(s)

Prasad R, Metherell LA, Clark AJ, Storr HL. Deficiency of ALADIN impairs redox homeostasis in human adrenal cells and inhibits steroidogenesis. *Endocrinology.* 2013;154(9):3209-3218. PMID: 23825130

Roucher-Boulez F, Brac de la Perriere A, Jacquez A, et al. Triple-A syndrome: a wide spectrum of adrenal dysfunction. *Eur J Endocrinol.* 2018;178(3):199-207. PMID: 29237697

Muscatelli F, Strom TM, Walker AP, et al. Mutations in the DAX-1 gene give rise to both X-linked adrenal hypoplasia congenita and hypogonadotropic hypogonadism. *Nature.* 1994;372(6507):672-676. PMID: 7990958

Kemp S, Huffnagel IC, Linthorst GE, Wanders RJ, Engelen M. Adrenoleukodystrophy - neuroendocrine pathogenesis and redefinition of natural history. *Nat Rev Endocrinol.* 2016;12(10):606-615. PMID: 27312864

Flokas ME, Tomani M, Agdere L, Brown B. Triple A syndrome (Allgrove syndrome): improving outcomes with a multidisciplinary approach. *Pediatric Health Med Ther.* 2019;10:99-106. PMID: 31695556

Polat R, Ustyol A, Tuncez E, Gurna T. A broad range of symptoms in Allgrove syndrome: single center experience in Southeast Anatolia. *J Endocrinol Invest.* 2020;43(2):185-196. PMID: 31435881

Patt H, Koehler K, Lodha S, et al. Phenotype-genotype spectrum of AAA syndrome from Western India and systematic review of literature. *Endocr Connect.* 2017;6(8):901-913. PMID: 29180348

5 ANSWER: B) Measure TSH

Although familial hypercholesterolemia due to a heterozygous pathogenic variant in the *LDLR* gene is quite common in the general population (2 or more per 1000 persons), and this patient's LDL-cholesterol and total cholesterol concentrations are compatible with such a diagnosis, it is important to exclude secondary causes of hypercholesterolemia before committing her to lifelong lipid-lowering therapy (Answers D and E), which may be associated with potential adverse effects. Also, patients with familial hypercholesterolemia are typically prescribed a statin, not ezetimibe.

Lack of family history does not exclude familial hypercholesterolemia. Genetic testing is generally not required to confirm the diagnosis, although this may change. Genetic testing (Answer A) should not be ordered until secondary causes of hypercholesterolemia have been excluded.

Hypothyroidism can present with hypercholesterolemia and normocytic anemia, and this must be excluded (Answer B). Indeed, this patient's TSH value was markedly elevated at 229 mIU/L (0.45-4.5 mIU/L), with a very low free T_4 concentration (<0.10 ng/dL [<1.3 pmol/L]). She was started on levothyroxine, 50 mcg daily, and the dosage has been gradually increased. Subsequent testing demonstrated that her primary hypothyroidism is due to Hashimoto thyroiditis based on very elevated TPO and thyroglobulin antibodies. Secondary hypercholesterolemia may also be observed in nephrotic syndrome, but she had no edema and her serum albumin level was normal. Her urinary protein excretion was too mild to be a cause of elevated cholesterol. Of note, hypothyroidism is associated with a decreased glomerular filtration rate. In severe cases, it may result in elevated serum creatinine and proteinuria, which are reversible upon correction of hypothyroidism. One month after this patient started levothyroxine, her creatinine corrected to 0.86 mg/dL (76.0 μmol/L) and her TSH concentration decreased to 20.5 mIU/L. A repeated lipid panel should be done once she is euthyroid.

Her diet is not optimal, and it is most likely contributing to her obesity. However, she does not seem to have high intake of saturated fats. She would benefit from seeing a dietitian (Answer C), but she will not need a diet low in saturated fat diet to control her hypercholesterolemia.

Educational Objective
Identify hypothyroidism as a secondary cause of hypercholesterolemia.

Reference(s)

Nordestgaard BG, Chapman MJ, Humphries SE, et al; European Atherosclerosis Society Consensus Panel. Familial hypercholesterolaemia is underdiagnosed and undertreated in the general population: guidance for clinicians to prevent coronary heart disease: consensus statement of the European Atherosclerosis Society. *Eur Heart J.* 2013;34(45):3478-3490a. PMID: 23956253

Chang Y-C, Chang CH, Yeh Y-C, Chuang L-M, Tu Y-K. Subclinical and overt hypothyroidism is associated with reduced glomerular filtration rate and proteinuria: a large cross-sectional population study. *Sci Rep.* 2018;8(1):2031. PMID: 29391480

Weerakkody RM, Lokuliyana PN. Severe hypothyroidism presenting as reversible proteinuria: two case reports. *J Med Case Rep.* 2019;13(1):270. PMID: 31455390

6. ANSWER: E) X-linked acrogigantism

Based on this patient's clinical presentation and laboratory results, she has gigantism. This is supported by the elevated IGF-1 concentration and random measurement of GH, consistent with GH excess. The lack of dysmorphic features on examination suggests that the gigantism is caused by a GH-producing pituitary adenoma rather than a syndromic overgrowth condition. The MRI finding of a pituitary macroadenoma also supports the diagnosis. The early presentation during infancy/early childhood makes X-linked acrogigantism (X-LAG) (Answer E) the most likely etiology.

X-LAG was described in 2014 when several individuals with gigantism and pituitary tumors but with no known pathogenic variants in the genes associated with pituitary adenomas were found to have microduplications on chromosome Xq26.3. Interestingly, in this study, the microduplications were found only in individuals with the early childhood form and not in individuals with onset in adolescence. Further analysis showed that the microduplications contain 4 protein-coding genes. One of these genes is *GPR101*, which encodes a G-protein–coupled receptor; pathogenic variants in *GPR101* have been found in some adults with acromegaly. Duplication of this gene in patients with childhood-onset gigantism results in overexpression and an increase in the synthesis of a G-protein–coupled receptor in the pituitary lesions of affected patients (pituitary adenomas [microadenomas or macroadenomas] with or without pituitary hyperplasia). Microduplication of Xq26.3 can be familial (inherited) or sporadic. These microduplications of the Xq26.3 region happen during chromosome replication and lead to gain of function of this specific G-protein–coupled receptor; therefore, this can occur in females despite being categorized as X-linked. In 1 study of 13 patients with Xq26.3 microduplication, 9 were female and had normal birth size.

Although McCune-Albright syndrome (Answer A) may also lead to GH excess and gigantism in childhood, other clinical findings are usually present, including typical café-au-lait spots and monostotic or polyostotic fibrous dysplasia.

Neurofibromatosis type 1 (Answer B) can also lead to gigantism as a result of excess GH secretion via a different mechanism. In this setting, GH secretion is not related to pituitary GH-producing adenomas, but rather it is postulated to be due to disruption of the somatostatin control of GH production.

Sotos syndrome (Answer C) is a syndromic overgrowth condition with a specific phenotype that includes prenatal onset of rapid growth, macrocephaly, hypertelorism, and variable degrees of intellectual disability. This condition is not associated with pituitary abnormalities.

Tatton-Brown-Rahman syndrome (Answer D) is characterized by prenatal and postnatal overgrowth with typical dysmorphic features that include increased head circumference, round face, heavy horizontal eyebrows, and narrow palpebral fissures. Affected individuals also have impaired intellectual development.

Educational Objective
Diagnose X-linked acrogigantism and identify the clinical features that can help distinguish it from other overgrowth conditions.

Reference(s)

Trivellin G, Daly AF, Faucz FR, et al. Gigantism and acromegaly due to Xq26 microduplications and GPR101 mutation. *N Engl J Med.* 2014;371(25):2363-2374. PMID: 25470569

Dénes J, Korbonits M. The clinical aspects of pituitary tumor genetics. *Endocrine.* 2021;71(3):663-674. PMID: 33543431

7 ANSWER: D) Nephrogenic syndrome of inappropriate antidiuresis

This male newborn has presented with irritability, possible seizure activity, and hyponatremia without physical signs of volume overload or dehydration. His serum osmolality is low, and there is evidence of increased natriuresis.

Arginine vasopressin (AVP) secretion from the posterior pituitary gland is regulated by plasma and interstitial osmotic pressure sensed by osmoreceptors in the hypothalamus, as well as by circulating blood volume sensed by carotid, aortic, and atrial baroreceptors. After AVP is released into the circulation, it binds to its receptor, AVPR2, on the basolateral or interstitial side of the renal collecting duct. AVPR2 is a G-protein–coupled receptor. Binding of AVP to the receptor results in activation of adenylyl cyclase, an increase in cAMP release, and activation of protein kinase. The protein kinase phosphorylates AQP2, which stimulates the translocation of subapical AQP2-containing vesicles to the apical (luminal) membrane. Water is then able to enter the apical side of the collecting duct and leave the cell to the interstitium on the basolateral side via AQP3 and AQP4 channels (*see figure*).

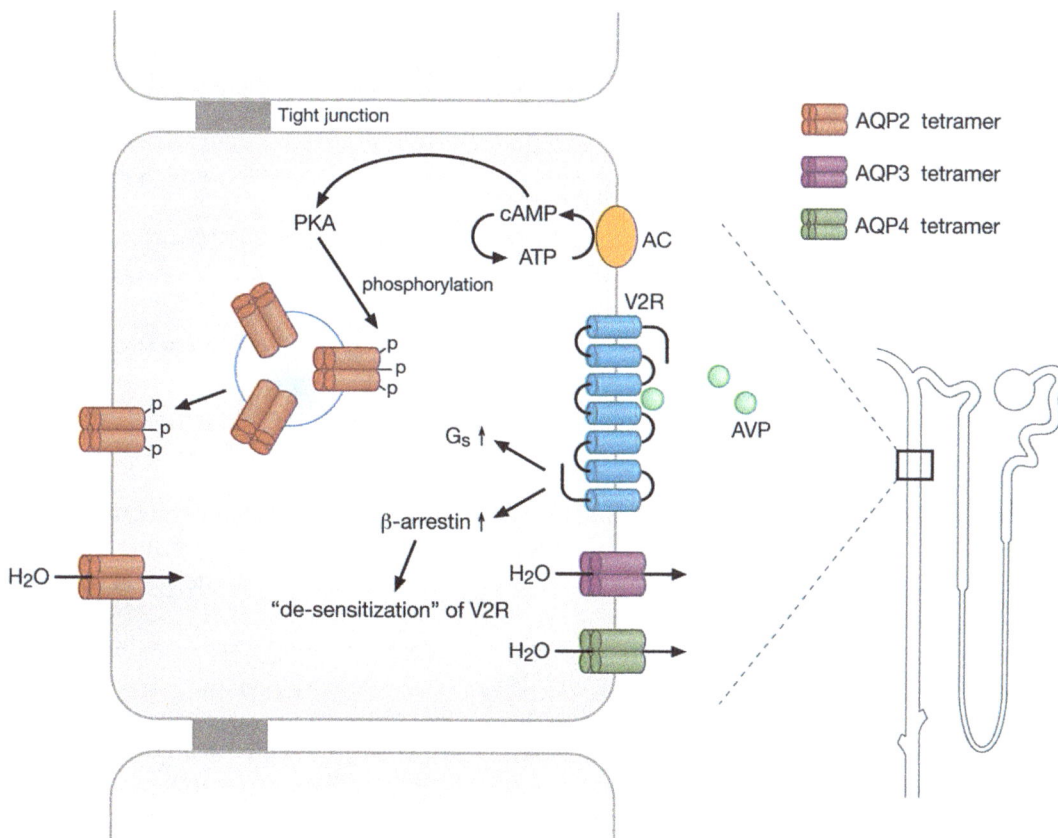

Reprinted from Moeller HB et al. Endocr Rev, 2013; 34(2). © Endocrine Society.

Nephrogenic syndrome of inappropriate antidiuresis is a rare X-linked disease caused by pathogenic variants in the *AVPR2* gene, which lead to constitutive activation of the AVPR2 receptor. The disorder most commonly presents with hyponatremia and seizures in neonates and infants. Low or undetectable AVP levels distinguish this condition from other causes of syndrome of inappropriate antidiuretic hormone secretion. Measurement of copeptin, a surrogate marker for AVP, would also be low or undetectable. Measurement of copeptin can be performed on serum or plasma by a sandwich immunoassay. This infant's presentation is consistent with inappropriate antidiuresis. The arginine vasopressin level is undetectable, making nephrogenic syndrome of inappropriate antidiuresis (Answer D) the most likely cause of his hyponatremia, not other forms of syndrome of inappropriate antidiuretic hormone secretion (Answer E). Genetic sequencing in this patient confirmed the presence of a pathogenic variant (Arg137Cys) in the *AVPR2* gene, which resulted in increased water reabsorption independent from AVP ligand binding.

In an individual with polyuria, a serum osmolality greater than 300 mOsm/kg with urine osmolality less than 300 mOsm/kg in the setting of polyuria establishes the diagnosis of diabetes insipidus (Answer C), which can be due to inadequate production of arginine vasopressin by the posterior pituitary gland (neurohypophyseal diabetes insipidus or central diabetes insipidus) or signaling defects of vasopressin in the kidneys (nephrogenic diabetes insipidus). The opposite phenotype of nephrogenic syndrome of inappropriate antidiuresis, due to inactivating pathogenic variants in the *AVPR2* receptor gene, is characterized by nephrogenic diabetes insipidus. This infant has a low serum osmolality and a low sodium level, so this answer is incorrect.

Congenital adrenal hyperplasia (Answer B), most commonly due to 21-hydroxylase deficiency, could present with hyponatremia, but mineralocorticoid deficiency would also cause hyperkalemia. Volume depletion would also be expected, but this infant has moist mucous membranes, normal pulse rate, and normal blood pressure.

Cerebral salt-wasting (Answer A) can be very difficult to distinguish from syndromes of inappropriate antidiuresis, but it would be a more likely etiology if there were evidence of circulatory volume depletion.

Educational Objective
Differentiate among clinical syndromes of inappropriate vasopressin secretion or action.

Reference(s)

Bardanzellu F, Pintus MC, Masile V, Fanos V, Marcialis MA. Focus on neonatal and infantile onset of nephrogenic syndrome of inappropriate antidiuresis: 12 years later. *Pediatr Nephrol*. 2019;34(5):763-775. PMID: 29546600

Vezzi V, Ambrosio C, Grò MC, et al. Vasopressin receptor 2 mutations in the nephrogenic syndrome of inappropriate antidiuresis show different mechanisms of constitutive activation for G protein coupled receptors. *Sci Rep*. 2020;10(1):9111. PMID: 32499611

Bichet DG, Granier S, Bockenhauer D. GNAS: a new nephrogenic cause of inappropriate antidiuresis. *J Am Soc Nephrol*. 2019;30(5):722-725. PMID: 30962326

Moeller HB, Rittig S, Fenton RA. Nephrogenic diabetes insipidus: essential insights into the molecular background and potential therapies for treatment. *Endocr Rev*. 2013;34(2):278-301. PMID: 23360744

Refardt J, Winzeler B, Christ-Crain M. Copeptin and its role in the diagnosis of diabetes insipidus and the syndrome of inappropriate antidiuresis. *Clin Endocrinol (Oxf)*. 2019;91(1):22-32. PMID: 31004513

8 **ANSWER: D) Recommend discontinuation of minocycline**
This patient presents with symptomatic thyrotoxicosis of subacute onset. The differential diagnosis of thyrotoxicosis includes Graves disease, thyroiditis of multiple etiologies (including autoimmune, medication-induced, radiation-induced, and infectious), excessive ingestion of thyroid hormone, and autonomous thyroid nodules.

This patient has medication-associated thyroiditis caused by minocycline, a tetracycline antibiotic that is frequently used to treat acne and accumulates in the thyroid and other tissues. Minocycline-associated thyroiditis typically occurs 6 to 24 months after initiation of the drug and presents without thyroid enlargement or tenderness. Minocycline causes nonautoimmune thyroiditis, and thyroid autoantibodies are not present. If performed, thyroid scintigraphy shows decreased radioiodine uptake typical of thyroiditis. In addition to symptomatic treatment with β-adrenergic blockade, management consists of discontinuing minocycline (Answer D), after which thyroiditis generally resolves in 2 to 5 months, sometimes with a subsequent hypothyroid phase.

Treatment with methimazole (Answer E) would be indicated for Graves disease. However, this patient lacks typical findings of Graves disease, including TRAb (highly sensitive for Graves disease) and thyroid enlargement. Methimazole might also be considered for treatment of hyperthyroidism caused by an autonomous nodule, but an autonomous nodule causing hyperthyroidism is generally palpable and is therefore unlikely in this case.

Erythrocyte sedimentation rate (Answer A) may be elevated and may assist in the diagnosis of subacute (painful) thyroiditis, which is generally presumed to be of viral or postviral inflammatory etiology. However, subacute thyroiditis is usually accompanied by fever, viral symptoms, and thyroid pain or tenderness, all of which are absent in this case.

Large doses of biotin can confound the assessment of thyroid function due to interference with avidin-biotin binding used in certain laboratory assays. The direction of confounding of each analyte (falsely high or falsely low) depends on the specific assay, but in many assays, biotin can cause falsely low TSH and falsely high (free) T_4, T_3, and/or TRAb. Biotin use can usually be elicited by history and should be suspected particularly in patients who have laboratory evidence of thyroid abnormalities but are clinically euthyroid. In this patient with clinical thyrotoxicosis and no history of supplement use, the laboratory abnormalities are unlikely to be caused by biotin (Answer B). If interference from biotin supplementation is suspected, thyroid function tests can be repeated at least 3 days after discontinuation of the supplement; measurement of serum biotin is usually not necessary.

Exogenous thyroid hormone ingestion (Answer C) can cause thyrotoxicosis but is associated with serum thyroglobulin levels that are suppressed, not elevated as in this patient.

Educational Objective
Diagnose and manage minocycline-associated thyroiditis.

Reference(s)

Millington K, Charrow A, Smith J. Case series: minocycline-associated thyroiditis. *Horm Res Paediatr.* 2019;92(4):276-283. PMID: 31533103

Barbesino G. Misdiagnosis of Graves' disease with apparent severe hyperthyroidism in a patient taking biotin megadoses. *Thyroid.* 2016;26(6):860-863. PMID: 27043844

9 ANSWER: E) MIRAGE syndrome

MIRAGE syndrome (Answer E) stands for myelodysplasia, infection, growth restriction, adrenal hypoplasia, genital phenotypes, and enteropathy, which are present in this child. MIRAGE syndrome was first described as a new multisystem disorder in 2016 by Narumi et al. Eleven Japanese patients with adrenal hypoplasia and extraadrenal features (myelodysplasia, infection, growth restriction, genital phenotypes, and enteropathy) were shown to harbor heterozygous gain-of-function pathogenic variants in the *SAMD9* gene (sterile α motif domain–containing protein 9). All 11 patients had healthy, nonconsanguineous parents, suggesting de novo germline variants in *SAMD9*. In 1 patient, germline mosaicism was likely, as there was recurrence of the condition in a sibling. Heterozygous pathogenic variants in the *SAMD9* gene can also cause monosomy 7 myelodysplasia and leukemia syndrome 2.

SAMD9 is a growth suppressor gene on the long arm of chromosome 7 (7q21.2), which encodes a 1589–amino acid protein. Unlike gain-of-function pathogenic variants that result in growth-suppressive effects on the cell cycle leading to reduced cellular proliferation, biallelic inactivating pathogenic variants in *SAMD9* cause normophosphatemic familial tumoral calcinosis, a hereditary form of dystrophic calcification in the skin. The meaning of *SAMD9* variants when they are identified requires careful interpretation to demonstrate causality, as single nucleotide polymorphisms are common in the gene. Pathogenic variants in patients with MIRAGE syndrome have been shown to cluster in a key hotspot, which is often reported in gain-of-function changes. Mortality is high in patients with MIRAGE syndrome, and most patients die of invasive infections. Interestingly, 2 of 11 patients with MIRAGE syndrome due to *SAMD9* pathogenic variants were shown to have mosaic monosomy 7. In a separate cohort, Buonocore et al showed that 6 or 8 patients with MIRAGE syndrome developed monosomy 7, deletions of 7q, or secondary somatic loss-of-function (nonsense and frameshift) pathogenic variants in *SAMD9*. These studies support the concept that complex and dynamic somatic events lead to cells losing the *SAMD9* variant at the expense of losing all or part of chromosome 7 to evade the growth-restricting effects of the gain-of-function *SAMD9* variant–carrying cells. This mechanism is termed *adaptation-by-aneuploidy* in diseased cells.

Antley-Bixler syndrome (Answer A) is a rare craniosynostosis syndrome characterized by radiohumeral synostosis present from the perinatal period. P450 oxidoreductase deficiency leads to congenital adrenal hyperplasia and disordered sex development in both sexes. Antley-Bixler syndrome does not have the additional features of MIRAGE syndrome, and this patient does not have craniosynostosis.

Autoimmune polyendocrine syndrome type 1 (Answer B) is characterized by the triad of chronic mucocutaneous candidiasis, hypoparathyroidism, and adrenal insufficiency. The condition is inherited in an autosomal recessive manner due to pathogenic variants in the *AIRE* gene. The condition often presents later in life and is not associated with myelodysplasia, intrauterine growth restriction, or a gonadal phenotype.

Autoimmune polyendocrine syndrome type 2 (Answer C), or Schmidt syndrome, is characterized by the presence of autoimmune Addison disease in association with either autoimmune thyroid disease or type 1 diabetes mellitus, or both. This is a polygenic disorder that most commonly presents in middle-aged women.

IMAGe syndrome (Answer D) is characterized by intrauterine growth restriction, metaphyseal dysplasia (and short limbs), adrenal hypoplasia congenita, and genital anomalies due to gain-of-function variants in the gene encoding the paternally imprinted cell-cycle regulator CDKN1C. Although the prenatal growth restriction phenotype and adrenal phenotype are similar to what is observed in MIRAGE syndrome, children with IMAGe syndrome do not have enteropathies, bone marrow failure, or infections. The disorder of sex development phenotype may also be less severe.

Educational objective
Diagnose MIRAGE syndrome and explain the genetic etiology.

Reference(s)

Narumi S, Amano N, Ishii T, et al. SAMD9 mutations cause a novel multisystem disorder, MIRAGE syndrome, and are associated with loss of chromosome 7. *Nat Genet.* 2016;48(7):792-797. PMID: 27182967

Buonocore F, Kuhnen P, Suntharalingham JP, et al. Somatic mutations and progressive monosomy modify SAMD9-related phenotypes in humans. *J Clin Invest.* 2017;127(5):1700-1713. PMID: 28346228

Wong JC, Bryant V, Lamprecht T, et al. Germline SAMD9 and SAMD9L mutations are associated with extensive genetic evolution and diverse hematologic outcomes. *JCI Insight.* 2018;3(14):e121086. PMID: 30046003

10 ANSWER: C) Recombinant human GH and an aromatase inhibitor

GH therapy has been shown to increase final height in children with idiopathic short stature and was approved by the US FDA in 2003 for the management of idiopathic short stature in children whose height SDS is below –2.25. Idiopathic short stature is, however, a diagnosis that may include multiple unknown conditions with dissimilar underlying etiologies and varied pathogenic mechanisms leading to the expectation that not all children classified as having idiopathic short stature have the same type of response. The child in this vignette has progressed in puberty and skeletal maturation without normal growth exerting a negative impact on the prediction of adult height. The height prediction is likely to decline further, as pubertal progression will continue to advance his skeletal maturation. Hence, an intervention intended to slow down his epiphyseal closure would be expected to improve final height outcome.

Delaying epiphyseal fusion has been proposed as a strategy to prolong the period of growth in children with short stature with the intention of improving final height outcome. These interventions have been used alone or in combination with recombinant human GH therapy in different clinical studies targeting various populations of children, including those with idiopathic short stature undergoing pubertal development and even prepubertal children.

Based on case reports of inactivating pathogenic variants in the estrogen receptor gene and in the aromatase gene (*CYP19A1*), estrogen has been identified as a major factor in growth plate maturation, senescence, and fusion. This led to the idea of decreasing estrogen levels to delay growth plate senescence and fusion. Two main strategies have been used: GnRH analogues and aromatase inhibitors. GnRH analogues suppress gonadotropin (LH and FSH) secretion, leading to a hypogonadal state with consequential decline in both testosterone and estrogen levels. Aromatase inhibitors interfere with the aromatization of androgens (androstenedione and testosterone) to estrogens (estrone and estradiol, respectively), which consequently decreases estrogen levels with a reciprocal increase in testosterone.

The hypogonadal state achieved with GnRH analogues is associated with lack of virilization in boys and untoward effects on body composition and on calcium, protein, and lipid metabolism. Fat mass and percentage fat mass were noted to increase after treatment with GnRH analogues despite no significant changes in BMI, favoring an increase in adiposity that was not seen with the use of aromatase inhibitors for a similar length of time. Similarly, a significant increase in urinary calcium loss was observed in individuals receiving GnRH analogue therapy, while no significant changes were noted in urinary calcium excretion using stable tracers in children receiving aromatase inhibitors for 10 weeks. When assessed in leucine tracer studies, GnRH analogues exerted a catabolic effect, leading to a significant decrease in protein synthesis, while aromatase inhibitors did not induce a negative effect on protein kinetics. The reciprocal increase in testosterone levels that occurs with aromatase inhibitors may partly explain the differences in the metabolic effects of GnRH analogues and aromatase inhibitors. Another part of the explanation may be the degree of estrogen suppression induced by these 2 approaches. Although aromatase inhibitors have not been approved by the US FDA for this indication and their use would be off-label, the strategy that would provide the most benefit with the least untoward metabolic effects would be the simultaneous administration of recombinant human GH and an aromatase inhibitor (Answer C). An aromatase inhibitor alone (Answer A) without the concomitant administration of GH may delay the fusion of growth plates without the negative metabolic effects of GnRH analogues but its effect on height potential is inferior to the combination therapy. Even though the combination of a GnRH analogue with GH (Answer B) would also potentially improve the final height outcome, the negative metabolic effects of GnRH analogues make this option less desirable.

Oxandrolone (Answer D) is a nonaromatizable androgen that has been used to manage short stature associated with constitutional delay of puberty. Oxandrolone provides the anabolic effects of androgens with enhanced growth velocity and progression of secondary sexual characteristics while exerting minimal effect in growth plate fusion given that it cannot be aromatized to an estrogenic molecule. The child in this vignette is undergoing puberty and would not benefit from this intervention.

Exogenous testosterone (Answer E) can also be used in children with short stature associated with constitutional delay of puberty. There are concerns, however, that it can be aromatized to estradiol and may lead to faster closure of growth plates, limiting final height potential. Additionally, given that this patient is already in puberty, testosterone administration would not be indicated.

Educational Objective
Explain the metabolic effects that GnRH analogues and aromatase inhibitors have on protein, calcium kinetics, and body composition and describe strategies to delay epiphyseal fusion to improve final adult height in children with short stature.

Reference(s)
Leschek EW, Rose SR, Yanovski JA, et al; National Institute of Child Health and Human Development-Eli Lilly & Co Growth Hormone Collaborative Group. Effect of growth hormone treatment in adult height in peripubertal children with idiopathic short stature: a randomized, double-blind, placebo-controlled trial. *J Clin Endocrinol Metab.* 2004;89(7):3140-3148. PMID: 15240584

Mauras N, O'Brien KO, Klein KO, Hayes V. Estrogen suppression in males: metabolic effects. *J Clin Endocrinol Metab.* 2000;85(7):2370-2377. PMID: 10902781

Mauras N, Hayes V, Vieira NE, Yergey AL, O'Brien KO. Profound hypogonadism has significant negative effects on calcium balance in males: a calcium kinetic study. *J Bone Miner Res.* 1999;14(4):577-582. PMID: 10234579

Boot AM, De Muinck Keizer-Schrama S, Pols HA, Krenning EP, Drop SL. Bone mineral density and body composition before and during treatment with gonadotropin-releasing hormone agonist in children with precocious and early puberty. *J Clin Endocrinol Metab.* 1998;83(2):370-373. PMID: 9467543

Mauras N, Ross JL, Gagliardi P, et al. Randomized trial of aromatase inhibitors, growth hormone, or combination in pubertal boys with idiopathic short stature. *J Clin Endocrinol Metab.* 2016;101(12):4984-4993. PMID: 27710241

Miller BS, Ross J, Ostrow V. Height outcomes in children with growth hormone deficiency and idiopathic short stature treated concomitantly with growth hormone and aromatase inhibitor therapy: data from the ANSWER program. *Int J Pediatr Endocrinol.* 2020;2020:19. PMID: 33042202

11 ANSWER: E) Low serum iron

This child has autosomal dominant hypophosphatemic rickets (ADHR), a rare genetic disorder due to pathogenic variants in the *FGF23* gene located on chromosome 12q13, resulting in secretion of an intact molecule more resistant to cleavage by proteolytic enzymes. Thus, the molecule remains active in the body for longer durations, which results in increased renal phosphate wasting and inactivation of 1α-hydroxylase. Commercial assays measure both intact FGF-23 and the biologically inactive C-terminal fragments. Individuals with ADHR have a higher proportion of intact FGF-23.

Incomplete penetrance is characteristic of ADHR. Some individuals carry a pathogenic variant but remain normophosphatemic, whereas others have delayed onset of symptoms that can spontaneously resolve with normalization of serum phosphate. Thus, there is evidence of the disease waxing and waning throughout adulthood, similar to tumor-induced osteomalacia. In contrast to X-linked hypophosphatemic rickets, in which males usually have a more severe phenotype, males and females are affected equally by ADHR. Interestingly, observations that skeletal manifestations (osteomalacia, bone pain, weakness, and insufficiency fractures) became more prominent in women of childbearing age led to the discovery that iron suppresses FGF-23 secretion. Patients with ADHR who are iron deficient have higher levels of intact FGF-23 and lower serum phosphate concentrations, whereas individuals without ADHR maintain normal serum phosphate levels because increased FGF-23 secretion is coupled with increased proteolytic cleavage. A recently published study by Imel et al showed that correction of iron deficiency decreased intact FGF-23 secretion in patients with ADHR, normalizing the serum phosphate level and allowing them to discontinue phosphorus and calcitriol supplementation. Thus, the most likely additional finding is low serum iron (Answer E).

Serum alkaline phosphatase is likely to be elevated in conditions that result in increased osteoid formation but impaired mineralization. Hypophosphatasia, which may cause rachitic changes on x-ray and fractures, has the hallmark findings of low alkaline phosphatase (Answer D) and elevated urinary phosphoethanolamine (Answer C). Importantly, serum phosphate levels are not low.

Conductive hearing loss (Answer A) is associated with autosomal recessive hypophosphatemic rickets (type 2) due to pathogenic variants in the *ENPP1* gene.

Due to inhibition of 1α-hydroxylase activity, 1,25-dihydroxyvitamin D_3 (Answer B) levels are low or normal in FGF-23–mediated disease, whereas levels are significantly elevated in nutritional phosphate depletion.

Educational Objective
Explain how iron is involved in FGF-23 regulation and describe the phenotypic expression of autosomal dominant hypophosphatemic rickets.

Reference(s)
Econs MJ, McEnery PT. Autosomal dominant hypophosphatemic rickets/osteomalacia: clinical characterization of a novel renal phosphate-wasting disorder. *J Clin Endocrinol Metab*. 1997;82(2):674-681. PMID: 9024275

Imel EA, Peacock M, Gray AK, Padgett LR, Hui SL, Econs MJ. Iron modifies plasma FGF23 differently in autosomal dominant hypophosphatemic rickets and healthy humans. *J Clin Endocrinol Metab*. 2011;96(11):3541-3549. PMID: 21880793

Imel EA, Liu Z, Coffman M, Acton D, Mehta R, Econs MJ. Oral iron replacement normalizes fibroblast growth factor 23 in iron-deficient patients with autosomal dominant hypophosphatemic rickets. *J Bone Miner Res*. 2020;35(2):231-238. PMID: 31652009

12 ANSWER: B) Genetic testing for *ABCC8* or *KCNJ11* pathogenic variants

The patient in this vignette has a pathogenic variant in the *ABCC8* gene (Answer B). Defects in KATP channel can cause congenital hyperinsulinism and diabetes mellitus. A common heterozygous missense pathogenic variant has been described in published case reports. In infancy, individuals with an *ABCC8* pathogenic variant have a mild form of congenital hyperinsulinism due to reduction of KATP channel activity, and they are responsive to diazoxide. In early childhood, these pathogenic variants cause loss of insulin secretory capacity with glucose intolerance. Diabetes mellitus develops at older ages. The mechanism of this slow deterioration of insulin secretion is not clear. Chronic membrane depolarization has been suggested to result in increased intracellular calcium, which in turn activates apoptosis pathways. Alternatively, chronic insulin hypersecretion may result in endoplasmic reticulum stress, which also initiates apoptosis pathways. Whatever the mechanism, the insulin-secreting capacity of β cells diminishes over time with the development of diabetes mellitus.

Pathogenic variants in the *LEP* gene are associated with the most severe forms of obesity, and pathogenic variants in the *LEPR* gene induce less pronounced pathology with a similar phenotype. Disturbed expression of the *POMC* gene results in obesity and inhibition of the pituitary gland–adrenal cortex axis. Pathogenic variants in the *MC4R* gene inhibit the function of melanocortins in the hypothalamus, increase food consumption, and result in obesity. None of these genes (Answer A) is directly associated with neonatal hyperinsulinism and later with diabetes.

Antibody measurement (islet cell, insulin, glutamic acid decarboxylase 65, and ZnT8) (Answer C) is the logical next step in most patients presenting with diabetes mellitus. However, antibody titers would not offer an etiologic explanation in this case because the presentation and phenotype are not typical for type 1 diabetes.

PET and tandem CT of the pancreas (Answer E) couple the functional information of PET with the anatomic details of CT. Integrated PET/CT scanners produce both PET and contrast material-enhanced CT images of the pancreas in one setting. PET/CT offers an opportunity to depict pancreatic tumors. In selected cases, PET/CT findings may be used to help diagnose autoimmune pancreatitis mimicking a mass by revealing systemic involvement. It can help distinguish focal from diffuse pancreatic lesions in cases of hyperinsulinemic hypoglycemia. PET and tandem CT of the pancreas would not be helpful in this patient's evaluation.

Ordering oral glucose tolerance testing and measuring proinsulin, insulin, and C-peptide (Answer D) would not assist in determining the etiology of this patient's diabetes.

Educational Objective
Determine the underlying etiology of diabetes mellitus following a history of neonatal hypoglycemia.

Reference(s)
Glaser B, Ryan F, Donath M, et al. Hyperinsulinism caused by paternal-specific inheritance of a recessive mutation in the sulfonylurea-receptor gene. *Diabetes.* 1999;48(8):1652-1657. PMID: 10426386

Huopio H, Otonkoski T, Vauhkonen I, Reimann F, Ashcroft FM, Laakso M. A new subtype of autosomal dominant diabetes attributable to a mutation in the gene for sulfonylurea receptor 1. *Lancet.* 2003;361(9354):301-307. PMID: 12559865

Harding HP, Ron D. Endoplasmic reticulum stress and the development of diabetes: a review. *Diabetes.* 2002;51(Suppl 3):S455-S461. PMID: 12475790

Hussain K, Cosgrove KE. From congenital hyperinsulinism to diabetes mellitus: the role of pancreatic beta-cell KATP channels. *Pediatr Diabetes.* 2005;6(2):103-113. PMID: 15963039

13 ANSWER: D) Stimulates GH secretagogue receptor 1α in the hypothalamus and pituitary

Macimorelin is the only oral agent approved for GH-stimulation testing in adults. It mimics the endogenous ghrelin-mediated effects on GH secretion by binding to the GH secretagogue receptor 1α in the hypothalamus and pituitary (Answer D). It does not increase endogenous ghrelin (Answer B) or insulin secretion (Answer C) or inhibit somatostatin binding to its receptor (Answer A). Insulin, the gold standard agent to screen for adult GH deficiency, causes hypoglycemia-induced GH secretion (Answer E). Glucagon is also used for adult GH deficiency screening, as it stimulates endogenous insulin secretion. In fact, one of the main advantages of using macimorelin is that it does not increase the risk of hypoglycemia as does insulin tolerance testing and glucagon-stimulation testing. Also, the duration of macimorelin testing is shorter (1.5 hours) than the duration of insulin tolerance testing (2 to 3 hours) or glucagon-stimulation testing (3 to 4 hours). Unlike glucagon-stimulation testing, testing with macimorelin does not require BMI-adjusted peak GH cutoffs for patients with excess body weight (BMI >40 kg/m^2).

In a sample of 114 adults with stratified likelihood of having GH deficiency and 25 healthy adults, macimorelin had 92% sensitivity and 96% specificity when compared with the gold standard insulin tolerance test (using a GH cutoff value of 5.1 ng/mL for both tests). There was 94% negative agreement and 82% positive agreement between the 2 tests. Also, the macimorelin test had a reproducibility of 94%, and there were no substantial differences in peak GH levels upon repeating the test. No serious adverse effects were noted with macimorelin.

Macimorelin can cause QT prolongation and thus concomitant use with drugs that prolong the QT interval should be avoided. Macimorelin has not been tested in certain populations such as elderly patients (>65 years), pediatric patients, or patients with morbid obesity (BMI >40 kg/m^2). Concomitant use of strong CYP3A4 inducers can decrease macimorelin plasma levels significantly and thereby lead to a false-positive result. Strong CYP3A4 inducers should be discontinued, and enough time should be allowed for adequate washout of CYP3A4 inducers before the test is administered.

Educational Objective
Explain the mechanism of action of the only approved oral agent (macimorelin) for GH-stimulation testing to screen for adult GH deficiency.

Reference(s)
Garcia JM, Biller BMK, Korbonits M, et al. Macimorelin as a diagnostic test for adult GH deficiency. *J Clin Endocrinol Metab.* 2018;103(8):3083-3093. PMID: 29860473

Garcia JM, Biller BMK, Korbonits M, et al. Sensitivity and specificity of the macimorelin test for diagnosis of AGHD. *Endocr Connect.* 2021;10(1):76-83. PMID: 33320108

14 ANSWER: C) Perform postnatal chromosome testing on cord blood or peripheral blood to guide decision-making

Klinefelter syndrome occurs in 1 of every 600 male births. Approximately 20% of patients with Klinefelter syndrome are diagnosed prenatally. With the introduction of noninvasive prenatal screening, prenatal identification is becoming more common. Prenatal diagnosis of chromosomal anomalies results in a high degree of parental distress, and it is important to recognize the limitations of noninvasive prenatal screening. Screening for chromosomal aneuploidy via cell-free DNA methods is highly sensitive and specific, but abnormalities should always be verified by postnatal testing. Thus, postnatal chromosome testing on cord blood or peripheral blood (Answer C) should be recommended.

A limited number of studies in persons with Klinefelter syndrome all demonstrate normal activation of the hypothalamic-pituitary-gonadal axis ("minipuberty of infancy"), with some differences. LH concentrations are normal but FSH concentrations are typically higher. Testosterone concentrations are often normal but are more likely to be in the lower end of the reference range. Reduced penile length/growth in infancy throughout childhood is more common in Klinefelter syndrome, but this is not universal, and it typically normalizes at the time of puberty. A short course of testosterone can be considered if micropenis is present (<2 standard deviations below the mean for age). This treatment is not dependent on assessment of LH, FSH, or testosterone levels (Answer B).

Two observational studies have suggested that testosterone treatment in infancy may reduce neurodevelopmental deficits in Klinefelter syndrome. However, in both studies, significant ascertainment bias was likely present, and most participants were treated after minipuberty. One randomized study of testosterone replacement (20 participants total) demonstrated improvement in adiposity, linear growth, and penile length in the treatment group at 5 months of age. Larger studies that assess benefits beyond 5 months of age are needed and are ongoing. Given the limited data and lack of FDA indication, testosterone treatment for this purpose (Answer A) cannot be recommended as standard of care.

While testosterone levels have been shown to be lower in prepubertal boys with Klinefelter syndrome (age 4 to 9.5 years), low-dosage testosterone replacement in childhood does not appear to have significant benefit. A double-blind, randomized controlled trial of patients treated with oxandrolone for 24 months (0.06 mg/kg) in boys aged 4 to 12 years showed some improvement in visual-motor function but no significant effects on most aspects of cognition (general cognition, verbal skills, working memory). As such, treatment with low-dosage androgen therapy (Answer D) in early childhood cannot be recommended.

Delays in speech and language, as well as hypotonia, hypermobility, pes planus, and genu valgum leading to motor delays, are all seen with greater frequency in Klinefelter syndrome. Approximately 50% to 75% of boys with Klinefelter syndrome demonstrate a specific reading and/or language disability and 60% to 86% require special education services. Proactive counseling should be provided to address both endocrine and neurodevelopmental concerns at the time of Klinefelter syndrome diagnosis and referrals to screen for and address delays should be recommended. Thus, waiting to follow-up until puberty (Answer E) is incorrect.

Educational Objective
Provide appropriate counseling regarding use of testosterone therapy in Klinefelter syndrome.

Reference(s)
Aksglade L, Davis SM, Ross JL, Juul A. Minipuberty in Klinefelter syndrome: Current status and future directions. *Am J Med Genet C Semin Med Genet.* 2020;184(2):320-326. PMID: 32476267

Samango-Sprouse C, Keen C, Sadeghin T, Gropman A. The benefits and limitations of cell-free DNA screening for 47, XXY (Klinefelter syndrome). *Prenat Diagn.* 2017;37(5):497-501. PMID: 28346690

15 ANSWER: B) Recommend nutrition consultation and follow-up in 6 months to assess weight, linear growth, and pubertal development

The peak GH response during GH-stimulation testing is blunted in individuals with obesity. Regardless of the cutoff peak used to diagnose GH deficiency, the higher the BMI, the more likely it is that the GH peak does not reach the cutoff, thus leading to an erroneous diagnosis of GH deficiency. In addition, the peak GH response normalizes after weight loss. The child in this vignette has obesity (BMI at the 97th percentile). This raises concerns about the reliability of GH-stimulation testing to diagnose GH deficiency. Also, her IGF-1 value is not significantly low. She displays linear growth deceleration that brought her height from the 5th percentile to below the 3rd percentile. Breast development is currently Tanner stage 2. The slowing of her growth velocity is most likely the result of physiologic prepubertal deceleration. Therefore, the most appropriate course of action is to encourage the family to work on lifestyle and dietary modification to achieve weight loss and then reevaluate her linear and ponderal growth and pubertal development before initiating GH therapy (thus, Answer B is correct and Answer C is incorrect).

An insulin-tolerance test (Answer A) is not needed now. The possibility of repeating a GH-stimulation test could be considered if, after weight loss and adequate pubertal progression, her growth velocity is subnormal.

The TSH concentration is frequently mildly elevated in the setting of obesity and does not represent thyroid dysfunction. TSH levels seem to be proportional to the degree of obesity and normalize with weight loss. The patient in this vignette has a minimally increased TSH level and a normal free T_4 level. This is not consistent with hypothyroidism, so starting levothyroxine (Answer E) is incorrect.

Tanner stage 2 breast development is appropriate for this patient's age and is not consistent with precocious puberty. This is also supported by the finding of normal skeletal maturation for age. The use of a GnRH analogue (Answer D) would not be the most appropriate next step in this child's management.

Educational Objective
Identify the pitfalls of interpreting results of GH-stimulation tests in children with obesity.

Reference(s)
Stanley T, Levitsky LL, Grinspoon SK, Misra M. Effect of body mass index on peak growth hormone response to provocative testing in children with short stature. *J Clin Endocrinol Metab.* 2009;94(12):4875-4881. PMID: 19890023

Argente J, Caballo N, Barrios J, et al. Multiple endocrine abnormalities of the growth hormone and insulin-like growth factor axis in prepubertal children with exogenous obesity: effect of short- and long-term weight reduction. *J Clin Endocrinol Metab.* 1997;82(7):2076-2083. PMID: 9215275

Biondi B. Thyroid and obesity: an intriguing relationship. *J Clin Endocrinol Metab.* 2010;95(8):3614-3617. PMID: 20685890

16   ANSWER: C) Start levothyroxine, 25 mcg daily

This newborn has a mild and compensated form of congenital hypothyroidism, and her TSH rose when measurement was repeated on day of life 17. In light of the importance of thyroid hormones in infant brain development and cognition, it would not be prudent to wait another 2 weeks to repeat thyroid function testing before starting levothyroxine (Answer B). A sporadic form of congenital hypothyroidism is unlikely given her eutopic thyroid gland. Sporadic forms are usually observed in patients with an ectopic or athyrotic gland. In forms of congenital hypothyroidism more severe than in this patient, the starting levothyroxine dosage recommended in newborns is 10 to 15 mcg/kg per day. The levothyroxine dosage of 37.5 mcg daily (13.4 mcg/kg per day) (Answer D) is higher than would be required in such a mild form of congenital hypothyroidism, and 44 mcg daily (15.7 mcg/kg per day) (Answer E) is even higher. Starting levothyroxine, 25 mcg daily (Answer C), is correct (8.9 mcg/kg per day). Infants with overt but mild congenital hypothyroidism (free T_4 below the reference range but >0.78 ng/dL [>10 pmol/L] in combination with elevated TSH) should be treated with the lowest initial levothyroxine dosage (10 mcg/kg per day). In infants with pretreatment free T_4 concentrations within the age-specific reference range, an even lower starting dosage may be considered (5 to 10 mcg/kg per day).

Measuring thyroid antibodies and, if negative, ordering a congenital hypothyroidism genetic panel (Answer A) does not include a treatment recommendation and is incorrect. However, this answer option raises 2 important points. The first point is that transplacental transfer of TSH-receptor antibodies can cause congenital hypothyroidism of varying severity with a eutopic gland. TPO antibodies do not cause congenital hypothyroidism. The second point is that one should not delay starting levothyroxine until the results are back.

Whole-genome sequencing may miss certain pathogenic variants that are detected in a dedicated panel in which the depth of genetic study is deeper. Thus, the use of specific panels may be warranted in some cases, even if whole-genome sequencing is negative.

This infant was diagnosed with Say-Barber-Biesecker-Young-Simpson syndrome, a rare autosomal dominant condition due to a pathogenic variant in the *KAT6B* gene. Many of this infant's dysmorphic features fit this syndrome. A mild form of congenital hypothyroidism has often been described in Say-Barber-Biesecker-Young-Simpson syndrome, and some cases may be transient. Being aware of such associations is important when counseling families about the cause and expected course of their child's hypothyroidism.

Reference(s)

van Trotsenburg P, Stoupa A, Léger J, et al. Congenital hypothyroidism: a 2020-2021 consensus guidelines update-an ENDO-European Reference Network initiative endorsed by the European Society for Pediatric Endocrinology and the European Society for Endocrinology. *Thyroid.* 2021;31(3):387-419. PMID: 33272083

Campeau PM, Lu JT, Dawson BC, et al. The KAT6B-related disorders genitopatellar syndrome and Ohdo/SBBYS syndrome have distinct clinical features reflecting distinct molecular mechanisms. *Hum Mutat.* 2012;33(11):1520-1525. PMID: 22715153

17 ANSWER: D) Setmelanotide

Approved pharmacotherapeutic options for the treatment of pediatric obesity are limited. In 2020, the US FDA approved the use of setmelanotide (Answer D), a melanocortin 4 receptor agonist, for weight management in patients 6 years and older with severe obesity due to 1 of 3 rare conditions: proopiomelanocortin (POMC) deficiency, proprotein subtilisin/kexin type 1 (PCSK1) deficiency, and leptin receptor (LEPR) deficiency. Patients must have a confirmed genetic diagnosis with a documented *POMC, PCSK1,* or *LEPR* gene variant that is considered to be pathogenic, likely pathogenic, or of uncertain significance. A significant proportion of patients in clinical trials who took setmelanotide lost at least 10% or more of their body weight (80% of patients with POMC or PCSK1 deficiency and 46% of patients with LEPR deficiency). Setmelanotide is a proopiomelanocortin-derived peptide that is a melanocortin 4 receptor agonist. It works by binding to and activating melanocortin 4 receptors in the paraventricular nucleus and the lateral hypothalamic area, which leads to appetite suppression. Setmelanotide is given as a once-daily subcutaneous injection. In several clinical trials, setmelanotide significantly decreased participants' maximal hunger scores. The most common adverse reactions are injection site reactions, hyperpigmentation, headache, and gastrointestinal adverse effects.

Metformin (Answer A) is approved for the treatment of type 2 diabetes mellitus in patients 10 years and older. While metformin has been used off label for the treatment of pediatric obesity, most studies have shown only modest benefit in BMI reduction compared with that of placebo with heterogeneous results among studies.

Orlistat (Answer B) is FDA-approved as a weight-loss medication in adolescents who are 12 years and older. It works by inhibiting gastric and pancreatic lipases, resulting in decreased absorption of dietary fat. Its use is often limited by its adverse effect profile. Patients may experience significant gastrointestinal adverse effects such as steatorrhea, diarrhea, abdominal pain, and fecal spotting. Orlistat can increase risk for acute kidney injury and could increase risk for osteoporosis through impaired absorption of calcium and vitamin D.

Extended-release topiramate/phentermine capsules (Answer E) are FDA-approved for the treatment of obesity in patients 12 years and older. Phentermine alone is FDA-approved for short-term obesity treatment in patients 16 years and older. Topiramate is an anticonvulsant drug that is FDA approved for seizures in children 2 years and older. It has been used for obesity treatment in adults with good efficacy, but it is not FDA-approved by itself for weight loss. Potential safety issues of the combination therapy include nephrolithiasis, tachycardia, and teratogenicity. Patients may notice dry mouth, constipation, paresthesias, difficulty sleeping, dizziness, and altered taste; the likelihood of adverse effects is dosage dependent. Due to concerns that topiramate can increase risk for suicidal ideation, appropriate counseling before initiating this medication is important and patients must be closely monitored for emergence of or worsening depression, suicidal thoughts/behavior, and/or changes in mood or behavior. It is not recommended for use in patients who have a history of suicide attempts or those with active suicidal ideation.

Semaglutide (Answer C) is a GLP-1 receptor agonist that is approved for obesity treatment in pediatric patients 12 years and older. Semaglutide is given as a once-weekly subcutaneous injection. Common adverse effects include gastrointestinal symptoms (abdominal pain, nausea, vomiting, diarrhea), headache, and fatigue.

Educational Objective

Recommend setmelanotide, a melanocortin 4 receptor agonist, for treatment of chronic obesity in patients diagnosed with proopiomelanocortin deficiency, proprotein subtilisin/kexin type 1 deficiency, or leptin receptor deficiency.

Reference(s)

Clément K, van den Akker E, Argente J, et al; Setmelanotide POMC and LEPR Phase 3 Trial Investigators. Efficacy and safety of setmelanotide, an MC4R agonist, in individuals with severe obesity due to LEPR or POMC deficiency: single-arm, open-label, multicentre, phase 3 trials. *Lancet Diabetes Endocrinol.* 2020;8(12):960-970. PMID: 33137293

Srivastava G, Fox CK, Kelly AS, et al. Clinical considerations regarding the use of obesity pharmacotherapy in adolescents with obesity. *Obesity (Silver Spring).* 2019;27(2):190-204. PMID: 30677262

18 ANSWER: B) 47,XYY

This patient's karyotype is 47,XYY, which is a relatively common sex chromosomal disorder associated with tall stature in males, with an incidence of 1 in 1000 live male births. Unlike boys with 47,XXY (Klinefelter syndrome) (Answer A) who often have small, firm testes, boys with 47,XYY syndrome may have macroorchidism. Other features typically seen in boys with 47,XYY syndrome include macrocephaly and learning disabilities such as speech delay and dyslexia. There is also an increased incidence of attention-deficit/hyperactivity disorder and autism spectrum disorder. Contrary to what was previously thought, most boys with a 47,XYY karyotype do not have aggressive behavior. Testosterone and gonadotropin levels are frequently normal; however, there is a lack of pubertal rise in inhibin B in adolescent boys with a 47,XYY karyotype. Although genital abnormalities such as micropenis, cryptorchidism, and hypospadias have been reported, most boys with a 47,XYY karyotype have normal genitalia. Most affected boys have normal puberty, although some may have delayed puberty. There is an increased risk of infertility.

Patients with Marfan syndrome (Answer E), a connective tissue disorder due to autosomal dominant pathogenic variants in the *FBN1* gene, typically have other clinical features such as long arms and legs (decreased upper segment-to-lower segment ratio, arm span > height), joint hypermobility (thumb sign/wrist sign), chest wall deformities (pectus excavatum or carinatum), and heart murmur. GH excess (Answer D) can lead to tall stature and gigantism. This patient's normal IGF-1 level helps rule out GH excess as the cause of his tall stature. Boys with a 47,XYY karyotype have normal circulating levels of IGF-1 and IGFBP-3.

He has several physical characteristics that point toward a possible pathologic cause of tall stature. Thus, familial tall stature (Answer C) cannot be diagnosed without further evaluation.

Educational Objective

Identify the characteristic clinical features of 47,XYY syndrome as a cause of tall stature in male adolescents.

Reference(s)

Bardsley MZ, Kowal K, Levy C, et al. 47,XYY syndrome: clinical phenotype and timing of ascertainment. *J Pediatr.* 2013;163(4):1085-1094. PMID: 23810129

Davis SM, Bloy L, Roberts TPL, et al. Testicular function in boys with 47,XYY and relationship to phenotype. *Am J Med Genet C Semin Med Genet.* 2020;184(2):371-385. PMID: 32544298

Aksglaede L, Skakkebaek NE, Juul A. Abnormal sex chromosome constitution and longitudinal growth: serum levels of insulin-like growth factor (IGF)-I, IGF binding protein-3, luteinizing hormone, and testosterone in 109 males with 47,XXY, 47,XYY, or sex-determining region of the Y chromosome (SRY)-positive 46,XX karyotypes. *J Clin Endocrinol Metab.* 2008;93(1):169-176. PMID: 17940117

19 ANSWER: B) No intervention until after delivery

Prenatal dexamethasone treatment of fetuses with congenital adrenal hyperplasia (CAH) is controversial. Although prenatal treatment was introduced in the 1980s and is still practiced at some institutions, current international consensus does not advise prenatal administration of high-dosage dexamethasone (Answers C and D) because of safety concerns.

The concept of prenatal treatment is that dexamethasone given to the mother will cross the placenta into the fetal circulation to suppress ACTH-driven virilization of female external genitalia. The treatment protocol consists of administering dexamethasone at a dosage of 20 mcg/kg per day (maximum 1.5 mg daily). This is effective in ameliorating virilization of the external genitalia of female fetuses if treatment is started by gestational week 6 to 7. In most centers, this is before a fetal CAH diagnosis can be made. Prenatal diagnosis by chorionic villus sampling is performed during gestational weeks 10 to 11. If the fetus were female and had classic CAH, then the treatment would be continued until term. If not, treatment would be stopped. On average, 8 pregnancies at risk for CAH must be treated for every affected female who might benefit from treatment. There has not been a randomized controlled trial evaluating this scenario. Retrospective data on antenatal dexamethasone use in animals and humans delineated long-term complications affecting brain, cardiovascular, renal, reproductive, thyroid, and metabolic functions, as well as teratogenicity with birth defects such as cleft lip. Hence, various endocrine societies and others have stated that prenatal dexamethasone treatment for CAH is experimental and should only be performed in centers taking part in long-term research studies of these treated pregnancies.

Therefore, recommending chorionic villus sampling to determine fetal sex and genotype (Answer A) or urgent ultrasonography to determine fetal age (Answer E) and thus appropriate timing for diagnostic testing is not necessary. Recommending no intervention until after delivery (Answer B) is the best management now. Involvement of the obstetrics team is essential for careful interpretation and understanding of antenatal scans, as well as developing a coordinated approach to counseling the family and managing the baby at birth.

The child in this vignette has a diagnosis of late-presenting, classic, simple virilizing CAH. This patient's genotype with compound heterozygosity (c.293-13C>G and c.515T>A) is associated with severe simple virilizing CAH. As such, any female fetus in this family who inherits CAH is at risk for prenatal virilization.

Educational Objective
Explain the changing view of prenatal dexamethasone treatment in congenital adrenal hyperplasia.

Reference(s)

Liu SY, Lee CT, Tung YC, Chien YH, Hwu WL, Tsai WY. Clinical characteristics of Taiwanese children with congenital adrenal hyperplasia due to 21-hydroxylase deficiency detected by neonatal screening. *J Formos Med Assoc.* 2018;117(2);126-131. PMID: 28392195

Hannah-Shmouni F, Chen W, Merke DP. Genetics of congenital adrenal hyperplasia. *Endocrinol Metab Clin North Am.* 2017;46(2):435-458. PMID: 28476231

Claahsen-van der Grinten HL, Speiser PW, Ahmed SF, et al. Congenital adrenal hyperplasia - current insights in pathophysiology, diagnostics and management. *Endocr Rev.* 2022;43(1):91-159. PMID: 33961029

20 ANSWER: A) Calcitonin

This child has a small (<1 cm) thyroid nodule that is solid but has no other features concerning for malignancy. In the absence of other risk factors for malignancy, such a nodule generally does not require FNA and may be monitored by ultrasonography.

However, this patient has skin findings consistent with cutaneous lichen amyloidosis, a rare dermatologic condition that is associated with multiple endocrine neoplasia (MEN) type 2A, and specifically with pathogenic variants in codon 634 of the *RET* proto-oncogene. Cutaneous lichen amyloidosis is characterized by chronic pruritis leading to the formation of hyperpigmented, lichenified plaques, often beginning in infancy and most frequently localized to the upper back near the scapula (dermatomes T2-T6). The finding of cutaneous lichen amyloidosis in a child or adolescent with a thyroid nodule should raise the possibility of MEN type 2A, which is associated with medullary thyroid carcinoma. Therefore, measurement of serum calcitonin (Answer A) would be appropriate in this case. Of note, medullary thyroid cancer is less likely than papillary thyroid cancer to have classic ultrasonographic features of malignancy such as hypoechogenicity or calcifications.

Measurement of TPO antibodies (Answer D) is a diagnostic test for autoimmune thyroid disease, which can be associated with chronic idiopathic urticaria. However, this patient's dermatologic findings are not consistent with urticaria, and his thyroid ultrasound findings do not suggest autoimmune thyroid disease.

Measurement of TRAb (Answer E) is a diagnostic test for Graves disease, which can be associated with cutaneous findings of localized myxedema (Graves dermopathy). Typical findings are bilateral nonpitting induration of the skin that occurs most commonly in the lower legs (pretibial) or feet but can appear in other areas. The unilateral pruritic rash on the upper back present since infancy in this euthyroid patient is not consistent with Graves dermopathy.

Measurement of thyroglobulin (Answer C) is an important component of postoperative staging and surveillance for differentiated (follicular-cell–derived) thyroid cancer. However, measuring serum thyroglobulin is not useful or indicated in the evaluation of thyroid nodules.

Radioiodine uptake (Answer B) and scintigraphy should be performed in patients with a thyroid nodule who have a low TSH concentration, which suggests a possible autonomous thyroid nodule. Measuring radioiodine uptake is not indicated in this euthyroid patient.

Educational Objective

Recognize cutaneous lichen amyloidosis as a manifestation of multiple endocrine neoplasia type 2A.

Reference(s)

Verga U, Fugazzola L, Cambiaghi S, et al. Frequent association between MEN 2A and cutaneous lichen amyloidosis. *Clin Endocrinol (Oxf)*. 2003;59(2):156-161. PMID: 12864791

Wells SA Jr, Asa SL, Dralle H, et al; American Thyroid Association Guidelines Task Force on Medullary Thyroid Carcinoma. Revised American Thyroid Association guidelines for the management of medullary thyroid carcinoma. *Thyroid*. 2015;25(6):567-610. PMID: 25810047

Francis GL, Waguespack SG, Bauer AJ, et al; American Thyroid Association Guidelines Task Force. Management guidelines for children with thyroid nodules and differentiated thyroid cancer. *Thyroid*. 2015;25(7):716-759. PMID: 25900731

21 ANSWER: D) Low lumbar spine bone density

This young woman's clinical history initially raises concern for hypothalamic amenorrhea, but the elevated FSH and low estradiol are strongly suggestive of primary ovarian insufficiency. Repeating these laboratory tests in 1 month is necessary to confirm the diagnosis and commence treatment with estrogen replacement therapy. Estrogen deficiency primarily results in accelerated bone resorption; however, it also has a role in bone formation. During adolescence, estrogen deficiency may have a more pronounced and long-term impact on bone health given inadequate accrual of bone mass. Thus, assessment of bone health is recommended at diagnosis.

While estrogen is important for maintenance of both cortical and trabecular bone, low bone density at the lumbar spine (Answer D) can become apparent in as few as 6 months of inadequate hormone exposure. Changes in cortical bone, especially at weight-bearing sites such as the total hip (Answer E) are less sensitive to hormone changes and thus the Z-score may remain in the normal range. Stress fractures are due to excessive mechanical strain on an otherwise healthy bone. Thus, this clinical history alone does not increase the likelihood of identifying an impairment in bone strength.

Bone turnover markers in pediatric patients are of limited clinical utility given the wide range of normal results. Estrogen deficiency increases bone resorption, and because of the coupling of resorption with formation, there may be a compensatory increase in bone formation markers. Therefore, bone-specific alkaline phosphatase (Answer C) is unlikely to be low. Hypophosphatasia may present with metatarsal stress fractures in adults, although this patient's clinical history of excessive training is sufficient to account for these injuries. Osteocalcin is also a marker of bone formation; elevation coincides with the pubertal growth spurt. Although possible, having elevated osteocalcin (Answer A) is less likely than having low bone density at the lumbar spine.

Elevated total T_4 (Answer B) is most commonly associated with estrogen replacement due to increased thyroid-binding globulin, and it would not be an expected finding in primary ovarian insufficiency.

Learning Objective

Describe the skeletal effects of estrogen deficiency during adolescence.

Reference(s)

Kurtoglu-Aksoy N, Akhan SE, Bastu E, et al. Implications of premature ovarian failure on bone turnover markers and bone mineral density. *Clin Exp Obstet Gynecol*. 2014;41(2):149-153. PMID: 24779240

Hewlett M, Mahalingaiah S. Update on primary ovarian insufficiency. *Curr Opin Endocrinol Diabetes Obes*. 2015;22(6):483-489. PMID: 26512773

22 ANSWER: A) Assess the need to order a stimulated thyroglobulin measurement and whole-body ^{123}I scan 6 months postoperatively

The adolescent in this vignette has papillary thyroid cancer that is considered intermediate risk for recurrence or persistent locoregional disease based on TNM staging with extensive N1a disease (T1b,N1a,Mx). Individuals with minimal N1b (lateral neck) disease, which does not apply in this patient's case, also qualify as being at intermediate risk. Patients at intermediate risk should maintain a TSH concentration between 0.1 and 0.5 mIU/L. The TSH cutoff of less than 0.1 mIU/L (Answer B) is reserved for patients at high risk.

Patients at intermediate risk have a very low risk of distant metastases but are at increased risk for incomplete lymph node resection and persistent cervical disease. Neck ultrasonography is recommended 6 months after thyroidectomy to assess for locoregional lymphadenopathy or for incomplete resection of the thyroid, which may occur in the hands of a surgeon with low case volume. Ordering ultrasonography (Answer E) or CT (Answer D) this early (2 months after surgery) is therefore incorrect. CT is often useful preoperatively to help the surgeon plan for the appropriate dissection. The purpose of postoperative staging is to assess for evidence of persistent locoregional disease and to identify patients who are likely to benefit from additional therapy with [131]I. The pediatric guidelines recommend a TSH-stimulated thyroglobulin measurement and a diagnostic ^{123}I whole-body scan in most patients at intermediate risk—but not all—and in all patients at high risk. In most patients at intermediate risk, ordering a stimulated thyroglobulin measurement with whole-body ^{123}I scan within 12 weeks postoperatively (Answer C) would be correct. However, for patients with an unstimulated (TSH-suppressed) thyroglobulin concentration less than 0.1 ng/mL (<0.1 µg/L), it is rare for a stimulated thyroglobulin measurement to be greater than 2.0 ng/mL (>2.0 µg/L), which indicates persistent disease. Therefore, in this patient, who had a thyroglobulin value less than 0.1 ng/mL (<0.1 µg/L) and a small tumor, one can wait until a repeated unstimulated thyroglobulin measurement and neck ultrasonography are performed 6 months postoperatively and reassess the need for stimulated thyroglobulin measurement and whole-body scan (Answer A). If the thyroglobulin concentration is rising, or there is lymphadenopathy noted via neck ultrasonography, then there would be value in measuring stimulated thyroglobulin and performing a whole-body scan. The whole-body scan would help distinguish between metastatic lymph nodes vs reactive lymph nodes that are common in pediatric patients but are not always easy to identify clearly on ultrasonography, especially if the lymph nodes are small.

Educational Objective
Define intermediate-risk papillary thyroid cancer in pediatric patients and explain how to stage it postoperatively.

Reference(s)

Chindris AM, Diehl NN, Crook JE, Fatourechi V, Smallridge RC. Undetectable sensitive serum thyroglobulin (<0.1 ng/mL) in 163 patients with follicular cell-derived thyroid cancer: results of rhTSH stimulation and neck ultrasonography and long-term biochemical and clinical follow-up. *J Clin Endocrinol Metab*. 2012;97(8):2714-2723. PMID: 22639286

Francis GL, Waguespack SG, Bauer AJ, et al; American Thyroid Association Guidelines Task Force. Management guidelines for children with thyroid nodules and differentiated thyroid cancer. *Thyroid*. 2015;25(7):716-759. PMID: 25900731

23   ANSWER: B) Forearm x-ray

The bone age x-ray of this girl, who was referred for short stature, shows metaphyseal lucency of the medial side of the distal radius (*arrow*), epiphyseal hypoplasia of the medial side of the distal radius (*arrowhead*), and decreased carpal angle (≤117°), all of which are consistent with SHOX deficiency (*see image 1*).

SHOX deficiency is the most common monogenic cause of short stature, with a population incidence up to 1 in 300. SHOX deficiency may be caused by large deletions, microdeletions, or missense or nonsense pathogenic variants in the *SHOX* gene, which is present in the pseudoautosomal region (PAR1) of the short arm of chromosomes X and Y. There is no correlation between the severity of phenotype and the underlying genotype. SHOX deficiency is the cause of short stature in girls with Turner syndrome, who lack one X chromosome.

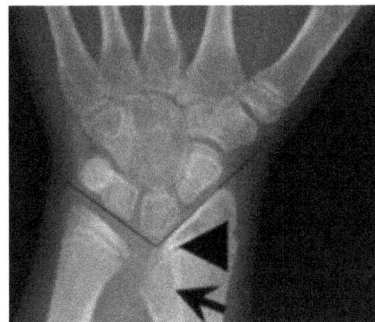

Image 1. Reprinted from Marchini A et al. *Endocr Rev*, 2016; 37(4). © Endocrine Society.

SHOX deficiency causes mesomelic short stature and Madelung deformity (also known as Leri-Weill dyschondrosteosis). Reference curves are available to assess arm span minus height and arm span-to-height ratio for boys and girls 2 to 17 years of age. This patient has an arm span minus height of 6 cm (–2 SD) and an arm span-to-height ratio of 0.954 (less than –2 SD), suggestive of short arm length (mesomelia). Thus, the anthropometric measurements and radiographic findings in this case are highly suggestive of SHOX deficiency. In such patients, radiograph of the forearm (Answer B) to look for Madelung deformity is the best next step, followed by genetic testing. Madelung deformity of the wrist and forearm denotes bilateral shortening and bowing of the radius, distal dislocation of the ulna, and wedged carpal bones (*see images 2 and 3 on the following page*).

This patient does not have any features suggestive of chronic systemic illness as the cause of her short stature. Thus, ordering a basic metabolic panel, complete blood cell count, and erythrocyte sedimentation rate (Answer A) would not help in clinching the diagnosis. Thyroid function testing (Answer C), GH stimulation testing (Answer D), pituitary MRI (Answer E) would not help diagnose SHOX deficiency, as affected patients do not have pituitary abnormalities or dysfunction.

Note: Image in the stem reprinted from Marchini A et al. Endocr Rev. 2016;37(4). © Endocrine Society.

Images 2 and 3. Reprinted from Kant SG et al. J Clin Endocrinol Metab, 2011; 96(2). © Endocrine Society

Educational Objective
Diagnose SHOX deficiency based on history and clinical and radiologic features.

Reference(s)

Marchini A, Ogata T, Rappold GA. A track record on SHOX: from basic research to complex models and therapy. *Endocr Rev.* 2016;37(4):417-448. PMID: 27355317

Kant SG, van der Kamp HJ, Kriek M, et al. The jumping *SHOX* gene--crossover in the pseudoautosomal region resulting in unusual inheritance of Leri-Weill dyschondrosteosis. *J Clin Endocrinol Metab.* 2011;96(2):E356-E359. PMID: 21068148

Blum WF, Ross JL, Zimmermann AG, et al. GH treatment to final height produces similar height gains in patients with SHOX deficiency and Turner syndrome: results of a multicenter trial. *J Clin Endocrinol Metab.* 2013;98(8):E1383-E1392. PMID: 23720786

Gerver WJM, Gkourogianni A, Dauber A, Nilsson O, Wit JM. Arm span and its relation to height in a 2- to 17-year-old reference population and heterozygous carriers of ACAN variants. *Horm Res Paediatr.* 2020;93(3):164-172. PMID: 32575104

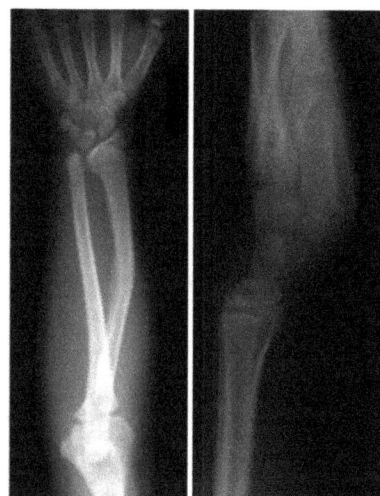

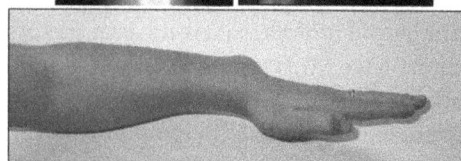

24 ANSWER: D) The practice of not counting carbohydrates or administering insulin for the carbohydrates consumed

This vignette demonstrates the challenges of "reactive" insulin management, which is common among teenagers and young adults. The practice results in a wide range of blood glucose excursions. Due to frequent hypoglycemia episodes, hemoglobin A_{1c} can be relatively close to target range (<7.0% [<53 mmol/mol]), which is deceiving. Although there are no universal recommendations for initiating pump therapy, most diabetes centers prefer not to initiate pump therapy if the hemoglobin A_{1c} level is 10.0% or higher (≥86 mmol/mol), especially without adequate glucose monitoring. This patient's hemoglobin A_{1c} value of 8.6% (70 mmol/mol) (Answer B) (and she is wearing a continuous glucose monitor) would not be a reason to avoid pump therapy.

Another common expectation is the ability to accurately count carbohydrates since all pumps require input of carbohydrate amounts before consumption. In this vignette, the patient is portrayed as unable to count carbohydrates and does not have the management skill of administering insulin before carbohydrate consumption (Answer D), which would be a major challenge for insulin pump therapy. She would benefit from educational session(s) that would focus on accurate carbohydrate counting skills, augmented by Internet-based applications and resources. This patient should demonstrate the learned skills reflected in daily management by improving her glucose sensor tracings before initiating insulin pump therapy.

Fear of hypoglycemia (Answer A) is not a risk factor for proceeding to insulin pump therapy, but it is a major obstacle in achieving reasonable glycemic control since fear drives irrational and intentional elevation of blood glucose for a false sense of security.

Reacting to hyperglycemia with a correction insulin bolus dose (Answer C) is considered a required management skill and not a reason to avoid insulin pump therapy.

Quickly advancing to insulin pump therapy without properly addressing all management concerns (Answer E) may result in deteriorating diabetes control and increased risk of comorbidities such as diabetic ketoacidosis.

Educational Objective
Identify gaps in education and important factors to consider before transitioning patients with type 1 diabetes mellitus to insulin pump therapy.

Reference(s)

Danne T, Phillip M, Buckingham BA, et al. ISPAD clinical practice consensus guidelines 2018: insulin treatment in children and adolescents with diabetes. *Pediatric Diabetes.* 2018;19(Suppl 27):115-135. PMID: 29999222

Olivier P, Lawson ML, Huot C, Richardson C, Nakhla M, Romain J. Lessons learned from a pilot RCT of simultaneous versus delayed initiation of continuous glucose monitoring in children and adolescents with type 1 diabetes starting insulin pump therapy. *J Diabetes Sci Technol.* 2014;8(3):523-528. PMID: 24876616

25 ANSWER: A) Fasting glucose and insulin

This girl has evidence of a prolactinoma and hyperparathyroidism in the setting of a family history of multiple endocrine neoplasia (MEN) type 1. MEN type 1 is an autosomal dominant disorder due to pathogenic variants in the tumor suppressor gene *MEN1*. The most common tumors associated with MEN type 1 are parathyroid tumors, pancreatic islet tumors, and anterior pituitary tumors. Less than 3% of patients with pituitary tumors have MEN type 1. Parathyroid tumors resulting in hyperparathyroidism occur in approximately 90% of patients with MEN type 1. Parathyroid tumors develop at a younger age in patients with MEN type 1 (20-25 years of age) than in those with sporadic hyperparathyroidism, and all glands may be overactive. Anterior pituitary tumors occur in 30% to 40% of patients with MEN type 1, and they can be prolactinomas, somatotropinomas, corticotropinomas, and nonfunctioning adenomas. Pancreatic islet tumors (also called pancreatic neuroendocrine tumors), including gastrinomas, insulinomas, glucagonomas, vasoactive intestinal polypeptidomas (VIPomas), and nonfunctioning pancreatic neuroendocrine tumors, occur in 40% to 70% of patients with MEN type 1. Other associated tumors include adrenocortical tumors (estimated penetrance 40%), pheochromocytomas (<1%), bronchopulmonary neuroendocrine tumors (2%), thymic neuroendocrine tumors (2%), gastric neuroendocrine tumors (10%), lipomas (30%), angiofibromas (80%), collagenomas (70%), and meningiomas (8%). Suggested screening for patients with MEN type 1 is shown (*see table*).

Table. Suggested Biochemical and Radiologic Screening in Individuals at High Risk of Multiple Endocrine Neoplasia Type 1

Tumor	Age to begin, y	Biochemical test annually (plasma or serum)	Imaging test (time interval)
Parathyroid	8	Calcium, PTH	None
Pancreatic neuroendocrine tumors			
Gastrinoma	20	Gastrin (± gastric pH)	None
Insulinoma	5	Fasting glucose, insulin	None
Other pancreatic neuroendocrine tumors	<10	Chromogranin A, pancreatic polypeptide, glucagon, vasoactive intestinal peptide	MRI, CT, or endoscopic ultrasonography (annually)
Anterior pituitary	5	Prolactin, IGF-1	MRI (every 3 years)
Adrenal	<10	None unless symptoms or signs of functioning tumor and/or tumor >1 cm identified on imaging	MRI or CT (annually with pancreatic imaging)
Thymic and bronchial carcinoid	15	None	CT or MRI (every 1-2 years)

Reprinted from Thakker RV et al. *J Clin Endocrinol Metab*, 2012; 97(9). © Endocrine Society.

Insulinomas (β-islet–cell tumors) account for 10% to 30% of all pancreatic tumors in MEN type 1 and occur more often in younger patients (<40 years), many of them diagnosed in individuals younger than 20 years. An insulinoma may be the first manifestation of MEN type 1 in 10% of patients. Current clinical guidelines recommend screening for insulinoma with fasting glucose and insulin measurements (Answer A) beginning at age 5 years.

Serum calcitonin levels (Answer D) are elevated in the setting of medullary thyroid carcinoma, which is a feature of MEN type 2.

Serum vasoactive intestinal peptide (VIP) measurement (Answer E) is recommended to screen for other pancreatic neuroendocrine tumors; however, VIPomas are very rare (<1%) in MEN type 1, so screening for an insulinoma would be the prioritized next step.

Plasma metanephrines (Answer B) are elevated in the setting of pheochromocytoma, which is rare in MEN type 1 and more commonly a feature of MEN type 2.

Asymptomatic adrenocortical tumors, including cortical adenomas, hyperplasia/nodular hyperplasia, multiple adenomas, cysts, and carcinomas occur in 20% to 73% of patients with MEN type 1 and are typically nonfunctioning. Fewer than 10% are hormonally active, with primary hyperaldosteronism and ACTH-independent Cushing syndrome occurring most commonly. Current clinical care guidelines recommend annual MRI or CT screening, but only recommend biochemical testing if a mass larger than 1 cm is seen on imaging or if there are signs of hypersecretion. This child has no signs or symptoms of oversecretion, so measuring aldosterone and renin (Answer C) is incorrect.

Educational Objective
Describe the association of prolactinoma with other tumors in patients with multiple endocrine neoplasia type 1.

Reference(s)

Thakker RV, Newey PJ, Walls GV, et al; Endocrine Society. Clinical practice guidelines for multiple endocrine neoplasia type 1 (MEN1). *J Clin Endocrinol Metab.* 2012;97(9):2990-3011. PMID: 22723327

Al-Salameh A, Baudry C, Cohen R. Update on multiple endocrine neoplasia type 1 and 2. *Presse Med.* 2018;47(9):722-731. PMID: 29909163

26 ANSWER: C) *SLC16A2* (formerly *MCT8*) (solute carrier family 16 member 2)

This child has classic clinical and laboratory features of Allan-Herndon-Dudley syndrome. This rare X-linked condition is caused by a genetic defect in the *SLC16A2* gene (Answer C) that encodes the thyroid hormone transporter monocarboxylate transporter 8 (MCT8). Because MCT8 is required for the transport of thyroid hormone into the central nervous system, MCT8 deficiency leads to profound neurologic sequelae, including those present in this patient. In addition, MCT8 deficiency leads to a unique biochemical pattern of low free T_4, normal TSH, and elevated T_3. Therefore, in this clinical scenario, measurement of T_3 is critical to distinguish MCT8 deficiency from central hypothyroidism. The mechanisms underlying this biochemical pattern are not fully understood but may include increased peripheral activation of T_4 to T_3 by type 1 iodothyronine deiodinase. Elevated T_3 concentrations cause thyroid hormone excess in tissues that are not dependent on MCT8 for thyroid hormone uptake, leading to symptoms of poor weight gain, increased SHBG concentrations, and tachycardia. Treatment of MCT8 deficiency is challenging. Levothyroxine monotherapy is contraindicated because it worsens peripheral thyrotoxicosis. Experimental treatments with thyroid hormone analogues that do not require MCT8 for central nervous system transport (such as DITPA and TRIAC) have shown promise for improving peripheral thyrotoxicosis but have minimal effect on the neurologic symptoms when initiated postnatally. Whether prenatal initiation of these agents can improve neurologic outcomes remains to be determined.

Autosomal recessive pathogenic variants in *SECISBP2* (Answer B) have been described in a few patients. Pathogenic variants in *SECISBP2* impair the normal synthesis of iodothyronine deiodinases. The function of type 2 deiodinase appears to be most affected, and impaired T_4 to T_3 conversion leads to a biochemical pattern of elevated T_4, normal-to-high TSH, and low T_3. Mild short stature and delayed bone age may be present during childhood.

Pathogenic variants in the *THRB* gene (Answer E) cause resistance to thyroid hormone β, which is characterized biochemically by elevated T_4 and T_3 levels with normal-to-high TSH due to impairment of the central negative feedback that is normally mediated by the TRβ2 receptor isoform. Additional clinical features include goiter, symptoms of hypothyroidism in TRβ-predominant tissues (slow growth, delayed bone age), and symptoms of thyroid hormone excess in TRα-predominant tissues (tachycardia, hyperactivity). This disorder is usually autosomal dominant but may occur de novo.

Rare genetic defects of *THRA* (Answer D) cause resistance to thyroid hormone α. Because TRα is not involved in central thyroid hormone feedback, TRα deficiency causes subtle, if any, biochemical thyroid abnormalities. Typically, TSH is normal, T_4 is low-normal, and T_3 is high-normal. Additional subtle laboratory findings include low reverse T_3 and elevated ratios of T_3 to reverse T_3 and of T_3 to T_4. Clinical features are primarily those of hypothyroidism, including poor growth with skeletal dysplasia, macrocephaly, developmental delay, constipation, bradycardia, and macrocytic anemia. Most reported cases have been caused by autosomal dominant de novo pathogenic variants.

Type 3 iodothyronine deiodinase (Answer A) inactivates both T_4 and T_3 to bioinactive metabolites. Although a mouse model of genetic type 3 deiodinase deficiency exists, to date no human case has been described. However, massive overexpression of type 3 deiodinase in large infantile hepatic hemangiomas can cause consumptive hypothyroidism with elevated TSH and low T_4 and T_3 levels.

Table. Syndromes of Impaired Sensitivity to Thyroid Hormone

Genetic disorder	TSH	T_4 / free T_4	T_3	Other laboratory features	Clinical features
SLC16A2 (MCT8)	Normal	Low	High	Low reverse T_3	Severe developmental delay, muscle weakness, low body weight, dyskinesia
SECISBP2	Normal/high	High	Low	High reverse T_3	Short stature, delayed bone age
THRB	Normal/high	High	High	...	Goiter, tachycardia, hyperactivity, slow growth, deafness
THRA	Normal	Normal (low-normal)	Normal (high-normal)	Low reverse T_3	Poor growth, skeletal dysplasia, developmental delay, constipation, macrocytic anemia

Educational Objective
Diagnose monocarboxylate transporter 8 (MCT8) deficiency based on clinical and laboratory findings.

Reference(s)
Groeneweg S, van Geest FS, Abacı A, et al. Disease characteristics of MCT8 deficiency: an international, retrospective, multicentre cohort study. *Lancet Diabetes Endocrinol.* 2020;8(7):594-605. PMID: 32559475

Bianco AC, Dumitrescu A, Gereben B, et al. Paradigms of dynamic control of thyroid hormone signaling. *Endocr Rev.* 2019;40(4):1000-1047. PMID: 31033998

27 ANSWER: A) Ectopic posterior pituitary with interrupted pituitary stalk

This patient had severe hypoglycemia resulting in seizures, raising the suspicion for pituitary hormone deficiencies. Pituitary anatomy is usually best evaluated using sagittal and coronal slices of T1-weighted images in cerebral MRI. Normal morphology (Answer D) of the anterior pituitary, pituitary stalk, and the posterior pituitary bright spot in the sagittal section is shown (*see image 1, arrow*). The neurohypophysis is not seen in the coronal slice, as it is anterior to it.

Given the MRI findings, this patient most likely has multiple pituitary hormone deficiencies from ectopic posterior pituitary with interrupted pituitary stalk (Answer A). In the images in the vignette, the patient's anterior pituitary is small, the pituitary stalk is not visualized, and the posterior pituitary bright spot is present ectopically at the median eminence (*see image 2*).

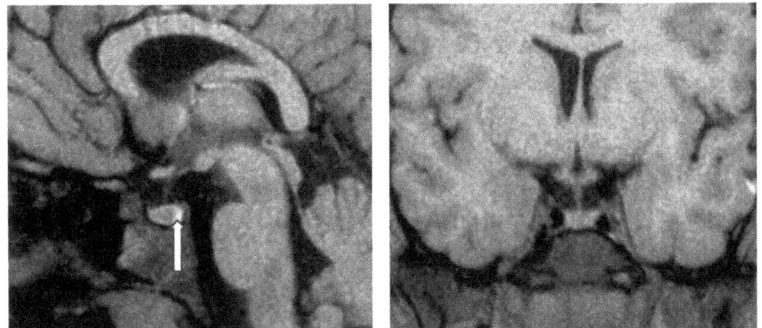

Image 1. Reprinted from Chen S et al. *J Clin Endocrinol Metab*, 1999; 84(7). © Endocrine Society.

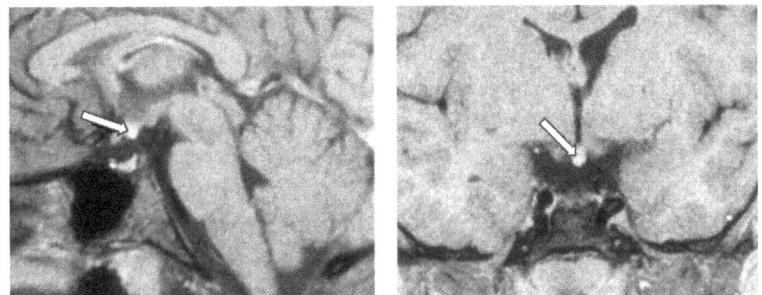

Image 2. Reprinted from Chen S et al. *J Clin Endocrinol Metab*, 1999; 84(7). © Endocrine Society.

Ectopic posterior pituitary within the pituitary stalk (Answer B) (*see image 3*) occurs when the posterior pituitary gland is incompletely descended anywhere along the path of the pituitary stalk. The image shows small pituitary sella, anterior pituitary hypoplasia (*arrow*), and ectopic posterior lobe within the middle third (*arrowhead*) of the pituitary stalk (*arrow*). When the stalk is visualized, the clinical presentation is more often isolated GH deficiency rather than multiple pituitary hormone deficiencies.

Pituitary macroadenomas (Answer E) frequently show invasion into the sellar floor and extension into the parasellar structures (*see image 4*), which was not observed in this patient's imaging.

In individuals with Langerhans-cell histiocytosis (Answer C), central diabetes insipidus could be a presenting feature due to invasion of the hypothalamus and/or the pituitary stalk by the histiocytes (*see image 5, arrow*). Anterior and posterior pituitary anatomy is preserved.

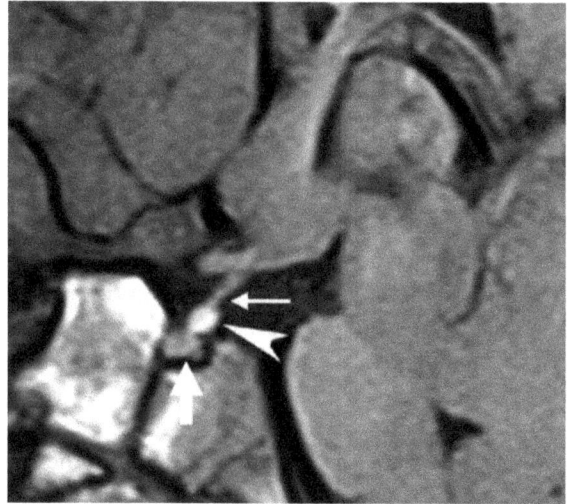

Image 3. Reprinted from di Iorgi N et al. *J Clin Endocrinol Metab*, 2007; 92(10). © Endocrine Society.

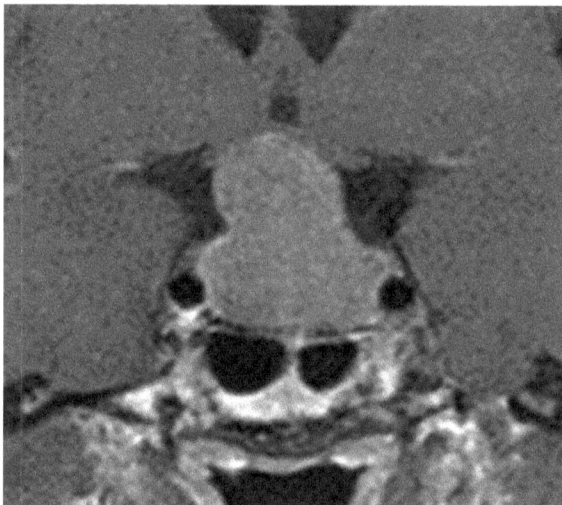

Image 4. Reprinted from Drummond J et al. *J Clin Endocrinol Metab*, 2019; 104(7). © Endocrine Society.

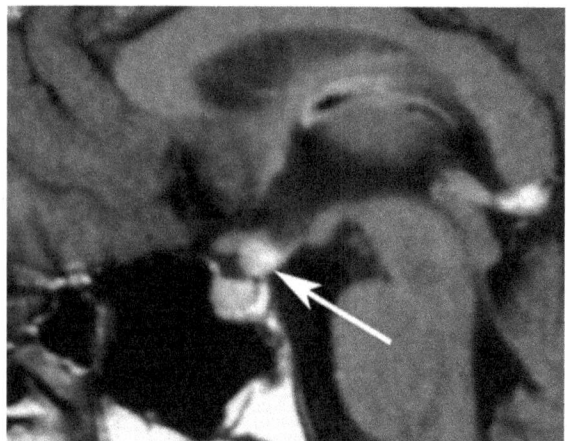

Image 5. Reprinted from Marchand I et al. *J Clin Endocrinol Metab*, 2011; 96(9). © Endocrine Society.

Note: Image in the stem reprinted from Chen S et al. *J Clin Endocrinol Metab.* 1999;84(7). © Endocrine Society.

Educational Objective
Identify abnormal anatomy of an ectopic pituitary gland and interrupted stalk on brain MRI.

Reference(s)
Chen S, Léger J, Garel C, Hassan M, Czernichow P. Growth hormone deficiency with ectopic neurohypophysis: anatomical variations and relationship between the visibility of the pituitary stalk asserted by magnetic resonance imaging and anterior pituitary function. *J Clin Endocrinol Metab*. 1999;84(7):2408-2413. PMID: 10404812

di Iorgi N, Secco A, Napoli F, et al. Deterioration of growth hormone (GH) response and anterior pituitary function in young adults with childhood-onset GH deficiency and ectopic posterior pituitary: a two-year prospective follow-up study. *J Clin Endocrinol Metab*. 2007;92(10):3875-3884. PMID: 17666476

Marchand I, Barkaoui MA, Garel C, Polak M, Donadieu J; Writing Committee. Central diabetes Insipidus as the inaugural manifestation of Langerhans cell histiocytosis: natural history and medical evaluation of 26 children and adolescents. *J Clin Endocrinol Metab*. 2011;96(9);9:E1352-E1360. PMID: 21752883

Drummond J, Roncaroli F, Grossman AB, Korbonits M. Clinical and pathological aspects of silent pituitary adenomas. *J Clin Endocrinol Metab*. 2019;104(7):2473-2489. PMID: 30020466

28 ANSWER: B) Pancreatic autoantibodies

The prevalence of overweight and obesity has increased substantially in recent decades among children and adolescents. Historically, patients with type 1 diabetes have been described as lean and this helped distinguish them from patients with type 2 diabetes. However, overweight and obesity in patients with type 1 diabetes are now very common. There has been more than a 2-fold increase in overweight/obesity since the 1990s in youth with type 1 diabetes. Data from the T1D Exchange Clinic Registry found that of 5529 adolescents with type 1 diabetes, 22.9% met criteria for overweight and 13.1% met criteria for obesity. The patient in this vignette has had significant worsening of her glycemic control despite adherence to diet and metformin therapy. She has significant hyperglycemia and is also ketotic. She has had weight loss, which is most likely secondary to her marked hyperglycemia. Therefore, it is crucial to evaluate the possibility that she has autoimmune type 1 diabetes. Autoantibodies are markers of β-cell autoimmunity (Answer B) and they are frequently found in patients with type 1 diabetes.

Heterozygous activating pathogenic variants in the *KCNJ11* gene (Answer E) are a common cause of permanent neonatal diabetes, which is diagnosed within the first 6 months of life. These infants often have a history of intrauterine growth retardation and can have failure to thrive after birth. Approximately 30% of cases of permanent neonatal diabetes are due to pathogenic variants in the *KCNJ11* gene. These variants result in K-ATP channels that are permanently open at the level of the β cell, leading to reduced insulin secretion and resultant hyperglycemia. More recently, pathogenic variants in *KCNJ11* have also been associated with later-onset diabetes mellitus; thus, *KCNJ11* testing should be considered for any patient who is undergoing testing for a possible diagnosis of maturity-onset diabetes of the young (MODY). Affected patients may respond to oral sulfonylurea therapy.

C-peptide is a byproduct made when insulin is produced in the pancreas, and its measurement can help assess pancreatic β-cell function. Low levels of C-peptide are seen in patients with type 1 diabetes and with suboptimal glycemic control, which this patient has. Elevated C-peptide levels (Answer A) occur when insulin production is high, which is common in the setting of type 2 diabetes with accompanying insulin resistance.

Inactivating heterozygous pathogenic variants in the *GCK* gene (Answer D) cause maturity-onset diabetes of the young, also known as MODY 2. Affected patients typically have mild fasting hyperglycemia and hemoglobin A_{1c} values in the range of 5.8% to 7.6% (40-60 mmol/mol), so they would not be expected to have the degree of hyperglycemia that the patient in this vignette has.

Pathogenic variants in the insulin gene (*INS*) (Answer C) can result in permanent neonatal diabetes mellitus, but they have also been found to be a rare cause of MODY type 10. These variants affect the gene that encodes preproinsulin, the biologically inactive precursor of insulin. Patients with MODY type 10 have reduced β-cell mass, progressive loss of insulin secretion, and ultimately diabetes mellitus that is variable in onset. While this patient has a family history of diabetes mellitus, which could suggest a possible inherited disorder, autoimmune type 1 diabetes is far more common and therefore is the most likely explanation for the clinical scenario presented here.

Educational Objective
Describe the common presence of overweight or obesity in patients with type 1 diabetes mellitus.

Reference(s)
Minges KE, Whittemore R, Grey M. Overweight and obesity in youth with type 1 diabetes. *Annu Rev Nurs Res.* 2013;31:47-69. PMID: 24894137

Minges KE, Whittemore R, Weinzimer SA, Irwin ML, Redeker NS, Grey M. Correlates of overweight and obesity in 5529 adolescents with type 1 diabetes: the T1D Exchange Clinic Registry. *Diabetes Res Clin Pract.* 2017;126:68-78. PMID: 28214669

29 ANSWER: C) Methamphetamine use

This patient has no goiter, bruit, or eye findings suggestive of Graves disease. She also has negative thyroid antibodies and thyroid-stimulating immunoglobulin, and her TSH is not suppressed. Thus, hashitoxicosis (Answer B) and Graves disease (Answer A) are incorrect diagnoses. She does not have any neck tenderness and her TSH is not suppressed, so subacute thyroiditis (Answer E) is incorrect.

Oral contraceptive pills (Answer D) may raise SHBG and having low T_3 uptake and elevated total T_4 would fit, but she would be euthyroid with a normal free T_4 level and not tachycardic.

Methamphetamine use (Answer C) results in dysregulation of the hypothalamic-pituitary-thyroid axis, leading to high T_4 without the expected suppressed TSH that would normally be seen in hyperthyroidism. There are also reports of elevated free T_3 in methamphetamine users, although that was not measured in this patient. Methamphetamines contain iodine and lithium, which can cause primary thyroid dysfunction (goiter or hypothyroidism), but this is less common than the central dysfunction evident in this vignette.

Educational Objective

Describe the dysregulation of the hypothalamic-pituitary-thyroid axis caused by methamphetamine use.

Reference(s)

Li SX, Yan SY, Bao YP, et al. Depression and alterations in hypothalamic-pituitary-adrenal and hypothalamic-pituitary-thyroid axis function in male abstinent methamphetamine abusers. *Hum Psychopharmacol.* 2013;28(5):477-483. PMID: 23913817

Morley JE, Shafer RB, Elson MK, et al. Amphetamine-induced hyperthyroxinemia. *Ann Intern Med.* 1980;93(5):707-709. PMID: 6782925

30 ANSWER: B) Continued monitoring for pubertal progression

Transient activation of the hypothalamic-pituitary-gonadal axis in healthy infants of both sexes is defined as minipuberty. At birth, gonadotropins are low in both sexes, and they begin rising at 1 to 2 weeks of age. In male infants, serum LH peaks between the second and tenth week of life before both LH and FSH decrease to a prepubertal range by 6 months of age. In girls, LH concentrations generally decrease at the same time as in boys, but prolonged minipuberty in girls has been recognized and FSH levels can remain elevated for up to 3 to 4 years. As such, a baseline FSH concentration (Answer D) is not helpful in distinguishing minipuberty from central precocious puberty.

As compared with central precocious puberty, breast development in isolated premature thelarche is characterized by normal height velocity and lack of maturation of the areola and nipple. However, testing to distinguish central precocious puberty from premature thelarche in this age range can be challenging. While the LH concentration in this vignette appears concerning, a basal LH concentration greater than 0.3 mIU/mL in girls younger than 3 years is poorly predictive of central precocious puberty. Although consensus statements on precocious puberty recommend use of the same threshold values in the interpretation of GnRH-stimulation tests in all children younger than 8 years (stimulated LH >5.0 mIU/mL or LH-to-FSH ratio greater than either 0.66 or 1.0), girls younger than 3 years without central precocious puberty frequently have stimulated LH values above 5.0 mIU/mL, and as high as 20.0 mIU/mL. Thus, GnRH-stimulation testing (Answer E) may not be helpful in predicting progression.

While the finding of both pubic hair and breast development is concerning, the patient in this vignette is lacking enough evidence (ie, accelerated growth or virilization) to indicate the presence of a significant underlying adrenal disorder. Given her presentation, cosyntropin-stimulation testing (Answer C) is unlikely to reveal congenital adrenal hyperplasia and would not help establish the diagnosis of central precocious puberty.

Observational studies suggest that the incidence of central precocious puberty in girls younger than 2 years presenting with thelarche is most likely only 2% to 4%. In this vignette, the patient's history does not suggest that there has been significant progression of breast development or accelerated growth, and there are no findings to suggest a central nervous system abnormality that would increase concern for central precocious puberty. As such, it would be most appropriate to monitor for progression and accelerated growth (Answer B) before pursing treatment. The decision to proceed with central nervous system imaging and GnRH agonist treatment (Answer A) should be determined based on a combination of biochemical results and clinical findings to avoid unnecessary treatment. Given the low likelihood of central precocious puberty in this patient, central nervous system imaging and treatment with a GnRH agonist would not be warranted without additional information to help determine whether the patient indeed has central precocious puberty.

Educational Objective

Interpret biochemical data in a patient younger than 2 years who presents with signs of precocious puberty.

Reference(s)

Bizzarri C, Cappa M. Ontogeny of hypothalamus-pituitary gonadal axis and minipuberty: an ongoing debate? *Front Endocrinol (Lausanne).* 2020;11:187. PMID: 32318025

Kaplowitz P, Bloch C; Section on Endocrinology, American Academy of Pediatrics. Evaluation and referral of children with signs of early puberty. *Pediatrics.* 2016;137(1). PMID: 26668298

Kuiri-Hänninen T, Sankilampi U, Dunkel L. Activation of the hypothalamic-pituitary-gonadal axis in infancy: minipuberty. *Horm Res Paediatr.* 2014;82(2):73-80. PMID: 25012863

31

ANSWER: C) Genetic testing of resected tumor tissue for a molecularly targetable driver variant

This adolescent was diagnosed with papillary thyroid carcinoma with distant metastases to the lungs. Initial therapy with radioactive iodine (RAI) is indicated for distantly metastatic papillary thyroid carcinoma. Many metastatic thyroid cancers in pediatric patients respond favorably to RAI therapy, but some cases may be refractory to RAI. Thyroid cancer is considered RAI-refractory if it does not concentrate RAI on scintigraphy and/or shows evidence of clinical progression despite RAI therapy. This patient's pulmonary metastases showed no uptake after the second RAI treatment, and subsequent disease progression was demonstrated by a rising thyroglobulin level and enlarging lung nodules. Therefore, this patient has progressive, RAI-refractory disease.

In recent years, molecular therapies have been developed that directly target specific genetic variants that underlie many thyroid cancers. Specifically, small-molecule inhibitors are now available to target cancers driven by *RET*, *NTRK1/3*, and *BRAF* variants. In one study, a pathogenic variant in one of these genes was identified in two-thirds of children and adolescents with distantly metastatic papillary thyroid carcinoma (*RET*, 40%; *NTRK1/3*, 19%; *BRAF*, 9%). Although some of these molecular therapies are not yet approved for use in children and data on their efficacy in children are limited, adult data and initial pediatric experience suggest that these agents may be effective and should be considered in pediatric patients with progressive, RAI-refractory papillary thyroid carcinoma that possesses a targetable driver variant. Therefore, the optimal management of this patient should include genetic testing of the resected thyroid cancer to identify a targetable driver variant (Answer C) that may respond to molecular therapy.

Further RAI therapy (Answers D and E) is not indicated for RAI-refractory thyroid cancer, as it unlikely to be effective and has adverse effects. External beam radiation (Answer B) may be applied to certain clinically significant, RAI-refractory thyroid cancer lesions that are localized but cannot be surgically resected (eg, bone metastasis). However, external beam radiation has limited efficacy, potentially significant adverse effects, and would not be applied to a wide anatomic field (ie, both lungs).

Cytotoxic chemotherapy with doxorubicin with or without cisplatin (Answer A) has limited efficacy for the treatment of thyroid cancer but may be used in select cases not amenable to other therapies. Identifying a driver variant targetable by molecular therapy is more likely than cytotoxic chemotherapy to result in effective treatment.

Educational Objective
Identify and manage radioactive iodine–refractory thyroid cancer in pediatric patients.

Reference(s)
Francis GL, Waguespack SG, Bauer AJ, et al; American Thyroid Association Guidelines Task Force. Management guidelines for children with thyroid nodules and differentiated thyroid cancer. *Thyroid.* 2015;25(7):716-759. PMID: 25900731

Nies M, Vassilopoulou-Sellin R, Bassett RL, et al. Distant metastases from childhood differentiated thyroid carcinoma: clinical course and mutational landscape. *J Clin Endocrinol Metab.* 2021;106(4):e1683-e1697. PMID: 33382403

Bauer AJ. Pediatric thyroid cancer: genetics, therapeutics and outcome. *Endocrinol Metab Clin North Am.* 2020;49(4):589-611. PMID: 33153669

Haugen BR, Alexander EK, Bible KC, et al. 2015 American Thyroid Association management guidelines for adult patients with thyroid nodules and differentiated thyroid cancer: the American Thyroid Association Guidelines Task Force on Thyroid Nodules and Differentiated Thyroid Cancer. *Thyroid.* 2016;26(1):1-133. PMID: 26462967

32

ANSWER: A) Cosyntropin-stimulation test

While survival rates for childhood cancer now exceed 80%, both the treatments and underlying diseases predispose patients to a wide range of health risks, including endocrine disorders. Radiation exposure to the hypothalamus, pituitary, thyroid, and gonads increases the risk of endocrinopathies (*see image*). Hypothalamic-pituitary dysfunction depends on the radiation dose, age at exposure, and time elapsed since exposure. Endocrine disorders can occur several months to many years after treatment; therefore, it is essential that childhood cancer survivors undergo lifetime surveillance for endocrinopathies. In those treated with radiation exposure to the hypothalamus and pituitary, GH deficiency is the most common endocrine disorder, followed by TSH deficiency, LH/FSH deficiency, ACTH deficiency, and central precocious puberty.

ACTH deficiency is a less common late effect of radiation therapy, but it occurs more often after 30 Gy or more is administered to the hypothalamic-pituitary region, in the presence of other hypothalamic-pituitary deficits, and after a longer period has elapsed since diagnosis and treatment. Signs of ACTH deficiency can be subtle and therefore may be missed, resulting in increased morbidity and mortality. This patient has fatigue and low blood pressure, as well as several risk factors for ACTH deficiency. Thus, it is essential to assess his hypothalamic-pituitary-adrenal axis. An 8-AM serum cortisol measurement can be a first screen for ACTH deficiency, but a cosyntropin-stimulation test may be needed to confirm whether cortisol values are low or intermediate. Therefore, a cosyntropin-stimulation test (Answer A) is the best diagnostic test to perform now.

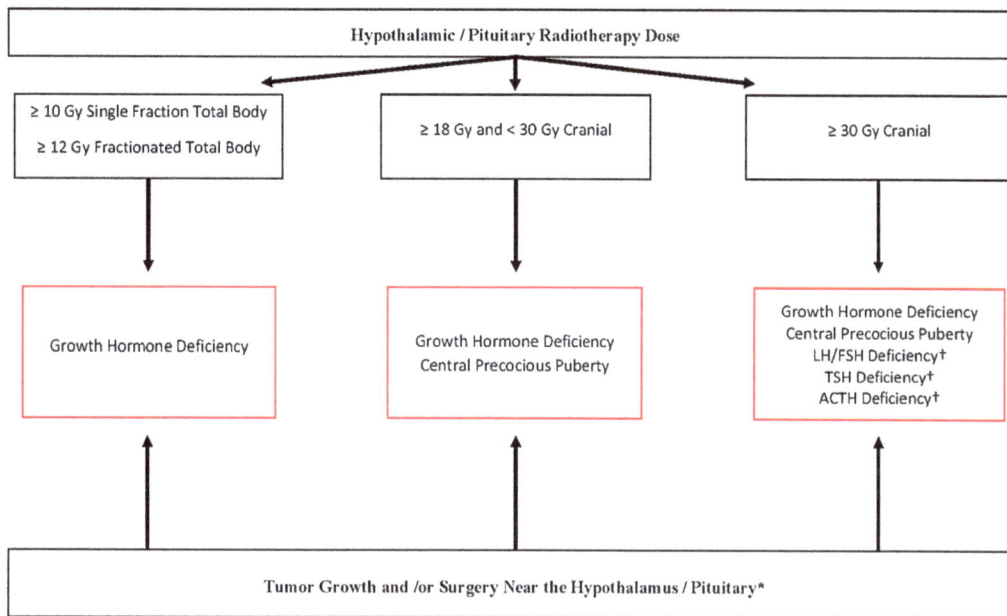

†Deficiencies in LH/FSH, TSH and / or ACTH may appear after treatment with lower doses of radiotherapy with longer follow-up.
*Tumor and surgery –induced damage may acutely cause multiple hypothalamic-pituitary deficits in addition to central diabetes insipidus.

Reprinted from Sklar CA et al. *J Clin Endocrinol Metab*, 2018; 103(8). © Endocrine Society.

This patient has a known history of GH deficiency and central precocious puberty. His short stature is most likely multifactorial, due to GH deficiency, early puberty, and decreased spinal growth (resulting in a decreased upper-to-lower segment ratio) as a result of spinal irradiation. GH deficiency may account for his increased abdominal adiposity and may be contributing to his fatigue. An IGF-1 value (Answer D) is not always a reliable indicator of GH deficiency in this setting; therefore, provocative GH-stimulation testing should be considered. While GH deficiency may be contributing to this patient's fatigue, it is most important to rule out ACTH deficiency.

While this young man is certainly at risk for gonadotropin deficiency (Answer B) and/or gonadal dysfunction due to gonadotoxic chemotherapy, it is unlikely to account for his fatigue and low blood pressure. Low or declining levels of testosterone in males and estradiol in females, in the setting of low or "normal" LH and FSH levels, suggest gonadotropin deficiency.

TSH deficiency is a common late effect of radiation therapy, but TSH levels (Answer E) can be normal in that setting. This patient's free T_4 concentration is normal, so central hypothyroidism is not present.

Although hyperprolactinemia (Answer C) can occur after radiation, it is rarely symptomatic and would not account for his fatigue.

Educational Objective
Recognize the possibility of progressive loss of or decrease in function of anterior pituitary hormones after radiation exposure.

Reference(s)

Sklar CA, Antal Z, Chemaitilly W, et al. Hypothalamic-pituitary and growth disorders in survivors of childhood cancer: an Endocrine Society clinical practice guideline. *J Clin Endocrinol Metab*. 2018;103(8):2761-2784. PMID: 29982476

van Santen, Hanneke M., Wassim Chemaitilly, Lillian R. Meacham, Emily S. Tonorezos, Sogol Mostoufi-Moab. Endocrine health in childhood cancer survivors. *Pediatric Clinics*. 2020;67(6):1171-1186. PMID: 33131540

33 ANSWER: B) Decreases gastric emptying and has effects on hypothalamic nuclei involved in the regulation of appetite

Liraglutide is an example of a GLP-1 analogue. It is a derivative of GLP-1, which is a polypeptide incretin hormone that is secreted by the L cells that line the gastrointestinal tract. In response to food, L cells secrete GLP-1 and peptide YY. GLP-1 has multiple effects, including promotion of insulin release from pancreatic β cells, reduction in plasma glucagon, decreased gastric emptying, and increased satiation. Delayed gastric emptying results in gastric stretch that sends vagal afferent signals to the solitary nucleus of the medulla and onward to the hypothalamus to induce satiety, or the area postrema, to cause nausea. Gastrointestinal adverse effects such as nausea, vomiting, and diarrhea are common, but they are usually transient. Liraglutide also directly stimulates proopiomelanocortin neurons and inhibits neuropeptide Y and Agouti-related peptide neurons of the arcuate nucleus with subsequent appetite suppression, as well as effects on other central nervous system pathways leading to reduced food-seeking behaviors. Both appetite suppression and delayed gastric emptying are thought to contribute to the weight loss seen with GLP-1 analogues (Answer B). Native GLP-1 has a half-life of less than 2 minutes; thus, liraglutide was designed with improved pharmacokinetics such that its half-life is 13 hours, which allows for once-daily dosing.

Phentermine is a sympathomimetic stimulant that acts centrally at the level of the hypothalamus to stimulate release of norepinephrine, leading to suppressed appetite (Answer E), and it may also lead to increased metabolism. Outside the central nervous system, it releases norepinephrine and epinephrine, which causes fat cells to break down stored fat as well. Phentermine is approved for short-term use in patients with obesity who are older than 16 years.

Setmelanotide is a melanocortin 4 receptor agonist approved for weight management in patients 6 years and older with severe obesity due to proopiomelanocortin deficiency, PCSK1 deficiency, and leptin receptor deficiency. Setmelanotide binds to and activates melanocortin 4 receptors in the paraventricular nucleus of the hypothalamus and in the lateral hypothalamic area, which are important in the regulation of appetite, with resultant appetite suppression (Answer A).

Orlistat is an FDA-approved weight-loss medication in adolescents who are 12 years and older. It works by inhibiting gastric and pancreatic lipases, which are responsible for the breakdown of dietary triglycerides. As a result, there is decreased absorption of approximately 30% of dietary fat (Answer D).

While not approved as a weight-loss medication, metformin is approved for the treatment of type 2 diabetes mellitus in pediatric patients 10 years or older. Metformin acts on the liver to decrease glucose production, increases glucose use in the gut, increases GLP-1 secretion, and may alter the microbiome. From a molecular standpoint, metformin inhibits the mitochondrial respiratory chain in the liver, which leads to activation of AMPK (adenosine monophosphate-activated protein kinase) and enhanced insulin sensitivity (Answer C).

Educational Objective
Explain the mechanism of action for GLP-1 analogues when used for weight loss.

Reference(s)
Kelly AS, Auerbach P, Barrientos-Perez M, Gies I, et al; NN8022-4180 Trial Investigators. A randomized, controlled trial of liraglutide for adolescents with obesity. *N Engl J Med.* 2020;382(22):2117-2128. PMID: 32233338

Crane J, McGowan B. The GLP-1 agonist, liraglutide, as a pharmacotherapy for obesity. *Ther Adv Chronic Dis.* 2016;7(2):92-107. PMID: 26977279

34 ANSWER: D) Start pamidronate

Hypercalcemia is a frequent occurrence in acutely immobilized patients, especially when it occurs during periods of rapid bone turnover such as the pubertal growth spurt. While the mechanisms leading to hypercalcemia are still being elucidated, sudden loss of mechanical stimulation leads to increased bone resorption mediated by osteoclasts, as well as reduced bone formation due to the inhibitory effects of sclerostin. Sclerostin is a hormone secreted by osteocytes to suppress LRP5/Wnt signaling in osteoblasts. This patient's low alkaline phosphatase concentration at a time when he should be undergoing a peak growth spurt suggests uncoupling of bone formation with bone resorption.

While hyperhydration is usually the first step to treat hypercalcemia, caution is needed in patients with diabetes insipidus on fixed fluid intake due to the risk of developing hyponatremia. In fact, this was attempted with this patient and desmopressin was given as needed to prevent hyponatremia. Despite this approach, a positive fluid balance occurred, leading to dependent edema without significant reduction in serum calcium levels.

Pamidronate (Answer D) is the best next step, as bisphosphonate infusions very effectively treat hypercalcemia by suppressing bone resorption. Because of its long half-life, patients with hypercalcemia due to immobilization do not typically require repeated doses of intravenous bisphosphonates. Denosumab (Answer C), a RANK-ligand inhibitor, also suppresses bone resorption by decreasing osteoclast activity. Denosumab has recently been explored as a treatment for hypercalcemia due to immobilization, especially in individuals with impaired kidney function. However, denosumab should be used with caution in children who are still actively growing, as there have been case reports of severe rebound hypercalcemia when the medication is discontinued.

Cinacalcet (Answer B) is a calcimimetic that is useful for treating hypercalcemia due to PTH-dependent mechanisms. Cinacalcet binds to the calcium-sensing receptor (CaSR) and reduces synthesis and secretion of PTH. As this patient's PTH is low, cinacalcet is not recommended.

Assessing formula recipes (Answer E) is reasonable to ensure the patient is not receiving excess calcium; however, reducing the concentration to below the recommended daily allotment for age is unlikely to significantly affect his serum calcium levels.

Adrenal insufficiency can cause hypercalcemia due to volume contraction and increased proximal tubular calcium resorption. High-dosage steroids can sometimes reduce enteral calcium absorption by inhibiting 1,25-dihydroxyvitamin D formation such as in the case of subcutaneous fat necrosis or other granulomatous processes. However, this patient is on adequate hydrocortisone replacement and is unlikely to have high 1,25-dihydroxyvitamin D levels due to PTH suppression. Increasing his steroid dosage (Answer A) is unlikely to have the desired effect of reducing serum calcium concentrations.

Educational Objective
List risk factors for hypercalcemia due to immobilization and recommend appropriate treatment interventions based on symptom severity.

References
Stokes VJ, Nielsen MF, Hannan FM, Thakker RV. Hypercalcemic disorders in children. *J Bone Miner Res.* 2017;32(11):2157-2170. PMID: 28914984

35 ANSWER: E) Start oral calcium and remeasure calcium 4 hours later

Patients who undergo total thyroidectomy are at higher risk for postoperative hypoparathyroidism and hypocalcemia if they also have central neck dissection, due to parathyroid stunning. In pediatric patients, nearly one-half of those who experience hypocalcemia develop this condition 12 to 24 hours postoperatively, so a normal initial calcium concentration, as in this vignette, does not guarantee against developing hypocalcemia. Since she had extensive neck dissection, she is at higher risk of developing hypocalcemia. Waiting until the next morning (Answer C) may be too late and would delay treatment of hypocalcemia should it occur. A PTH cutoff of 10.0 pg/mL or higher (≥10.0 ng/L) in adults seems a robust way to predict who may be discharged home safely without developing hypocalcemia. However, recent data by Jiang et al suggest that a threshold of 26.0 pg/mL or greater (≥26.0 ng/L) may be needed in pediatric patients. Therefore, using the adult PTH cutoff of 10.0 pg/mL (10.0 ng/L) or even 15.0 pg/mL (15.0 ng/L) to recommend discharge cannot be advocated, so discharging the patient home (Answer A) is incorrect.

Measuring calcium at midnight 10 hours after surgery would be one way to monitor this adolescent, but there is no literature advocating repeated PTH measurement (Answer B). Starting calcitriol alone (Answer D) is insufficient to prevent hypocalcemia, as it often takes at least 24 hours to see an effect on calcium levels.

The pediatric guidelines for children with thyroid cancer recommend starting calcium (Answer E) with or without calcitriol. There is currently a lack of clear guidelines on how to approach this issue in children. Despite receiving 400 mg of elemental calcium 5 hours after surgery, this patient's calcium concentration dropped to 8.0 mg/dL (2.0 mmol/L) 4 hours later, and 1 mcg of calcitriol was added. With calcitriol and repeated calcium administration every 4 hours, she was able to avoid a further decrease in her calcium levels, and her concentration normalized by the next day.

Educational Objective
Identify risk factors for postoperative hypoparathyroidism and guide diagnosis and management.

Reference(s)

Francis GL, Waguespack SG, Bauer AJ, et al; American Thyroid Association Guidelines Task Force. Management guidelines for children with thyroid nodules and differentiated thyroid cancer. *Thyroid.* 2015;25(7):716-759. PMID: 25900731

Jiang W, Lee E, Newfield RS. The utility of intact parathyroid hormone level in managing hypocalcemia after thyroidectomy in children. *Int J Pediatr Otorhinolaryngol.* 2019;125:153-158. PMID: 31323353

36 ANSWER: B) *LZTR1* (leucine zipper like transcription regulator 1)

The patient in this vignette has multiple findings that support a clinical diagnosis of Noonan syndrome. However, a few aspects of his history make his case atypical, including being large for gestational age, as well as having unaffected consanguineous parents. Noonan syndrome is usually an autosomal dominant genetic disorder (although there is an autosomal recessive form), and it occurs in 1 in 1000 to 2500 live births. Clinical manifestations include proportioned postnatal short stature; dysmorphic features such as ocular hypertelorism, palpebral ptosis, high-arched palate, low-set, retrorotated ears, low posterior hairline, webbed neck, pectus carinatum or excavatum, and widely spaced nipples; developmental delay of variable degree; congenital heart defects such as pulmonic stenosis and hypertrophic cardiomyopathy; coagulation disorders; cryptorchidism; and predisposition to myeloproliferative disorders.

Multiple gene abnormalities have been associated with Noonan syndrome, and the number of genes is still expanding (*see table*). Presently, 20% to 30% of patients clinically diagnosed with Noonan syndrome do not have an identifiable genetic etiology.

Table. Genes Associated With Noonan Syndrome

OMIM #	Type of Noonan syndrome	Gene	Inheritance	Growth
163950	Noonan syndrome 1 (NS 1)	PTPN11	Autosomal dominant	Failure to thrive, postnatal short stature
605275	Noonan syndrome 2 (NS 2)	LZTR1	Autosomal recessive	Large for gestational age, postnatal short stature
609942	Noonan syndrome 3 (NS 3)	KRAS	Autosomal dominant	Postnatal short stature
610733	Noonan syndrome 4 (NS 4)	SOS1	Autosomal dominant	Postnatal short stature
611553	Noonan syndrome 5 (NS 5)	RAF1	Autosomal dominant	Postnatal short stature
613224	Noonan syndrome 6 (NS 6)	NRAS	Autosomal dominant	Postnatal short stature
613706	Noonan syndrome 7 (NS 7)	BRAF	Autosomal dominant	Neonatal short stature
615355	Noonan syndrome 8 (NS 8)	RIT1	Autosomal dominant	Failure to thrive
616559	Noonan syndrome 9 (NS 9)	SOS2	Autosomal dominant	Postnatal short stature
616564	Noonan syndrome 10 (NS 10)	LZTR1	Autosomal dominant	Postnatal short stature
618499	Noonan syndrome 11 (NS 11)	MRAS	Autosomal dominant	Postnatal short stature
618624	Noonan syndrome 12 (NS 12)	RRAS2	Autosomal dominant	Large for gestational age, failure to thrive
619087	Noonan syndrome 13 (NS 13)	MAPK1	Autosomal dominant	Postnatal short stature
607721	Noonan syndrome-like disorder with anagen hair 1 (NSLH1)	SHOC2	Autosomal dominant	Large for gestational age, failure to thrive
611706	Noonan syndrome-like disorder with anagen hair 2 (NSLH2)	PPP1CB	Autosomal dominant	Failure to thrive, postnatal short stature
613563	Noonan syndrome-like disorder +/- juvenile myelomonocytic leukemia (NSLL)	CBL	Autosomal dominant	Postnatal short stature
601321	Neurofibromatosis-Noonan syndrome (NFNS)	NF1	Autosomal dominant	Postnatal short stature

Created using data from OMIM resources, https://omim.org/

The most common genetic abnormality found in individuals with Noonan syndrome (accounting for approximately 50% of cases) is a gain-of-function missense pathogenic variant in the *PTPN11* gene (protein tyrosine phosphatase nonreceptor type 11) (Answer D) inherited in an autosomal dominant fashion that leads to excessive activation of the RAS/MAPK pathway. Pathogenic variants in the *SOS1* gene (SOS Ras/Rac guanine nucleotide exchange factor 1) (Answer E) and *RAF1* gene (Raf-1 proto-oncogene, serine/threonine kinase) account for approximately 10% of cases, respectively, and pathogenic variants in the *KRAS* gene (KRAS proto-oncogene, GTPase) account for approximately 2% of cases. These 3 forms of Noonan syndrome are inherited in an autosomal dominant manner and are not associated with large birth size. Thus, they are unlikely to be the etiology of this patient's Noonan syndrome.

This patient most likely has an autosomal recessive disorder given that he is the child of unaffected, consanguineous parents. In addition, he has a history of being large for gestational age (based on birth weight and birth length) with postnatal growth deceleration leading to short stature. One of his siblings has similar features, making a sporadic form of Noonan syndrome less likely. In the absence of clinical manifestations in his parents and in 4 of his 5 siblings, an autosomal recessive mode of inheritance is most likely. Pathogenic variants in the *LZTR1* gene (leucine zipper like transcription regulator 1) (Answer B) are the most likely culprit. Noonan syndrome associated with the *LZTR1* gene is the only form of Noonan syndrome with autosomal recessive inheritance and large size at birth. Of note, Noonan syndrome type 10 is also associated with abnormalities in the same gene, but it is inherited in an autosomal dominant fashion and is not associated with being large for gestational age.

Other types of Noonan syndrome that can present with large size at birth include type 12 due to pathogenic variants in the *RRAS2* gene (RAS related 2) and Noonan syndrome-like disorder with anagen hair type 1 due to pathogenic variants in the *SHOC2* gene (SHOC2 leucine rich scaffold protein), but these types are inherited in an autosomal dominant manner.

Pathogenic variants in the *NF1* gene (neurofibromin 1) (Answer C) are responsible for neurofibromatosis–Noonan syndrome), and pathogenic variants in the *CBL* gene (Cbl proto-oncogene) (Answer A) are responsible for Noonan syndrome-like disorder with or without juvenile myelomonocytic leukemia. Both are inherited in an autosomal dominant manner. In addition, the child in this vignette does not have clinical features of neurofibromatosis or myeloproliferative disorders.

Educational objective
Describe the most common etiologies of Noonan syndrome and recognize that being that large-for-gestational age can be a distinguishing feature of certain forms of Noonan syndrome.

Reference(s)
Yart A, Edouard T. Noonan syndrome: an update on growth and development. *Curr Opin Endocrinol Diabetes Obes.* 2018;25(1):67-73. PMID: 29120925

Tidyman WE, Rauen KA. The RASopathies: Developmental syndromes of Ras/MAPK pathway dysregulation. *Curr Opin Genet Dev.* 2009;19(3):230-236. PMID: 19467855

Online Mendelian Inheritance in Man, OMIM. McKusick-Nathans Institute of Genetic Medicine, Johns Hopkins University (Baltimore, MD). Accessed July 5, 2021. https://omim.org/

37 ANSWER: D) No treatment but monitor blood glucose with either a glucose meter (fasting and 1 hour postprandial) or glucose sensor

Abnormalities of glucose metabolism in cystic fibrosis represent a continuum; however, the predominant abnormality is postprandial, not preprandial, hyperglycemia. Insulin is currently recommended as the treatment of choice for cystic fibrosis–related diabetes, but its use is associated with a number of limitations, including hypoglycemia.

The patient in this vignette does not have a clearly defined abnormality in her response to a standardized glucose challenge with 75 g of glucose solution. Responses are defined in the *table*.

Description	Fasting plasma glucose	30- to 90-Minute glucose	2-Hour glucose
Normal glucose tolerance	≤126 mg/dL (SI: ≤7.0 mmol/L)	<140 mg/dL (SI: <7.8 mmol/L)	<140 mg/dL (SI: <7.8 mmol/L)
Indeterminate glucose tolerance	≤126 mg/dL (SI: ≤7.0 mmol/L)	≥200 mg/dL (SI: ≥11.1 mmol/L)	<140 mg/dL (SI: <7.8 mmol/L)
Impaired glucose tolerance	Any value	Any value	≥140 mg/dL (SI: ≥7.8 mmol/L) but <200 mg/dL (SI: <11.1 mmol/L)
Cystic fibrosis–related diabetes	Any value	Any value	≥200 mg/dL (SI: ≥11.1 mmol/L)

Patients with mid–oral glucose tolerance testing glucose values of 140 mg/dL or higher (≥7.8 mmol/L) and less than 200 mg/dL (<11.1 mmol/L) are defined as having a borderline abnormality of glucose tolerance. There are no clear guidelines for how to treat this type of metabolic derangement. However, these patients are at high risk for progression to fasting or postprandial hyperglycemia, and home glucose monitoring (Answer D) is recommended.

There is reasonable consensus that patients with fasting hyperglycemia should be treated with insulin, but the patient in this vignette has normal fasting glucose. Thus, basal insulin (Answer B), mealtime bolus insulin (Answer C), and a basal-bolus insulin regimen (Answer A) are incorrect. Deciding how to treat patients who do not have fasting hyperglycemia is more problematic because so few data are available. There are also limited data that oral agents such as repaglinide (Answer E) may be used initially and could be as effective as rapid-acting insulin when given before meals. Yet, this choice would be premature to consider without further home glucose monitoring, which is needed to assess the glycemic response to real-life meal and snack consumption since oral glucose tolerance testing may not be representative of glucose excursions.

Educational Objective
Interpret oral glucose tolerance test results in patients with cystic fibrosis and describe the criteria for starting treatment of cystic fibrosis–related diabetes.

Reference(s)
Moran A, Pillay K, Becker D, Granados A, Hameed S, Acerini CL. ISPAD clinical practice consensus guidelines 2018: management of cystic fibrosis-related diabetes in children and adolescents. *Pediatric Diabetes*. 2018;19(Suppl 27):64-74. PMID: 30094886

Piona C, Volpi S, Zusi C, et al. Glucose tolerance stages in cystic fibrosis are identified by a unique pattern of defects of beta-cell function. *J Clin Endocrinol Metab*. 2021;106(4):e1793-e1802. PMID: 33331877

Moran A, Milla C. Abnormal glucose tolerance in cystic fibrosis: why should patients be screened? *J Pediatr*. 2003;142(2):97-99. PMID: 12584525

38 ANSWER: B) Increased binding affinity of albumin for T_4

This child has elevated serum T_4 with normal TSH. Despite the elevated T_4 levels, he is clinically euthyroid. This suggests that free T_4 levels are likely normal and that his biochemical findings may be caused by an abnormality of thyroid hormone binding. The most common abnormality that might explain these findings is familial dysalbuminemic hyperthyroxinemia caused by a variant in the gene encoding albumin (usually at Arg218) that increases the binding affinity of albumin for T_4 (Answer B), and in some cases for T_3. The prevalence of familial dysalbuminemic hyperthyroxinemia varies among populations but is present in up to 2% of individuals of Hispanic ancestry. Because free T_4 levels are normal, individuals with familial dysalbuminemic hyperthyroxinemia are euthyroid and treatment is not indicated.

The clinical and biochemical findings in this patient could be consistent with other disorders of thyroid hormone binding, but these are less common than familial dysalbuminemic hyperthyroxinemia. Rare variants in the gene encoding prealbumin (transthyretin) may increase its binding affinity for T_4 (Answer C). Thyroxine-binding globulin excess is caused by duplication of the thyroxine-binding globulin gene that leads to increased circulating thyroxine-binding globulin concentrations (Answer A). Thyroxine-binding globulin excess occurs in about 1 in 6000 to 1 in 40,000 individuals. Alterations of thyroxine-binding globulin that cause increased binding affinity for T_4 (Answer D) have not been reported as a cause of apparent thyroxine-binding globulin excess.

Pathogenic variants that decrease the function of thyroid hormone receptor β (Answer E) impair the central negative feedback of thyroid hormones that is normally mediated by the TRβ2 receptor isoform. This leads to elevated T_4 (and T_3) levels with normal or high TSH. However, affected patients are not euthyroid. Tissues expressing predominant TRβ are functionally hypothyroid, while tissues expressing predominantly TRα are thyrotoxic, leading to clinical manifestations of slow growth, delayed bone age, tachycardia, and hyperactivity. Goiter is also common due to elevated TSH levels.

Educational Objective
Diagnose familial dysalbuminemic hyperthyroxinemia.

Reference(s)

Benvenga S. Thyroid hormone transport proteins and the physiology of hormone binding. In: Braverman LE, Cooper DS, eds. *Werner & Ingbar's The Thyroid*. 10th ed. Wolters Kluwer Health; 2013:93-103.

DeCosimo DR, Fang SL, Braverman LE. Prevalence of familial dysalbuminemic hyperthyroxinemia in Hispanics. *Ann Intern Med*. 1987;107(5):780-781. PMID: 3662294

39   ANSWER: B) Activation of adenylate cyclase

Hormones act by binding to specific receptor proteins. This binding generally induces conformational changes that induce signal transduction pathways, which result in a physiologic response. Four major receptor superfamilies have been identified and include the G protein–coupled receptors (GPCRs), cytokine receptors, receptor tyrosine kinases (RTKs), and nuclear receptors (*see table*). Pathogenic variants that influence receptor function can lead to a variety of endocrine disorders.

Hormone receptor class	Receptors	Signal transduction pathways
G protein–coupled receptors	ACTH, melanocortins, V2 vasopressin, LH, FSH, TSH, GnRH, TRH, GHRH, CRF, somatostatin, glucagon, oxytocin, gastric inhibitory peptide, Type 1 PTH, free fatty acid, GPR 54, orexin, ghrelin, melanin-concentrating, calcitonin, GLP-1, calcium-sensing	Cyclic AMP and phosphatidylinositol signal pathways
Type 1 cytokine receptors	GH, prolactin, leptin	Activation JAK-STAT pathway
Receptor tyrosine kinases	Insulin, IGF-1, fibroblast growth factor	Activation of tyrosine kinase
Nuclear receptors	Thyroid hormone, vitamin D_3, peroxisome proliferator–activated γ, hepatic nuclear factor 4A, glucocorticoid, androgen, estrogen, mineralocorticoid, DAX1	Activation of gene transcription through hormone response elements
TGF-β	Bone morphogenic proteins, growth factors, antimullerian hormone, activin	Smad phosphorylation

The patient in this vignette has recurrent vaginal bleeding with ovarian cyst formation and an elevated estradiol level. Her LH and FSH levels are prepubertal. While no information is given about café-au-lait macules or fibrous dysplasia, this girl may have McCune-Albright syndrome, which is due to activating pathogenic variants in the *GNAS* gene that result in constitutive activation of the stimulatory α-subunit of the G-protein (Answer B). GPCRs include ACTH and other melanocortins, V2 vasopressin, LH, FSH, TSH, GnRH, TRH, GHRH, corticotropin-releasing factor, somatostatin, glucagon, oxytocin, gastric inhibitory peptide, type 1 PTH, free fatty acid, GPR 54, orexin, ghrelin, melanin-concentrating, calcitonin, GLP-1, and calcium-sensing receptors. Two principal signal transduction pathways involve the GPCRs: the cyclic AMP signal pathway and the phosphatidylinositol signal pathway. Binding of a ligand to the receptor results in G-protein activation, which in turn triggers the production of second messengers. When activated by the GTP-bound α-subunit, adenylyl cyclase catalyzes synthesis of the second messenger cAMP from ATP.

The RTK superfamily includes receptors for insulin, IGF-1, and fibroblast growth factor. These receptors generally require dimerization to be activated. Activation of RTKs (Answer C) leads to phosphorylation of tyrosine, resulting in activation of the tyrosine kinases, which induce the transfer of phosphate from ATP to tyrosine residues in the cytosolic portion of the receptor and in cytosolic proteins that serve as docking sites for second messengers.

GH, prolactin, and leptin bind to type 1 cytokine receptors. First, the ligand binds a monomeric receptor, then interacts with a second receptor to induce receptor dimerization and activation. Activated receptors then stimulate members of the Janus family of tyrosine kinases (JAK kinases) to phosphorylate tyrosine residues on both the kinase itself and the cytoplasmic region of the receptors. Signal transducers and activators of transcription (STATs) then dock on the phosphorylated cytoplasmic receptor domains or JAK kinases and undergo tyrosine phosphorylation. The phosphorylated STATs dissociate and translocate to the nucleus where they bind and alter the activity of regulatory regions of target DNA (Answer A).

Thyroid hormone, vitamin D_3, peroxisome proliferator–activated receptor γ, hepatocyte nuclear factor 4A, glucocorticoid, androgen, estrogen, mineralocorticoid, and DAX1 bind to nuclear receptors. These receptors bind to specific consensus DNA sequences called hormone response elements and exert control of gene expression either in a stimulatory or inhibitory fashion. For example, the thyroid hormone receptor acts as a repressor in the absence of hormone, but when bound to hormone, it is converted into an activator that stimulates transcription of thyroid hormone–inducible genes (Answer E).

Bone morphogenetic proteins, growth and differentiation factors, antimullerian hormone, and activin bind to TGF-β receptors. Activation of these serine/threonine kinase receptors induces signaling by formation of Smad complexes that are translocated to the nucleus where they act as transcription factors (Answer D).

Educational Objective
Explain the signal transduction mechanism pathways of the hormone receptors.

Reference(s)
Kublaoui B, Levine MA. Receptor transduction pathways mediating hormone action. In: Sperling M, ed. *Sperling Pediatric Endocrinology.* 5th ed. Elsevier; 2021:30-85.

40 ANSWER: C) Indirect calorimetry

Indirect calorimetry (Answer C) is the gold standard to measure resting energy expenditure (REE). REE is the energy expended by an individual over 24 hours during a nonactive period and is the largest component of total energy expenditure. With indirect calorimetry, oxygen consumption (VO_2) and carbon dioxide production (VCO_2) are measured to calculate the metabolic rate. Indirect calorimetry measurements allow providers to personalize nutrition support by better identifying an individual's metabolic needs, whether hypometabolic or hypermetabolic. Because indirect calorimetry can be obtained in both mechanically ventilated and spontaneously breathing patients, it has many potential clinical applications. In patients who are breathing on their own, a ventilated hood or a fitted face mask is used to collect both inspired and expired gases.

One of the limitations of indirect calorimetry is the fact that traditional iterations are often very costly and technically complex. They require a warm-up period, extensive calibration, and ability to attain steady state; thus, they are very operator dependent. In recent years, handheld indirect calorimetry devices have been developed whose advantages include portability and a low degree of required technical expertise. The clinical status of a patient is also important to consider when deciding on the proper timing of indirect calorimetry or its interpretability. During the acute phase of illness, the body produces and uses endogenous substrates, which can make interpretation of REE by indirect calorimetry difficult. Other factors that can affect accuracy of indirect calorimetry include patient pain or agitation, febrile state, need for supplemental oxygen, or inability to tolerate a face mask/hood.

Basal metabolic rate (BMR) (Answer D) is sometimes used interchangeably with the term REE. However, using strict definitions, BMR refers to the minimal amount of energy expended by an organism for homeostatic processes. Total energy expenditure is the sum of basal metabolic rate, diet-induced thermogenesis, and activity-induced energy expenditure. While BMR is a large component of total energy expenditure (about 60%-80% in nonhospitalized patients), it is the lowest level of energy expenditure and can be as much as 10% lower compared with REE. Measuring the basal metabolic rate also requires a strict set of conditions, whereas measuring REE has fewer restrictions. BMR is measured through gas analysis (either direct or indirect calorimetry) in the morning after a patient has slept for at least 8 hours overnight. Additionally, patients must remain in a reclined position in a darkened room, not have exercised for the past 24 hours, and have fasted for at least 12 hours. To meet all of these conditions, patients typically are required to spend the night in the testing facility.

Although different predictive equations (using anthropometric data and clinical conditions) have been developed to estimate REE, the accuracy of these equations is very low and none is considered clinically acceptable compared with indirect calorimetry. The Owen equation (Answer E) is one such predictive equation that underestimates REE by as much as 13%. The Owen equation is as follows:

- Males: weight (kg) × 10.2 + 879 = kcal/d
- Females: weight (kg) × 7.18 + 795 = kcal/d

Direct calorimetry (Answer B) measures heat production or heat loss by the body. While it is very accurate for quantifying metabolic rate, it is costly, the engineering is complex, patients must remain in a confined space for extended periods, and appropriate facilities are scarce, which limits its feasibility and usefulness.

Accelerometry (Answer A) is an objective measurement of physical activity. The output is given in the form of "counts" per unit time and converted to energy expenditure units through the use of specific predictive equations. Unfortunately, current equations have significant limitations when it comes to translating accelerometer counts into energy expenditure.

Educational Objective
Explain the benefits and limitations of indirect calorimetry as a tool for improving nutritional management of pediatric obesity.

Reference(s)
Delsoglio M, Achamrah N, Berger MM, Pichard C. Indirect calorimetry in clinical practice. *J Clin Med.* 2019;8(9):1387. PMID: 31491883

Achamrah N, Delsoglio M, De Waele E, Berger MM, Pichard C. Indirect calorimetry: the 6 main issues. *Clin Nutr.* 2021;40(1):4-14. PMID: 32709554

Ndahimana D, Kim E-K. Measurement methods for physical activity and energy expenditure: a review. *Clin Nutr Res.* 2017;6(2):68-80. PMID: 28503503

41 ANSWER: E) Provide counseling on risk of type 2 diabetes mellitus

Several cohort studies have shown an inverse correlation between age at menarche and risk of developing type 2 diabetes mellitus. While it is not completely clear as to what extent this risk is mediated by BMI, a large British birth cohort study indicated that early menarche is associated with an increased risk of type 2 diabetes independent of BMI at 2 years of age and 7 years of age. While progression to menarche is often slower in girls who present with puberty at this age, the advanced stage of this patient's breast development indicates she is likely to undergo menarche at an early age. Her elevated BMI and high likelihood of early menarche are probably both risk factors for development of type 2 diabetes; therefore, the family should be counseled about this risk (Answer E).

The data presented in the vignette are sufficient to diagnose central precocious puberty without the need for GnRH-stimulation testing (Answer B). LH concentrations greater than 0.2 to 0.3 mIU/mL (the threshold depends on the assay used) can identify children with progressive central precocious puberty with high sensitivity and specificity. GnRH-stimulation testing may be helpful for children who appear to have ongoing pubertal progression but have basal LH concentrations less than 0.3 mIU/mL. Genetic testing for causes of central precocious puberty (Answer A) can identify a genetic etiology in some cases. However, in the absence of features of specific genetic syndromes associated with central precocious puberty, genetic testing is not recommended in current guidelines and a positive result is unlikely to influence management decisions.

TSH (Answer D) should be measured in girls if chronic primary hypothyroidism is suspected as the cause of pubertal development. Several mechanisms have been proposed, including overproduction of gonadotropins due to loss of negative feedback in the pituitary and cross-reactivity of TSH with the FSH receptor. While primary hypothyroidism should be considered in any girl with precocious puberty, this is very unlikely in the patient presented given her tall stature and accelerated growth, which would not be expected in a patient with chronic hypothyroidism.

Pelvic ultrasonography (Answer C) may be helpful in distinguishing between central precocious puberty and variants such as premature thelarche when other testing is not definitive. However, there is most likely considerable overlap in uterine and ovarian volumes between patients with and without central precocious puberty. In this vignette, the diagnostic testing was clearly consistent with central precocious puberty, making pelvic ultrasonography unnecessary.

Educational Objective
Counsel a family regarding the risk of type 2 diabetes mellitus in a child with central precocious puberty.

Reference(s)
Pierce MB, Kuh D, Hardy R. The role of BMI across the life course in the relationship between age at menarche and diabetes, in a British Birth Cohort. *Diabet Med.* 2012;29(5):600-603. PMID: 21999522

Bangalore Krishna K, Fuqua JS, Rogol AD, et al. Use of gonadotropin-releasing hormone analogs in children: update by an International Consortium. *Horm Res Paediatr.* 2019;91(6):357. PMID: 31319416

42

ANSWER: C) Measure blood pressure while the patient is laying down and standing

Adequacy of mineralocorticoid replacement should be closely monitored in all patients requiring treatment with the mineralocorticoid 9α-fludrocortisone. Measurement of blood pressure (Answer C) is an essential part of monitoring, as low blood pressure or a postural drop may indicate the need for an increase in the mineralocorticoid dosage, while high blood pressure maybe be indicative of overtreatment. Only after blood pressure measurement should a decision be made regarding a possible increase in the mineralocorticoid dosage (Answer A). Without knowing the timing of the blood samples and medication taken, it would be inappropriate to increase the hydrocortisone dosage (Answer B). Head MRI (Answer E) and a complete blood cell count (Answer D) may have merit after a full examination, but neither is the best next step now.

The parameters used to monitor optimal 9α-fludrocortisone replacement are relatively poorly studied. Pofi et al highlighted some of these issues in a recent article that describes how plasma renin activity measurements were unrelated to mineralocorticoid dosages in patients with primary adrenal insufficiency. In this study, serum electrolytes (notably potassium) were most closely and strongly related to the mineralocorticoid dosage at baseline and in the longitudinal analysis. However, others advocate the benefit of plasma renin activity measurement, as children with regularly measured plasma renin activity have lower blood pressure than do those without documentation of plasma renin activity. This lack of agreement on the relationship with mineralocorticoid dosage may be due to variability and difficulty at the time of sampling, as well as the fact that some glucocorticoids (hydrocortisone and prednisolone) have mineralocorticoid effects, so overtreatment with glucocorticoid could mask the need for mineralocorticoid.

The Endocrine Society clinical practice guideline on primary adrenal insufficiency suggests that mineralocorticoid replacement should be tailored primarily based on clinical assessment (salt craving, postural hypotension, or edema) and blood electrolyte measurements. The 2018 Endocrine Society clinical practice guideline on congenital adrenal hyperplasia recommends regular assessments of growth velocity, weight, and blood pressure; physical examination; and biochemical measurements (serum sodium, potassium, and plasma renin activity) to assess the adequacy of mineralocorticoid. In newborns and young infants, sufficient sodium supplementation is essential because of the low sodium content in diets at this age and the relative renal tubular resistance to the effects of aldosterone in early infancy.

Prospective studies are clearly needed to assess this issue; however, current consensus is that mineralocorticoid replacement should aim to achieve normotension, normokalemia, and a plasma renin activity concentration in the upper reference range, and that suppression or normalization of the plasma renin activity concentration is associated with mineralocorticoid overtreatment.

Educational Objective
Guide mineralocorticoid replacement and monitoring in adrenal insufficiency.

Reference(s)

Speiser PW, Arlt W, Auchus RJ, et al. Congenital adrenal hyperplasia due to steroid 21-hydroxylase deficiency: an Endocrine Society clinical practice guideline. *J Clin Endocrinol Metab.* 2018;103(11): 4043-4088. PMID: 30272171

Nimkarn S, Lin-Su K, Berglind N, Wilson RC, New MI. Aldosterone-to-renin ratio as a marker for disease severity in 21-hydroxylase deficiency congenital adrenal hyperplasia. *J Clin Endocrinol Metab.* 2007;92(1):137-142. PMID: 17032723

Pofi R, Prete A, Thornton-Jones V, et al. Plasma renin measurements are unrelated to mineralocorticoid replacement dose in patients with primary adrenal insufficiency. *J Clin Endocrinol Metab.* 2020;105(1):dgz055. PMID: 31613957

Bonfig W, Roehl FW, Riedl S, et al; AQUAPE CAH Study Group. Blood pressure in a large cohort of children and adolescents with classic adrenal hyperplasia (CAH) due to 21-hydroxylase deficiency. *Am J Hypertens.* 2016;29(2):266-272. PMID: 26071487

Bornstein SR, Allolio B, Arlt W, et al. Diagnosis and treatment of primary adrenal insufficiency: an Endocrine Society clinical practice guideline. *J Clin Endocrinol Metab.* 2016;101(2):364-389. PMID: 26760044

Husebye ES, Allolio B, Arlt W, et al. Consensus statement on the diagnosis, treatment and follow-up of patients with primary adrenal insufficiency. *J Intern Med.* 2014;275(2):104-115. PMID: 24330030

Claahsen-van der Grinten HL, Speiser PW, Ahmed SF, et al. Congenital adrenal hyperplasia - current insights in pathophysiology, diagnostics and management. *Endocr Rev.* 2022;43(1):91-159.PMID: 33961029

43

ANSWER: E) Screen for social determinants of health

This patient has been on hormone replacement therapy for central hypothyroidism, central adrenal insufficiency, and GH deficiency. Current dosages of levothyroxine (2.8 mcg/kg per day), hydrocortisone (16 mg/m² per day), and GH (0.32 mg/kg per week) are adequate or higher than typical daily requirements. Despite that, she is short with obesity and poor growth, which is most consistent with poor adherence to treatment recommendations. Therefore, increasing the dosage of levothyroxine (Answer C), GH (Answer A), or hydrocortisone (Answer B) would most likely not result in better health outcomes. However, these findings raise red flags for risk factors in social determinants of health (Answer E) in this family.

Social determinants of health are the conditions in the environments where people are born, live, learn, work, play, worship, and age that affect a wide range of health, functioning, and quality-of-life outcomes and risks. Social determinants of health can be grouped into 5 domains: (1) economic stability, (2) education access and quality, (3) health care access and quality, (4) neighborhood and built environment, and (5) social and community context. Categories of social determinants of health include, but are not limited to, safe housing and transportation, family financial support, language and literacy skills, access to nutritious food and good quality of air/water, child maltreatment, family mental illness, substance abuse in the household, and intimate partner violence. Understanding the presence of and complexities of social determinants of health is vital for providers to be able to help patients and their families in need. Thus, it is important to screen for social determinants of health using appropriate tools and to offer referral to applicable local and regional resources to improve the adverse effects of social determinants of health in these families.

Reporting the family to child protection services (Answer D) is not the best next step without understanding the underlying cause of the family's poor adherence to treatment and follow-up recommendations.

Educational Objective
Screen for social determinants of health to identify actions to improve health outcomes in children.

Reference(s)

Chung EK, Siegel BS, Garg A, et al. Screening for social determinants of health among children and families living in poverty: a guide for clinicians. *Curr Probl Pediatr Adolesc Health Care.* 2016;46(5):135-153. PMID: 27101890

Garg A, Byhoff E, Wexler MG. Implementation considerations for social determinants of health screening and referral interventions. *JAMA Netw Open.* 2020;3(3):e200693. PMID: 32154884

US Department of Health and Human Services. Healthy People 2030. Social Determinants of Health. Available at: https://health.gov/healthypeople/objectives-and-data/social-determinants-health. Accessed December 2021

44

ANSWER: C) Normal saline intravenous bolus: 20 mL/kg

This patient has presented in the hyperglycemic hyperosmolar state associated with new-onset diabetes mellitus. The best way to determine the effective osmolality is with the following formula:

$$[\text{sodium ion (mEq/L)} \times 2 + \text{glucose (mg/dL)} / 18]$$

The patient's effective osmolality is as follows:

$$(148 \times 2) + (852 / 18) = 343.3 \text{ (which is greater than 320 mOsm/kg, indicating the hyperosmolar state)}$$

He also has severe hyperglycemia with inconsistently mild to moderate ketosis for the degree of hyperglycemia. This fits with the diagnostic criteria for the hyperglycemic hyperosmolar state, including a plasma glucose concentration greater than 600 mg/dL (>33.3 mmol/L), effective osmolality greater than 320 mOsm/kg, and the relative absence of ketoacidosis. Patients presenting in the hyperglycemic hyperosmolar state have an increased anion gap metabolic acidosis as the result of concomitant ketoacidosis and/or an increase in serum lactate levels or renal failure.

Several medications that alter carbohydrate metabolism can precipitate the development of diabetic ketoacidosis and the hyperglycemic hyperosmolar state, including glucocorticoids, β-adrenergic blockers, thiazide diuretics, certain chemotherapeutic agents, and atypical antipsychotics.

The goal of initial fluid therapy is to expand the intravascular and extravascular volume and restore normal renal perfusion. The rate of fluid replacement should be more rapid than is recommended for diabetic ketoacidosis.

The initial bolus should be at least 20 mL/kg of isotonic saline (0.9% NaCl) (thus, Answer C is correct and Answer B is incorrect), and a fluid deficit of approximately 12% to 15% of body weight should be assumed. Additional fluid boluses should be given, if necessary, to restore peripheral perfusion. Thereafter, 0.45% to 0.75% NaCl should be administered to replace the deficit over 24 to 48 hours. The goal is to promote a gradual decline in the serum sodium concentration and osmolality.

Early insulin administration (Answers A, D, and E) is unnecessary to treat the hyperglycemic hyperosmolar state. Fluid administration alone causes a marked decline in the serum glucose concentration as a result of dilution, improved renal perfusion leading to glucosuria, and increased tissue glucose uptake with improved circulation. The osmotic pressure that glucose exerts within the vascular space contributes to the maintenance of blood volume. A rapid fall in the serum glucose concentration and osmolality after insulin administration may lead to circulatory compromise and thrombosis unless fluid replacement is adequate. Affected patients also have extreme potassium deficits; a rapid insulin-induced shift of potassium to the intracellular space can trigger an arrhythmia.

In general, deficits of potassium, phosphate, and magnesium are greater in the hyperglycemic hyperosmolar state than in diabetic ketoacidosis. Potassium replacement (40 mmol/L of replacement fluid) should begin as soon as the serum potassium concentration is within the normal range and adequate kidney function has been established. Severe hypophosphatemia may lead to rhabdomyolysis, hemolytic uremia, muscle weakness, and paralysis. Although administration of phosphate is associated with a risk of hypocalcemia, an intravenous solution that contains a 50:50 mixture of potassium phosphate and another suitable potassium salt (potassium chloride or potassium acetate) generally permits adequate phosphate replacement while avoiding clinically significant hypocalcemia.

Educational Objective
Establish the diagnosis of the hyperglycemic hyperosmolar state and differentiate how treatment deviates from the management of diabetes ketoacidosis.

Reference(s)

Kitabchi AE, Umpierrez GE, Miles JM, Fisher JN. Hyperglycemic crises in adult patients with diabetes. *Diabetes Care.* 2009;32(7):1335-1343. PMID: 19564476

Lipscombe LL, Austin PC, Alessi-Severini S, et al. Atypical antipsychotics and hyperglycemic emergencies: multicentre, retrospective cohort study of administrative data. *Schizophr Res.* 2014;154(1-3):54-60. PMID: 24581419

Fayfman M, Pasquel FJ, Umpierrez GE. Management of hyperglycemic crises: diabetic ketoacidosis and hyperglycemic hyperosmolar state. *Med Clin North Am.* 2017;101(3):587-606. PMID: 28372715

Wolfsdorf JI, Glaser N, Agus M, et al. ISPAD clinical practice consensus guidelines 2018. Diabetic ketoacidosis and hyperglycemic hyperosmolar state. *Pediatric Diabetes.* 2018;19(Suppl 27):155-177. PMID: 29900641

45 ANSWER: D) Elevated TSH

This patient has PTH resistance or pseudohypoparathyroidism. Vitamin D deficiency and hypomagnesemia may mimic PTH resistance; thus, it is important to first rule this out. Pseudohypoparathyroidism type 1A and type 1B have similar biochemical profiles; however, they have different phenotypic manifestations. Pseudohypoparathyroidism type 1A manifests with features of Albright hereditary osteodystrophy (short stature, brachydactyly, truncal obesity, ectopic ossification, and intellectual disability) along with resistance to other hormones where receptor activation is mediated through *GNAS* signaling (TSH, GH-releasing hormone, gonadotropins). Individuals with pseudohypoparathyroidism type 1A have maternally inherited loss-of-function pathogenic variants in the *GNAS* gene. In contrast, individuals with pseudohypoparathyroidism type 1B have defects in the differentially methylated regions associated with the *GNAS* complex leading to altered imprinting or methylation of transcripts. Most cases of pseudohypoparathyroidism type 1B are due to de novo pathogenic variants; only 15% to 20% of reported cases are familial (autosomal dominant).

Resistance to PTH is a progressive condition; thus, it is not surprising that this patient had a normal serum calcium level at birth. PTH elevation occurs first, followed by elevation in serum phosphate levels. It may take several years for hypocalcemia to manifest with symptoms, although these symptoms are common during times of rapid skeletal growth.

The lack of clinical features suggestive of Albright hereditary osteodystrophy indicates that the diagnosis is most likely pseudohypoparathyroidism type 1B. Bone age x-ray may reveal brachydactyly, as this occurs in 15% to 33% of individuals with pseudohypoparathyroidism type 1B, but also in 70% to 80% of those with pseudohypoparathyroidism type 1A. However, bone age x-rays are only recommended in patients with linear growth deceleration, which generally does not occur in patients with pseudohypoparathyroidism type 1B. Conversely, advanced bone age (Answer A) is seen in 70% to 80% of patients with pseudohypoparathyroidism type 1A, and 50% to 80% of these individuals develop GH deficiency due to resistance at the level of the GH-releasing hormone receptor. Therefore, elevated GH (Answer C) is not a manifestation and instead, screening with IGF-1 is recommended around age 3 to 6 years for children with pseudohypoparathyroidism type 1A. GH treatment may increase growth velocity in these individuals.

Ectopic ossifications (Answer B) are due to $G_s\alpha$ pathogenic variants in mesenchymal stem cells, which result in extraskeletal formation of osteoblasts forming islands of ectopic bone. Ectopic ossifications are unrelated to the serum calcium-phosphate product and are very uncommon in patients with pseudohypoparathyroidism. Conversely, chronic elevation of the calcium-phosphate product results in intracranial deposition of calcium, predominantly at the basal ganglia. Notably, this patient's evaluation for seizures documented normal findings on electroencephalography, but basal ganglia calcifications were noted on MRI, which prompted evaluation for a metabolic disorder. Other ectopic calcifications can occur, particularly in the eye, which may lead to cataracts. Thus, routine ophthalmology screening is recommended.

Cognitive impairment is rare in patients with pseudohypoparathyroidism type 1B, whereas up to 70% of individuals with pseudohypoparathyroidism type 1A present with lower intelligence quotient scores (Answer E), poorer executive function, delayed adaptive behavior skills, and increased behavior problems.

In pseudohypoparathyroidism type 1B, thyroid hormone resistance, manifesting as TSH at the high end of normal or mildly elevated (Answer D), is present in 30% to 100% of individuals. While there have been reports of other phenotypic features that overlap with pseudohypoparathyroidism type 1A, they are rare and thus an elevated TSH concentration is the most likely finding.

Educational Objective
Explain how the phenotypic manifestation of pseudohypoparathyroidism can guide diagnosis and subsequent screening for additional comorbidities.

Reference(s)
Mantovani G, Bastepe M, Monk D, et al. Diagnosis and management of pseudohypoparathyroidism and related disorders: first international consensus statement. *Nat Rev Endocrinol.* 2018;14(8):476-500. PMID: 29959430

Perez KM, Lee EB, Kahanda S, et al. Cognitive and behavioral phenotype of children with pseudohypoparathyroidism type 1A. *Am J Med Genet A.* 2018;176(2):283-289. PMID: 29193623

46   ANSWER: C) Fecal calprotectin measurement
This patient has growth deceleration, failure to thrive, and a normal BMI. He is grossly asymptomatic and has a normal erythrocyte sedimentation rate; however, he has aphthous stomatitis, inguinal lymphadenopathy, and anemia. The best next step is to evaluate for systemic disease, specifically, systemic inflammatory bowel disease. Of the choices provided, the only test that could be useful to evaluate for this condition is fecal calprotectin measurement (Answer C).

Inflammatory bowel disease usually presents with abdominal pain, diarrhea, bloating, and weight loss. However, the presentation of inflammatory bowel disease is usually different in children and many have nonspecific symptoms such as mild abdominal discomfort and growth impairment. Approximately 25% of cases of Crohn disease presents before age 17 years. However, it has been shown that only 25% of children with Crohn disease present with the usual triad of diarrhea, abdominal pain, and weight loss, which causes delays in diagnosis, usually for more than a year.

About 30% to 40% of patients younger than 18 years who have Crohn disease have impaired linear growth. A decreased growth rate is recorded in approximately 40% of affected patients before any other symptoms are noted (sometimes years before). About one-third of affected patients experience decreased height velocity before any weight loss and often present with a normal BMI. Erythrocyte sedimentation rate may also be normal at presentation, as illustrated by this case.

It is also very important to think about inflammatory bowel disease when evaluating children and adolescents with short stature or growth concerns because Crohn disease and ulcerative colitis have a high risk of complications requiring surgery and an increased risk of colorectal cancer, in addition to affecting growth and development.

With ELISA tests, fecal calprotectin (Answer C) has been validated for distinguishing between inflammatory bowel disease and noninflammatory bowel disease in pediatric populations. The sensitivities range from 95% to 100% at a cutoff of 50 μg/g, and the specificities range from 44% to 93%. Fecal calprotectin measurement is recommended by pediatric gastroenterologists as a cost-effective screening tool. This patient was referred to pediatric gastroenterology for additional evaluation and Crohn disease was diagnosed.

Serum biomarkers are being evaluated to improve the diagnosis of inflammatory bowel disease and to prevent unnecessary colonoscopies. Such biomarkers include anti-*Saccharomyces cerevisiae* antibodies for Crohn disease and antineutrophil cytoplasmic antibodies for ulcerative colitis. However, more research is needed in these areas.

Oral lesions can be the primary presenting sign preceding gastrointestinal symptoms in 5% to 10% of affected patients, and 10% of patients with ulcerative colitis and 20% to 30% of patients with Crohn disease have recurrent aphthous stomatitis. Interestingly, Bijelic et al found higher anti-*Saccharomyces cerevisiae* antibody levels in patients with recurrent aphthous stomatitis than in control participants.

An arginine and insulin-stimulation test (Answer A) to evaluate for GH deficiency is not indicated at this time because it is important to rule out inflammatory bowel disease first.

This patient is 11 years old, has no notable medical history suggestive of hypergonadotropic hypogonadism, is not tall, and does not have dysmorphic features or other conditions to suggest that FSH (Answer D) might be abnormal.

Although IGFBP-3 (Answer E) is a valuable tool in the evaluation of failure to thrive or in the evaluation of younger children with short stature, its measurement would not add additional information in this case because his IGF-1 concentration is normal.

Chromosome microarray analysis (Answer B) is not the best next step in the evaluation of short stature in this patient because his history, physical examination findings, and mild laboratory abnormalities should prompt the clinician to evaluate for inflammatory bowel disease first.

Educational objective
Diagnose Crohn disease as a cause of poor growth and identify clinical and laboratory clues to support this diagnosis.

Reference(s)
Oostdijk W, Grote FK, de Muinck Keizer-Schrama SMPF, Wit JM. Diagnostic approach in children with short stature. *Horm Res*. 2009;72(4):206-217. PMID: 19786792

Cezard JP, Touati G, Alberti C, Hugot JP, Brinon C, Czernichow P. Growth in paediatric Crohn's disease. *Horm Res*. 2002;58(Suppl 1):11-15. PMID: 12373007

Waugh N, Cummins E, Royle P, Kandala N-B, Shyangdan D, Arasaradnam R, Clar C, Johnston R. Faecal calprotectin testing for differentiating amongst inflammatory and non-inflammatory bowel diseases: systematic review and economic evaluation. *Health Technol Assess*. 2013;17(55):xv-xix, 1-211. PMID: 24286461

Bijelić B, Matić IZ, Besu I, et al. Celiac disease-specific and inflammatory bowel disease-related antibodies in patients with recurrent aphthous stomatitis. *Immunobiology*. 2019;224(1):75-79. PMID: 30446336

Zhou G, Song Y, Yang W, et al. ASCA, ANCA, ALCA and many more: are they useful in the diagnosis of inflammatory bowel disease? *Dig Dis*. 2016;34(1-2):90-97. PMID: 26982193

47 ANSWER: A) Contact a biochemist to review his results

In this vignette, the difference in cortisol measurements is due to the change in the cortisol assay used for each assessment. The assay used to assess this patient last year was the Roche Elecsys Cortisol I assay, while the current results were obtained with the Roche Elecsys Cortisol II immunoassay. The difference is the use of a monoclonal antibody rather than a polyclonal antibody in the immunoassay. Hence, the old cortisol cutoff of 18 μg/dL (500 nmol/L) as an indicator of adequate adrenal response no longer applies. Contacting a biochemist is necessary to review his results (Answer A) and determine which assay was used.

Starting hydrocortisone treatment at a dosage of either 12 mg/m² per day (Answer E) or 8 mg/m² per day (Answer D) or starting emergency hydrocortisone (Answer C) would be incorrect.

Contacting a geneticist (Answer B) is not required, as this patient has a genetic diagnosis of triple-A syndrome. Clinical heterogeneity in clinical features exists even within the same family despite the same pathogenic variant in the *AAAS* gene.

A cosyntropin-stimulation test is used to diagnose primary adrenal insufficiency. The 2016 Endocrine Society guidelines for the diagnosis of primary adrenal insufficiency suggest using a peak cortisol response of 18 μg/dL (500 nmol/L), which was previously reported to have a sensitivity of 0.92 (95% CI, 0.81-0.97). In the more recent 2018 CAH guidelines, in patients with nonclassic CAH, a suboptimal cortisol response to cosyntropin is stated to be less than 14 to 18 μg/dL (<386 to 500 nmol/L). A range is given because of corticosteroid-binding globulin variability and because newer assays that have greater specificity run lower. Raverot et al compared the 2 Roche assays and suggested that the difference is approximately 30% lower with the new Roche Elecsys Cortisol II assay compared with the older Roche Elecsys Cortisol I assay. The article recommends that for all suppression tests, the threshold of 1.8 μg/dL (50 nmol/L) may be retained, and for stimulation tests, the new cutoff should be 13.6 μg/dL (375 nmol/L). Other articles have suggested different cutoffs such as 14 to 15 μg/dL (386-414 nmol/L). Grassi et al found lower cortisol cutoff values of 12.7 μg/dL (350 nmol/L) and 13.3 μg/dL (367 nmol/L) using the Roche Elecsys Cortisol II assay and liquid chromatography–tandem mass spectrometry, respectively. Importantly, other assays are used internationally such as the Beckman Access assay. As such, all laboratories are recommended to base their cutoffs used in clinical practice on assay-specific normative data.

In this vignette, the laboratory confirmed that the cortisol results greater than 3.6 μg/dL (>100 nmol/L) were, on average, 25% lower when comparing the 2 Roche assays. Thus, a cortisol cutoff of 18 μg/dL (500 nmol/L) using the Roche Elecsys Cortisol I assay correlates to 13.6 μg/dL (375 nmol/L) with the Roche Elecsys Cortisol II assay. As a result, no treatment was recommended for this child, and he continued to be monitored in clinic.

Educational Objective
Summarize the ways in which cortisol immunoassays have changed in recent years and interpret results based on assay-specific values.

Reference(s)

Raverot V, Richet C, Morel Y, Raverot G, Borson-Chazot F. Establishment of revised diagnostic cut-offs for adrenal laboratory investigation using the new Roche Diagnostics Elecsys® Cortisol II assay. *Ann Endocrinol (Paris)*. 2016;77(5):620-622. PMID: 27449530

Bornstein SR, Allolio B, Arlt W, et al. Diagnosis and treatment of primary adrenal insufficiency: an Endocrine Society clinical practice guideline. *J Clin Endocrinol Metab*. 2016;101(2):364-389. PMID: 26760044

Speiser PW, Arlt W, Auchus RJ, et al. Congenital adrenal hyperplasia due to steroid 21-hydroxylase deficiency: an Endocrine Society clinical practice guideline. *J Clin Endocrinol Metab*. 2018;103(11):4043-4088. PMID: 30272171

Javorsky BR, Raff H, Carroll TB, et al. New cutoffs for the biochemical diagnosis of adrenal insufficiency after ACTH stimulation using specific cortisol assays. *J Endocr Soc*. 2021;5(4):bvab022. PMID: 33768189

Grassi G, Morelli V, Ceriotti F, et al. Minding the gap between cortisol levels measured with second-generation assays and current diagnostic thresholds for the diagnosis of adrenal insufficiency: a single-center experience. *Hormones (Athens)*. 2020;19(3):425-431. PMID: 32222957

Milenkovic T, Zdravkovic D, Savic N, et al. Triple A syndrome: 32 years experience of a single centre (1977-2008). *Eur J Pediatr*. 2010;169(11):1323-1328. PMID: 20499090

48   ANSWER: C) Germ-cell tumor

This boy presents with signs and symptoms of diabetes insipidus and has a mass involving the sella and suprasellar regions. Masses arising in these areas account for approximately 10% of all pediatric brain tumors. The proximity of these masses to critical brain structures, including the optic nerves and chiasm, the third ventricle, and the pituitary gland and infundibulum, can result in a variety of presenting features such as changes in visual acuity, loss of visual fields, hydrocephalus, and endocrine dysfunction.

Germ-cell tumors (Answer C), which include germinomas, nongerminomatous germ-cell tumors, and teratomas, account for approximately 3% of childhood brain tumors and are most commonly found in patients aged 10 to 20 years. Germ-cell tumors usually involve the suprasellar and pineal regions (pineal regions more common). Approximately 5% to 13% of affected patients have involvement of both regions at presentation. Germ-cell tumors that involve the suprasellar region commonly present with central diabetes insipidus, visual field defects, and other hypothalamic pituitary dysfunction. In males with tumors that produce β-hCG, pseudoprecocious puberty may be present due to β-hCG stimulation of Leydig cells, causing testosterone secretion. While no information regarding sex hormone levels is provided in this vignette, this boy does have development of secondary sexual characteristics, although not precocious in timing. Based on his age, presenting features, and MRI findings, a germ-cell tumor is the most likely diagnosis.

Craniopharyngiomas (Answer A) are the most commonly diagnosed tumors of the sellar/suprasellar region in children. Although histologically benign, they can cause a great deal of damage due to their proximity to critical brain structures. The peak incidence in childhood is between 5 and 14 years of age, and craniopharyngiomas are equally common in males and females. The most common presenting features are headache due to increased intracranial pressure, visual impairment, linear growth arrest, obesity, and endocrine dysfunction (eg, central diabetes insipidus, although deficiencies are more commonly seen postoperatively). Craniopharyngiomas typically contain both cystic and calcified components. Most are both suprasellar and intrasellar and involve the hypothalamus. Although craniopharyngioma should be considered in this patient, he does not have evidence of a cystic lesion or calcifications on MRI, making this diagnosis unlikely.

Chiasmatic gliomas (Answer B) are a subset of optic pathway gliomas that account for 2% to 5% of childhood brain tumors. They are typically found in patients aged 4 to 5 years and usually present with visual impairment, strabismus, and optic atrophy. Endocrine dysfunction can occur, typically central precocious puberty and GH deficiency. Very young children may present with failure to thrive and diencephalic syndrome. Diabetes insipidus is an uncommon presenting feature. This patient has diabetes insipidus and is older than one would expect at presentation.

Rathke cleft cysts (Answer E) arise from the ectopic remnants of the Rathke pouch (as do craniopharyngiomas). Although the incidence is unknown, they are quite rare. Cysts can be intrasellar, suprasellar, or both. A differentiating feature is that unlike craniopharyngiomas, Rathke cleft cysts are exclusively cystic. These cysts can be asymptomatic and found incidentally. They are more common in females. When symptomatic, they present with headache and visual impairment, and the most common presenting endocrinopathies are diabetes insipidus, central precocious puberty, or growth delay. This boy's lesion is not cystic, making a Rathke cleft cyst an unlikely diagnosis.

Langerhans-cell histiocytosis (Answer D) is due to proliferation of Langerhans cells and generally involves many organs throughout the body (eg, bone, skin). When the central nervous system is involved, there is infiltration of the pituitary. MRI generally shows thickening of the pituitary stalk. Clinically, endocrine dysfunction is common and includes central diabetes insipidus and anterior pituitary dysfunction, most commonly GH deficiency. Langerhans-cell histiocytosis is a rare neoplasm with an overall incidence of 4 and 9 cases per million, with males slightly more affected than females, most often presenting in the first 4 years of life. While Langerhans-cell histiocytosis should be included in this patient's differential diagnosis, his older age makes this much less likely.

Educational Objective
Construct the differential diagnosis for midline tumors in the hypothalamic/pituitary area.

Reference(s)
McCrea HJ, George E, Settler A, Schwartz TH, Greenfield JP. Pediatric suprasellar tumors. *J Child Neurol.* 2016;31(12):1367-1376. PMID: 26676303

Argyropoulou MI, Kiortsis DN. MRI of the hypothalamic-pituitary axis in children. *Pediatric Radiol.* 2005;35(11):1045-1055. PMID: 15928924

49 ANSWER: C) Metformin
The patient in this vignette has oligomenorrhea and biochemical hyperandrogenemia, which are the key criteria for diagnosis of polycystic ovary syndrome. Polycystic ovarian morphology is common for up to 5 years after menarche and is often a normal finding. Thus, ultrasonography (Answer E) would not be helpful for diagnosing polycystic ovary syndrome at this age.

She has impaired glucose tolerance as indicated by acanthosis nigricans and a hemoglobin A_{1c} level of 6.3% (45 mmol/mol). Endocrine Society guidelines recommend a hormonal contraceptive as first-line treatment in adolescents with polycystic ovary syndrome if the primary goal of therapy is to treat acne, hirsutism, or anovulatory symptoms. Metformin (Answer C) is recommended for adolescents with polycystic ovary syndrome and evidence of impaired glucose tolerance or metabolic syndrome. Treatment with a hormonal contraceptive (Answers A and B) can be helpful in terms of managing irregular menses. However, in this case, the history of complex migraines is a contraindication to hormonal contraceptive use.

This patient has multiple risk factors for developing metabolic syndrome and progressing to type 2 diabetes. The relationship between ethnic background and metabolic risk in women with polycystic ovary syndrome is complex. In 1 study of 702 women with polycystic ovary syndrome, Hispanic women had a greater degree of insulin resistance than nonHispanic White women, as well as a higher prevalence of metabolic syndrome compared with the prevalence in nonHispanic Black women. Other studies have shown an increased risk of type 2 diabetes in all women with polycystic ovary syndrome.

Given her ethnic background, family history, obesity, and insulin resistance, treatment with metformin would provide the most benefit to the patient in this case. She does not have significant hirsutism, so she does not need to start spironolactone (Answer D). Furthermore, a hormonal contraceptive should be used concurrently with spironolactone because of the risk of birth defects with this medication.

Educational Objective
Identify differences in metabolic risk associated with polycystic ovary syndrome across ethnicities.

Reference(s)
Engmann L, Jin S, Sun F, et al; Reproductive Medicine Network. Racial and ethnic differences in the polycystic ovary syndrome metabolic phenotype. *Am J Obstet Gynecol.* 2017;216(5):493.e1-493.e13. PMID: 28104402

Witchel SF, Burghard AC, Tao RH, Oberfield SE. The diagnosis and treatment of PCOS in adolescents: an update. *Curr Opin Pediatr.* 2019;31(4):562-569. PMID: 31299022

50 ANSWER: E) Restart insulin therapy

New-onset diabetes after transplant (NODAT) is a serious metabolic complication of kidney transplant. The incidence is 3% to 20% in children and adolescents who receive kidney transplants, and it is associated with increased mortality and morbidity from cardiovascular and infectious complications.

Patients with autosomal dominant polycystic kidney disease have an increased risk of developing NODAT. The pathogenesis is most likely due to increased insulin resistance that is directly associated with pathogenic variants underlying autosomal dominant polycystic kidney disease. Other etiologies with increased NODAT risk include cystinosis (secondary to impaired insulin secretion), hemolytic uremic syndrome (β-cell damage from an enterotoxin-mediated microangiopathic process), Bardet-Biedl and Alström syndromes (abnormalities in glucose metabolism), and bilateral cystic kidney diseases caused by pathogenic variants in the hepatocyte nuclear factor gene (*HNF1B*) (maturity-onset diabetes of the young type 5).

Developing hypomagnesemia during the posttransplant period correlates with glucose impairment, thought to be caused by the need for magnesium to preserve insulin secretion, cellular transport of glucose, and insulin–insulin receptor interactions. Close monitoring of blood glucose in the immediate posttransplant phase is necessary to detect early abnormalities in glucose metabolism that can be associated with surgical stress and the use of high-dosage glucocorticoids. Insulin therapy is required if hyperglycemia persists beyond the first week after transplant. If NODAT is confirmed, treatment should be based on the American Diabetes Association guidelines to maintain a fasting plasma glucose concentration of 90 to 130 mg/dL (5.0-7.2 mmol/L), a 2-hour plasma glucose concentration less than 200 mg/dL (<11.1 mmol/L), and a hemoglobin A_{1c} level less than 7.0% (<53 mmol/mol). It is important to consider that the hemoglobin A_{1c} concentration can be falsely reduced secondary to anemia and that red blood cell turnover can be increased with the use of erythropoietin.

The pathogenesis of NODAT is complex and multifactorial. The diabetogenic effect of glucocorticoids and calcineurin inhibitors (cyclosporine, tacrolimus, and pimecrolimus) is dosage- and duration-dependent and can be reversed with decreasing or discontinuing exposure. Immunosuppressants in patients with NODAT can be tailored on an individual basis and should balance the increased risk of rejection against long-term hyperglycemia and its complications.

Glucose concentrations should be routinely monitored in all pediatric patients who receive kidney transplant irrespective of the presence of hyperglycemia at hospital discharge. The 2003 International NODAT guidelines recommend fasting blood glucose screening for transplant recipients weekly for 1 month, then every 3 months for the first year, and annually thereafter. The overall management for NODAT is multifactorial and should involve lifestyle modifications with diet, exercise, and weight control, options for an alternative immunosuppressive regimen, and pharmacologic therapy to treat hyperglycemia. It is important to counsel patients regarding individualized nutrition therapy that encourages moderate carbohydrate intake to lower the glycemic burden, as well as moderation of fat consumption. Reduction in excess weight is recommended for all patients who are overweight or have obesity. In children, supervised exercise improves fasting insulin levels as early as 2 weeks before documented weight loss.

Pharmacologic intervention is necessary when lifestyle modifications fail to achieve adequate glycemic control. Hyperglycemia may develop acutely during the immediate posttransplant period and may require rapid intervention with insulin therapy. Given the concerns of safety and efficacy of using oral antihyperglycemic agents in pediatric patients with NODAT, as well as the theoretical potential of some of these agents to interact with immunosuppressants, insulin remains the gold standard therapy. Restarting insulin (Answer D) represents the most appropriate choice for this kidney transplant recipient.

This patient's average glucose readings depict significant hyperglycemia that is inconsistent with the measured hemoglobin A_{1c} for the reasons discussed above. Although lifestyle changes would most likely help improve glycemic control and are highly recommended, they would not be sufficient.

The evidence supporting the use of GLP-1 receptor agonist therapy (Answer A) remains very limited, yet promising. A major concern regarding GLP-1 receptor therapy in patients with NODAT is delayed gastric emptying, which could potentially affect absorption of co-administered medications with a narrow therapeutic index. Although GLP-1 receptor agonists are not metabolized by the liver or involved in cytochrome or transporter-mediated drug-drug interactions, there may be a delay in drug concentration.

Metformin (Answer B) and sulfonylurea therapy (Answer C) are not medically appropriate options in kidney transplant recipients as discussed above.

Offering no medical intervention (only monitoring) (Answer D) is not acceptable at this stage in a patient with severe hyperglycemia.

Educational Objective
Diagnose and manage new-onset diabetes after transplant.

Reference(s)

Garro R, Warshaw, B, Felner E. New-onset diabetes after kidney transplant in children. *Pediatr Nephrol*. 2015;30(3):405-416. PMID: 24894384

Cosio FG, Pesavento TE, Osei K, Henry ML, Ferguson RM. Post-transplant diabetes mellitus: increasing incidence in renal allograft recipients transplanted in recent years. *Kidney Int*. 2001;59(2):732-737. PMID: 11168956

Pham PTT, Pham PMT, Pham SV, Pham PAT, Pham PCT. New onset diabetes after transplantation (NODAT): an overview. *Diabetes Metab Syndr Obes*. 2011;4:175-186. PMID: 21760734

Al-Uzri A, Stablein DM, Cohn AR. Posttransplant diabetes mellitus in pediatric renal transplant recipients: a report of the North American Pediatric Renal Transplant Cooperative Study (NAPRTCS). *Transplantation*. 2001;72(6):1020-1024. PMID: 11579294

Greenspan LC, Gitelman SE, Leung MA, Glidden DV, Mathias RS. Increased incidence in post-transplant diabetes mellitus in children: a case–control analysis. *Pediatr Nephrol*. 2002;17(1):1-5. PMID: 11793126

Montada-Atin T, Prasad GVR. Recent advances in new-onset diabetes after kidney transplantation. *World J Diabetes*. 2021;12(5):541-555. PMID: 33995843

Davidson J, Wilkinson A, Dantal J, et al. International Expert Panel. New-onset diabetes after transplantation: 2003 International Consensus Guidelines. Proceedings of an international expert panel meeting. Barcelona, Spain, 19 February 2003. *Transplantation*. 2003;75(Suppl 10):SS3-SS24. PMID: 12775942

51 ANSWER: E) Reassure the family that no intervention is needed

The images show the characteristic appearance of ectopic thymic tissue both within the thyroid gland and in the neck inferior to the thyroid. This is a normal finding, and the family can thus be reassured that no intervention is needed (Answer E). On ultrasonography, thymic tissue has background homogenous decreased echogenicity and classic internal hyperechoic foci, giving a "speckled, starry sky" appearance.

The thymus has greatest activity in childhood. It typically grows in infancy and early childhood, reaches its peak size during puberty, and then slowly involutes and is replaced by fat tissue. Embryologically, the thymus develops primarily from the third pharyngeal pouch and then migrates caudally and medially to the mediastinum. Ectopic thymic tissue can be found anywhere along the pathway of descent including within the thyroid gland, as in this case. While the presence of intrathyroidal thymus is unusual, extension of thymic tissue into the neck above the manubrium is common and can be seen in up to two-thirds of children.

Ectopic intrathyroidal thymus can easily be confused with malignant thyroid nodules with the hyperechoic areas attributed to microcalcifications. However, some ultrasonographic features are helpful in distinguishing the 2 entities:

- Microcalcifications in malignant nodules often result in acoustic shadowing that is not present in thymic tissue
- Doppler imaging often shows increased vascularity in malignant nodules in contrast to normal or decreased vascularity in thymic tissue compared with the surrounding thyroid tissue
- Margins of malignant nodules may be ill-defined in contrast to the well-defined margins of ectopic thymic tissue
- If ectopic thymic tissue is present in the thyroid gland, it may also be connected inferiorly to thymic tissue in the neck. If a lesion is seen within the thyroid gland, it is useful to look for similar-appearing tissue inferiorly in the neck extending into the mediastinum. If present, the intrathyroidal tissue can more confidently be identified as thymic tissue (as in this case)

CT of the neck and chest (Answer C) is performed in children when evaluating for certain malignancies, but it is not a good imaging modality for the thyroid gland or masses within the thyroid gland.

If there were concerns that this intrathyroidal mass looked like a suspicious nodule, ultrasound-guided FNA biopsy (Answer D) would be the appropriate next step. This unfortunately occurs regularly when characteristic thymic tissue is not recognized. Biopsy, if performed, would most likely show numerous lymphocytes.

The serum calcitonin concentration (Answer B) is elevated in the setting of medullary thyroid cancer. In the absence of a family history of medullary thyroid cancer, measuring calcitonin is not the first step in the evaluation of thyroid nodules in children, even if the nodule looks suspicious.

Calcium, phosphate, and PTH (Answer A) are measured in children with symptoms of hypocalcemia or hypercalcemia and in individuals with a known familial risk for parathyroid disease. This patient has neither family history nor clinical features of parathyroid disease. The parathyroid gland on ultrasonography is often not easily visualized, but when overactive and enlarged it can be identified as an oval anechoic or hypoechoic mass.

Educational Objective
Identify ultrasound features of normal thymic tissue.

Reference(s)
Costa NS, Laor T, Donnelly LF. Superior cervical extension of the thymus: a normal finding that should not be mistaken for a mass. *Radiology.* 2010;256(1):238-242. PMID: 20505060

Wee T, Lee AF, Nadel H, Bray H. The paediatric thymus: recognizing normal and ectopic thymic tissue. *Clin Radiol.* 2021;76(7):477-487. PMID: 33762135

52   ANSWER: D) *MEN1*

The family history of autosomal dominant transmission of hyperparathyroidism along with tumors involving other endocrine organs (pituitary and pancreas) are the hallmark features of multiple endocrine neoplasia type 1 (MEN type 1). Parathyroid tumors occur in 95% of affected patients, frequently in the second decade of life. The *MEN1* gene (Answer D) encodes the menin protein, a nuclear protein involved in transcription regulation, cell division, and proliferation. Genetic testing should be offered to first-degree relatives of patients with confirmed *MEN1* pathogenic variants to allow for early screening of affected individuals. Recommendations for tumor surveillance include annual measurement of serum calcium, PTH, neuroendocrine tumor markers (gastrin, glucagon, pancreatic polypeptide, and chromogranin A), and pituitary tumor markers (prolactin and IGF-1). Screening should start between 5 and 10 years of age. In addition, imaging of the pituitary gland and abdomen is recommended to begin by age 10 years.

Pathogenic variants in the *RET* proto-oncogene (Answer E) lead to MEN type 2A and 2B. Parathyroid adenomas occur in 20% of individuals with *RET* pathogenic variants (usually in those with MEN type 2A). However, a more classic feature is medullary thyroid carcinoma. The patient in this vignette did have a relative with medullary thyroid cancer; however, this uncle is on her father's side, whereas the hyperparathyroidism condition is maternally inherited.

Loss-of-function pathogenic variants in the calcium-sensing receptor gene (*CASR*) (Answer A) can lead to familial hypercalcemia hypocalciuria type 1, which is more likely to present as parathyroid hyperplasia. While the name of this disorder implies that the urinary calcium-to-creatinine ratio should be low, approximately 20%

of individuals with this condition have ratios greater than 0.01. Twenty percent of individuals with familial hypercalcemia hypocalciuria type 1 also have elevated PTH concentrations, making it challenging to distinguish between this condition and primary hyperparathyroidism due to an adenoma. Historically, young patients with hypercalcemia due to familial hypercalcemia hypocalciuria type 1 have sometimes been inappropriately treated with subtotal parathyroidectomy, which does not cure hypercalcemia. Rarely, germline variants in the *CASR* gene lead to sporadic parathyroid adenomas. While the autosomal dominant transmission of hyperparathyroidism in this family may raise suspicion for a *CASR* pathogenic variant, the presence of other tumors (pituitary and pancreatic) makes MEN type 1 more likely.

Pathogenic variants in *CDC73* (Answer B) are found in the tissue of 65% to 100% of sporadic parathyroid carcinomas but in less than 4% of sporadic parathyroid adenomas. Twenty percent of individuals with sporadic parathyroid carcinomas have germline pathogenic variants in *CDC73*. Hyperparathyroidism–jaw tumor syndrome is due to pathogenic variants in the *CDC73* gene, which encodes the nuclear protein parafibromin, a tumor suppressor. Other features of this condition include fibro-osseous jaw tumors, uterine tumors, and kidney tumors. As this patient's family history is strongly suggestive of a familial predisposition and she had a parathyroid adenoma, not a carcinoma, a pathogenic variant in *CDC73* is unlikely.

Loss-of-function pathogenic variants in *CDKN1B* (Answer C) result in MEN type 4, a condition characterized by tumors in the parathyroids, pituitary, adrenal glands, kidneys, and gonads. The phenotype overlaps with that of MEN type 1. However, MEN type 4 accounts for only 3% of cases, making it less likely to explain the familial tumor syndrome in this vignette.

Educational Objective
Differentiate among the genetic causes of parathyroid tumors and prioritize testing based on family history.

Reference(s)
Shariq OA, Lines KE, English KA, et al. Multiple endocrine neoplasia type 1 in children and adolescents: clinical features and treatment outcomes. *Surgery*. 2022;171(1):77-87. PMID: 34183184

Thakker RV. Genetics of parathyroid tumours. *J Intern Med*. 2016;280(6):574-583. PMID: 27306766

53 **ANSWER: C)** *MCM4* **(minichromosome maintenance complex component 4)**
This child's adrenal insufficiency is most likely caused by pathogenic variants in the *MCM4* gene (minichromosome maintenance complex component 4) (Answer C). He has isolated glucocorticoid deficiency, has presented relatively late, has short stature, and was born to an Irish Traveller family with consanguineous parents. Pathogenic variants in *MCM4*, specifically a homozygous variant (c.71-1insG resulting in a severely truncated MCM4 protein [p.Pro24ArgfsX4]), cause adrenal insufficiency, short stature, and natural killer cell deficiency in the Irish Traveller community, a genetically isolated population in which consanguinity is common. The Irish Traveller community is an endogamous, nomadic, ethnic minority population that mainly lives on the island of Ireland with smaller populations in Europe and the United States. MCM4 (as a complex) is a replicative helicase essential for normal DNA replication and genomic stability in all eukaryotes. The original article by Hughes et al in 2012 describes 8 patients from 3 kindreds. Apart from those identified through screening, affected individuals usually present between ages 2.5 and 12 years. They typically have normal adrenal function, at least initially, followed by development of isolated glucocorticoid deficiency and elevated plasma ACTH but no mineralocorticoid involvement. Affected children are managed with hydrocortisone replacement alone. Short stature is common in this condition, and some children are born small-for-gestational-age. Some affected children have increased chromosomal breakage on screening but no other features of Fanconi anemia, and complete blood cell count is typically normal. In the Hughes et al article, 7 of 8 children had low levels of natural killer cells, and 1 child demonstrated increased susceptibility to recurrent pneumonitis.

In contrast, biallelic loss-of-function pathogenic variants in the *SGPL1* gene (Answer E) lead to adrenal insufficiency (with or without mineralocorticoid deficiency) associated with steroid-resistant nephrotic syndrome. Additional features include ichthyosis, neurologic involvement, lymphopenia, primary hypothyroidism, and gonadal dysfunction.

Heterozygous gain-of-function pathogenic variants in the *SAMD9* gene (Answer D) cause MIRAGE syndrome (myelodysplasia, infection, restriction of growth, adrenal hypoplasia, genital phenotypes, and enteropathy).

Biallelic loss-of-function pathogenic variants in the *AIRE* gene (Answer A) give rise to autoimmune polyendocrine syndrome type 1, which is characterized by the triad of chronic mucocutaneous candidiasis, hypoparathyroidism, and adrenal insufficiency. The condition often presents later in life and is not associated with intrauterine growth restriction or short stature. However, several cases have been associated with GH deficiency.

Gain-of-function pathogenic variants in the gene encoding the paternally imprinted cell-cycle regulator CDKN1C (Answer B) give rise to IMAGe syndrome (intrauterine growth restriction, metaphyseal dysplasia [and short limbs], adrenal hypoplasia congenita, and genitourinary anomalies). Similarities to the phenotype associated with *MCM4*, pathogenic variants in *CDKN1C* cause intrauterine growth restriction and short stature. However, adrenal hypoplasia presents within the first weeks to months with evidence of both glucocorticoid and mineralocorticoid deficiency, although later onset has been described. Affected males can have genital anomalies, including cryptorchidism, hypospadias, micropenis, and chordee, which are absent in this child.

Educational Objective
Diagnose primary adrenal insufficiency due to pathogenic variants in the *MCM4* gene.

Reference(s)
Hughes CR, Guasti L, Meimaridou E, et al. MCM4 mutation causes adrenal failure, short stature, and natural killer cell deficiency in humans. *J Clin Invest.* 2012;122(3):814-820. PMID: 22354170

Buonocore F, McGlacken-Byrne SM, Del Valle I, Achermann JC. Current insights into adrenal insufficiency in the newborn and young infant. *Front Pediatr.* 2020;8:619041. PMID: 33381483

Lynch SA, Crushell E, Lambert DM, et al. Catalogue of inherited disorders found among the Irish Traveller population. *J Med Genet.* 2018;55(4):233-239. PMID: 29358271

54 ANSWER: B) Activation of natriuretic peptide receptor 2

The child in the vignette has achondroplasia, which is an autosomal dominant disorder associated with gain-of-function pathogenic variants in the *FGFR3* gene. FGFR3 is a cell surface receptor with an extracellular domain, a transmembrane domain, and a tyrosine kinase intracellular domain. The ligands for the extracellular domain of FGFR3 include several fibroblast growth factors (2, 9, 18, and 23). Binding of the fibroblast growth factor to FGFR3 leads to dimerization of the receptor, transphosphorylation, and activation of the RAS-MAPK pathway, which, at the level of the chondrocyte, suppresses chondrocyte function by shortening the proliferative phase and speeding up final differentiation. In a separate pathway, activation of NPR2 (natriuretic peptide receptor type 2) by its endogenous ligand C-type natriuretic peptide leads to repression of the RAS-MAPK pathway, avoiding excess inhibition of chondrocyte differentiation and maintaining a balance in endochondral bone formation. In achondroplasia, activating variants in the *FGFR3* gene lead to the endogenous C-type natriuretic peptide being insufficient to counteract the accelerated RAS-MAPK pathway, resulting in excessive inhibition of chondrocyte function, poor endochondral bone formation, and severe, disproportionate short stature with greater compromise of the extremities.

Endogenous C-type natriuretic peptide has a very short half-life of 2.6 minutes. Vosoritide is a C-type natriuretic peptide analogue with a slightly longer half-life (27.9 minutes). It activates natriuretic peptide receptor type 2 (Answer B), exerting a negative effect on the overactive RAS-MAPK pathway, which in turn negatively affects chondrocyte proliferation. This "double-negative" effect translates into a positive net action on chondrocyte proliferation that potentiates endochondral bone growth and improves linear growth and, potentially, body proportions in individuals with achondroplasia.

FGFR3 pathogenic variants leading to achondroplasia produce constitutive activation of this receptor; therefore, a potential agent leading to its activation (Answer A) would not be desirable.

Although FGF-23 is a potential ligand for FGFR3, the main role of this ligand is to act as a phosphatonin, leading to increased renal excretion of phosphate. Monoclonal antibodies against FGF-23 (Answer D), such as burosumab, are new agents for the management of FGF-23 dependent–hypophosphatemic disorders such as X-linked hypophosphatemia or tumor-induced osteomalacia, but they would not have a significant effect on promoting chondrogenesis.

Although GH therapy has been used to manage the short stature associated with achondroplasia, it was shown to induce only a modest increase in growth velocity in the first year of treatment. Better results have been seen in the management of short stature in patients with hypochondroplasia when used during puberty. GH therapy, therefore, has never become standard of care and has not received approval by regulatory agencies for the management of short stature in achondroplasia. Suppression of somatostatin (Answer E), which would lead to increased endogenous GH secretion, and the administration of exogenous GH would enhance IGF-1 production (Answer C) and would not be the preferred choices.

Educational objective
Explain the mechanism of action of the novel C-type natriuretic peptide analogue, vosoritide, in the management of short stature associated with achondroplasia.

Reference(s)

Pauli RM. Achondroplasia: a comprehensive clinical review. *Orphanet J Rare Dis.* 2019;14(1):1-49. PMID: 30606190

Ornitz DM, Marie PJ. Fibroblast growth factor signaling in skeletal development and disease. *Genes Dev.* 2015;29(14):1463-1486. PMID: 26220993

Savarirayan R, Tofts L, Irving M, et al. Once-daily, subcutaneous vosoritide therapy in children with achondroplasia: a randomised, double-blind, phase 3, placebo-controlled, multicentre trial. *Lancet.* 2020;5:684-692. PMID: 32891212

Kochar IS, Rashim C. Use of growth hormone treatment in skeletal dysplasia – a review. *Pediatr Endocrinol Rev.* 2020;17(4):327-330. PMID: 32780956

55 ANSWER: E) Seek urgent surgical consultation

This patient has mesenteric ischemia, which is a rare complication of diabetic ketoacidosis. Given the high morbidity of acute mesenteric ischemia, rapid detection and surgical management are required; therefore, urgent surgical consultation (Answer E) is the best choice in this case. Both thrombotic and nonocclusive causes of acute mesenteric ischemia have been reported in diabetic ketoacidosis with worsening abdominal pain despite appropriate fluid resuscitation and improvement of ketoacidosis.

Acute mesenteric ischemia consists of the rapid, partial or complete, interruption of blood flow in the irrigation area of the superior or inferior mesenteric artery, which may result in intestinal infarction or hemorrhagic necrosis of the intestines. Intestinal ischemia is a rare condition in pediatric patients. It can be caused by a vascular occlusion due to a thromboembolic event or it can be nonocclusive due to mesenteric ischemia, induced by intestinal vasospasm. If untreated, acute mesenteric ischemia causes mesenteric infarction, intestinal necrosis, and an overwhelming inflammatory response that can be fatal. Early intervention can reverse this process, leading to full recovery, but diagnosing acute mesenteric ischemia is difficult. The failure to recognize acute mesenteric ischemia before intestinal necrosis has developed is responsible for high disease mortality.

When acute mesenteric ischemia is suspected, the patient should be on nothing-by-mouth status and receiving intravenous fluid therapy.

Placing the patient on a liquid diet (Answer A), ordering intravenous proton-pump inhibitor therapy (Answer B), or restarting an insulin drip (Answer D) would not be appropriate.

Abdominal MRI (Answer C) can be used as an imaging modality, but it would most likely delay the most needed clinical assessment or exploratory laparotomy approach by the surgical team. Contrast-enhanced magnetic resonance angiography can clearly map occlusive disease and collateral pathways in a manner similar to that of CT angiography. Newer imaging techniques have been developed and are in the testing stage for clinical use, such as 4-dimensional MRI flow sequences, which enable hemodynamic measurement. In neonates, the preferred imaging modality for diagnosing acute mesenteric ischemia is CT or ultrasonography, yet establishing the diagnosis based on imaging alone is difficult.

Although surgical therapy remains the treatment of choice for most cases of acute mesenteric ischemia, endovascular treatment (percutaneous transluminal angioplasty and stent placement) has emerged as a promising alternative in adult patients.

Educational Objective
Diagnose acute mesenteric ischemia as a rare complication of diabetic ketoacidosis.

Reference(s)

Zhao Y, Henghui Y, Yao C, et al. Management of acute mesenteric ischemia: a critical review and treatment algorithm. *Vasc Endovascular Surg.* 2016;50(3):183-192. PMID: 27036673

Une K, Sumi Y, Kurayoshi M, Nakanuno R, Nakahara M. Nonocclusive mesenteric ischemia during treatment for ketoacidosis associated with acute onset type 1 diabetes mellitus: a case report. *Clin Case Rep.* 2022;10(4):e05714. PMID: 35474982

56 ANSWER: B) Impaired posttranslational processing of the preprovasopressin precursor peptide

Central diabetes insipidus is caused by deficiency of vasopressin (also called antidiuretic hormone), a nonapeptide hormone produced by the hypothalamic paraventricular and supraoptic nuclei and secreted by the posterior pituitary in response to signals reflecting systemic volume depletion, including elevated serum osmolality and low intravascular volume. Vasopressin is one breakdown product of a 164–amino acid precursor peptide called preprovasopressin that also includes a signal peptide and 2 other peptides: the neurophysin II carrier protein and copeptin. Clinically, vasopressin deficiency leads to polyuria and polydipsia and can produce dehydration and hypernatremia if oral intake is impaired, as in this case where the patient developed an intercurrent vomiting illness. Central diabetes insipidus is treated with careful fluid replacement and vasopressin or synthetic analogues such as desmopressin.

Central diabetes insipidus can be congenital (caused by genetic variants or anatomical defects in hypothalamic/pituitary formation) or acquired (caused by neoplasm, infiltrative process, trauma, medication, and/or altered vasopressin clearance).

With respect to familial forms of diabetes insipidus, most demonstrate an autosomal dominant inheritance pattern, as in this vignette. When molecular testing yields an etiology, pathogenic variants in 1 allele of the *AVP* gene are identified, typically in either the sequence encoding the signal peptide or the neurophysin-II carrier protein. One case series is illustrative and included 5 kindreds with familial central diabetes insipidus with an autosomal dominant inheritance pattern. All families were found to have pathogenic variants in the *AVP* gene (2 families had a variant in the signal peptide coding region, and 3 families had a variant in the neurophysin II coding region). Follow-up in vitro studies demonstrated that these variants produced intracellular retention of the vasopressin prohormone. Over time, incomplete processing of the prohormone (Answer B) and subsequent intracellular retention leads to cellular toxicity, which most likely explains the progressive nature of the condition, as well as the autosomal dominant pattern of inheritance. Although age of onset and severity may vary in autosomal dominant familial diabetes insipidus, many individuals come to attention in the first decade of life and typically respond well to treatment with desmopressin, as in this vignette. Autosomal recessive forms of familial diabetes insipidus have also rarely been reported. For example, in one consanguineous kindred, affected individuals were homozygous for a pathogenic variant in an exon of the *AVP* gene encoding vasopressin itself, leading to deficiency of active vasopressin. Early-onset diabetes insipidus is sometimes a feature of Wolfram syndrome, which is caused by pathogenic variants in the *WFS1* gene. Inadequate transcription of the *AVP* gene encoding vasopressin (Answer C) or inadequate translation of vasopressin from *AVP* mRNA (Answer D), which might be expected to result from haploinsufficiency of vasopressin in the setting of autosomal recessive inheritance patterns, are inconsistent with the autosomal dominant inheritance pattern in this vignette.

Familial forms of nephrogenic diabetes insipidus demonstrate an X-linked pattern of inheritance when caused by pathogenic variants in the arginine vasopressin receptor type 2 gene (*AVPR2*). Affected boys often present in infancy. Because nephrogenic diabetes insipidus is caused by lack of responsiveness of the distal nephron to vasopressin, vasopressin or vasopressin analogues are not helpful; instead, treatment often includes thiazide diuretics. Thus, impaired action of vasopressin at its distal nephron receptor encoded by the *AVPR2* gene (Answer A) is incorrect.

Finally, pregnancy is the condition most often associated with increased vasopressin clearance (Answer E) via enhanced vasopressinase activity. In this vignette, the mother's DDAVP requirement increased during pregnancy, most likely because of enhanced placental vasopressinase activity. Some pregnant individuals develop gestational diabetes insipidus if vasopressinase activity is excessive and pituitary vasopressin production is insufficient to compensate, particularly if there are other risk factors (eg, liver disease and decreased vasopressinase degradation by the liver). However, vasopressin clearance is not the primary pathogenic mechanism of this family's condition.

Educational Objective
Describe the molecular pathogenic mechanisms underlying familial forms of central diabetes insipidus.

Reference(s)

Schernthaner-Reiter MH, Stratakis CA, Luger A. Genetics of diabetes insipidus. *Endocrinol Metab Clin North Am.* 2017;46(2):305-334. PMID: 28476225

Alvelos MI, Francisco A, Gomes L, et al. Familial neurohypophyseal diabetes insipidus: clinical, genetic and functional studies of novel mutations in the arginine vasopressin gene. *Pituitary.* 2021;24(3):400-411. PMID: 33433888

Willcutts MD, Felner E, White PC. Autosomal recessive familial neurohypophyseal diabetes insipidus with continued secretion of mutant weakly active vasopressin. *Hum Mol Genet.* 1999;8(7):1303-1307. PMID: 10369876

Perrotta S, Di Iorgi N, Ragione FD, et al. Early-onset central diabetes insipidus is associated with de novo arginine vasopressin-neurophysin II or Wolfram syndrome 1 gene mutations. *Eur J Endocrinol.* 2015;172(4):461-472. PMID: 25740874

Bockenhauer D, Bichet DG. Pathophysiology, diagnosis and management of nephrogenic diabetes insipidus. *Nat Rev Nephrol.* 2015;11(10):576-588. PMID: 26077742

57   ANSWER: A) Fanconi syndrome

This patient has Fanconi syndrome (Answer A). His history and laboratory test results are suggestive of global proximal tubular dysfunction. Fanconi syndrome is a global defect in the renal proximal tubule reabsorption of various electrolytes and substances resulting in excessive urinary excretion of amino acids, calcium, bicarbonate, glucose, phosphate, and uric acid. Individuals with Fanconi syndrome have clinical features suggestive of acidosis, dehydration, rickets, and poor growth. Fanconi syndrome has several inherited and acquired causes, including cystinosis, glycogen storage disease type 1, galactosemia, tyrosinemia, hereditary fructose intolerance, Wilson disease, Dent disease, heavy metal or drug toxicity, mitochondriopathy, or autoimmune disease (interstitial nephritis). This patient has associated hypercalciuria and most likely has nephrocalcinosis, making Dent disease a distinct possibility.

Dent disease is a rare genetic kidney disorder characterized by spillage of small proteins in the urine, hypercalciuria, nephrocalcinosis, and increased risk for recurrent nephrolithiasis. Dent disease is associated with mild renal tubular acidosis and typically low-normal serum potassium concentrations and hypophosphatemia that could result in chronic kidney disease. There are 2 types based on clinical presentation: type 1 is characterized by kidney involvement as mentioned above, while type 2 is characterized by, in addition to kidney impairment, mild intellectual disability, eye involvement, or diminished muscle tone (hypotonia). Genetic screening for Dent disease can identify pathogenic variants in the *CLCN5* (type 1) or *OCRL* (type 2) genes on the X chromosome. Approximately 30% of patients with Dent disease have no identifiable pathogenic variant. Dent disease is fully expressed only in males, although some female carriers may develop mild manifestations such as spillage of small proteins in the urine, hypercalciuria, or rarely kidney stones.

Nutritional vitamin D deficiency is still seen clinically in the 21st century, especially in dark-skinned children with limited exposure to sunlight and dietary vitamin D intake. Although this patient does have components of rickets, this appears to be secondary to his renal proximal tubular dysfunction and not the inciting disease process. Thus, nutritional vitamin D deficiency rickets (Answer C) is unlikely. If he had vitamin D–resistant rickets, his 1,25-dihydroxyvitamin D concentration would be expected to be much lower in type 1 (Answer D) or much higher in type 2 (Answer E). Some patients with type 2 vitamin D–resistant rickets have alopecia totalis. Urinary calcium is expected to be normal in the case of autosomal dominant/autosomal recessive/X-linked hypophosphatemic rickets.

Hereditary hypophosphatemic rickets with hypercalciuria (Answer B) is another consideration, although it would not produce a full Fanconi-type picture and PTH would be suppressed with a higher 1,25-dihydroxyvitamin D concentration.

Educational Objective
Identify the characteristic clinical features of Fanconi syndrome as a cause of short stature in boys.

Reference(s)

Foreman JW. Fanconi syndrome. *Pediatr Clin North Am.* 2019;66(1):159-167. PMID: 30454741

Elder CJ, Bishop NJ. Rickets. *Lancet.* 2014;383(9929):1665-1676. PMID: 24412049

Munns CF, Shaw N, Kiely M, et al. Global consensus recommendations on prevention and management of nutritional rickets. *J Clin Endocrinol Metab.* 2016;101(2):394-415. PMID: 26745253

58

ANSWER: A) American Indian male

In the United States, the prevalence of childhood obesity has more than tripled over the past 40 years. In 2017 to 2018, approximately 19.3% of all youth aged 2 to 19 years were categorized as having obesity. Unfortunately, recent data highlight that the COVID pandemic has only exacerbated the problem of childhood obesity. In a longitudinal cohort of 432,302 children aged 2 to 19 years, the monthly rate of BMI increase was almost double during the pandemic compared with rates during a prepandemic period. There are also substantial differences in the prevalence of childhood obesity, depending on racial/ethnic and/or sociodemographic factors. The prevalence of childhood obesity is substantially higher among racial and/or ethnic minorities in the United States than among White children.

American Indian (Answer A) and Native Alaskan children have the highest rates of pediatric obesity (approximately 30% of the population) compared with rates in all other racial/ethnic groups. NonHispanic Black youth, such as the boy in the vignette, have higher rates of pediatric obesity than nonHispanic White youth, with approximately one-quarter of children affected by obesity. Hispanic youth (Answer D) also have some of the highest rates of childhood obesity, with 24% to 25% of children being affected.

Asian children (Answers B and C) have the lowest prevalence of obesity among all children and adolescents. NonHispanic White children (Answer E) have the second lowest rates of obesity overall with 14% to 15% being affected.

When grouped by biological sex, Hispanic boys and nonHispanic Black girls have the highest rates of childhood obesity when comparing nonHispanic Black, nonHispanic White, Asian, and Hispanic children, although the prevalence is still lower than the prevalence among American Indian and Native Alaskan children.

Educational Objective

Describe differences in pediatric obesity rates in the United States with respect to race and ethnicity.

Reference(s)

Isong IA, Rao SR, Bind MA, Avendaño M, Kawachi I, Richmond TK. Racial and ethnic disparities in early childhood obesity. *Pediatrics*. 2018;141(1):e20170865. PMID: 29269386

Ogden CL, Fryar CD, Hales CM, Carroll MD, Aoki Y, Freedman DS. Differences in obesity prevalence by demographics and urbanization in US children and adolescents, 2013-2016. *JAMA*. 2018;319(23):2410-2418. PMID: 29922826

Lange SJ, Kompaniyets L, Freedman DS, et al. Longitudinal trends in body mass index before and during the COVID-19 pandemic among persons aged 2-19 years - United States, 2018-2020. *MMWR Morb Mortal Wkly Rep*. 2021;70(37):1278-1283. PMID: 34529635

59

ANSWER: E) MRI findings of hypoplastic adenohypophysis + ectopic posterior pituitary + interrupted pituitary stalk and clinical findings of multiple anterior pituitary hormone deficiencies

This patient's MRI shows 3 major findings: (1) an ectopic posterior pituitary (*) (the bright spot is not in the rear portion of the sella turcica but is located at the level of the median eminence); (2) an interrupted pituitary stalk (**); and (3) a hypoplastic adenohypophysis (***) (thus, Answer A is incorrect). There is no evidence of a suprasellar tumor suggestive of craniopharyngioma (Answer B) or Rathke cleft cyst (Answer D).

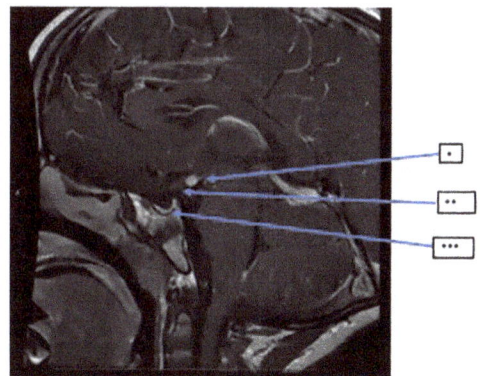

Embryologically, the pituitary gland originates from 2 different tissues: the neuroectoderm from the diencephalon and the oral ectoderm from the roof of the mouth. A caudal protrusion of the neuroectoderm of the diencephalon approaches a cranial invagination of the ectoderm of the roof of the mouth called the Rathke pouch. When these 2 structures are together, the original protrusion of the neuroectoderm localizes posteriorly (forming the posterior pituitary or neurohypophysis), while the Rathke pouch localizes anteriorly (forming the anterior pituitary or adenohypophysis), which eventually detaches from the roof of the mouth. The posterior pituitary is composed of neurons whose bodies are in some hypothalamic nuclei and whose axons extend through the pituitary stalk and end in the neurohypophysis. Posterior pituitary hormones (arginine vasopressin and oxytocin) are released directly to the systemic circulation from the neurohypophysis.

The cells of the adenohypophysis secrete pituitary hormones (GH, TSH, ACTH, LH, and FSH) in response to hypothalamic-releasing factors that reach them via a vascular network called the hypophyseal portal system that travels through the pituitary stalk. Prolactin, secreted by the lactotropes of the adenohypophysis, is inhibited by dopamine coming from the hypothalamus via the hypophyseal portal system.

Failed descent of the posterior pituitary (frequently referred to as ectopic posterior pituitary) has no negative effect on the ability to secrete oxytocin or arginine vasopressin; therefore, it does not lead to diabetes insipidus (Answer C). However, interruption of the formation of the pituitary stalk with subsequent absence or insufficiency of the hypophyseal portal system interferes with the normal trophic effect of the hypothalamic factors on the pituitary hormone–producing cells, frequently manifested radiologically with pituitary hypoplasia and clinically with multiple pituitary hormone deficiencies (Answer E).

The diagnosis of GH deficiency in children is not always straightforward. In neonates, the presence of hypoglycemia, prolonged direct hyperbilirubinemia, micropenis, and midline defects usually raises suspicion. In older infants and children, short stature with poor growth velocity is often the initial concern that elicits referral for evaluation. Although clinical assessment paired with measurements of IGF-1 and IGFBP-3 have been proposed by some to make the diagnosis, GH-stimulation tests have become commonly used to reach a "definite diagnosis" before initiating GH replacement therapy outside of the neonatal period.

MRI of the hypothalamic-pituitary area is useful to assess for the presence of anatomic abnormalities in children diagnosed with GH deficiency. Nevertheless, MRI of the brain and pituitary gland has been proposed by others as a first-line test in the diagnosis of GH deficiency.

Congenital hypopituitarism can be manifested by isolated GH deficiency or as multiple pituitary hormone deficiencies. Isolated GH deficiency is the most common form of isolated single pituitary hormone deficiency.

While some MRI abnormalities can be seen in isolated GH deficiency, they are more common in multiple pituitary hormone deficiencies.

Educational Objective
Explain the clinical and radiologic correlation of abnormalities of the pituitary axis with pituitary hormone deficiencies and recognize that ectopic posterior pituitary gland is usually not associated with posterior pituitary dysfunction/central diabetes insipidus.

Reference(s)

Dubois PM, Elamaroui A. Embryology of the pituitary gland. *Trends Endocrinol Metab.* 1995;6(1):1-7. PMID: 18406676

Argyropoulou M, Perignon F, Brauner R, Brunelle F. Magnetic resonance imaging in the diagnosis of growth hormone deficiency. *J Pediatr.* 1992;120(6):886-891. PMID:1593348

Xu C, Zhang X, Dong L, Zhu B, Xin T. MRI features of growth hormone deficiency in children with short stature caused by pituitary lesions. *Exp Ther Med.* 2017;13(6):3474-3478. PMID: 28587427

Maghnie M, Lindberg A, Koltowska-Häggström M, Ranke MB. Magnetic resonance imaging of CNS in 15,043 children with GH deficiency in KIGS (Pfizer International Growth Database). *Eur J Endocrinol* 2013;168(2):211-217. PMID: 23152438

Wilson DM, Frane J. A review of the use and utility of growth hormone stimulation testing in the NCGS: do we need to do provocative GH testing? *Growth Horm IGF Res.* 2005;15(Suppl A):S21-S25. PMID: 16039892

60 ANSWER: E) Variant in the *TACR3* gene

The patient in this vignette has a pathogenic variant in the *TACR3* gene (W275X) (Answer E) that is associated with hypogonadotropic hypogonadism. *TACR3* encodes the tachykinin receptor-3, which is required for normal GnRH pulse generation. Recent studies have shown that variants in the *TACR3* gene are as common as variants in *GNRHR* in cases of normosmic hypogonadotropic hypogonadism and that both males and females can be affected. Micropenis and cryptorchidism are common in male patients with *TACR3* variants but are not always identified. Spontaneous progression of puberty and fertility have been reported in 25% to 83% of families with pathogenic *TACR3* variants, which raises the question of whether milder *TACR3* variants could be a cause of constitutional delay of growth and puberty. In one cohort described by Gianetti et al, assessment after discontinuation of hormone treatment indicated normal function of the reproductive axis in 6 of 7 male patients and in 4 of 5 female patients. Homozygosity for inactivating variants in *TACR3* is most commonly described, but instances of some patients having a pathogenic variant on only 1 allele (specifically, the W275X variant) have been reported. *GNRHR* pathogenic variants are also a common cause of normosmic hypogonadotropic hypogonadism but are not associated with spontaneous resolution, as seen in this patient's father.

While inactivating pathogenic variants in the *NR0B1* (*DAX1*) gene (Answer C) are associated with normosmic hypogonadotropic hypogonadism, these individuals present in infancy with adrenal insufficiency secondary to adrenal hypoplasia.

Pathogenic variants in the *ANOS1* (*KAL1*) gene (Answer B) are present in 10% to 20% of individuals with Kallmann syndrome. Other features in addition to hypogonadotropic hypogonadism include synkinesia and unilateral renal agenesis in approximately 70% and 30% of affected individuals, respectively. While absence of these additional features does not rule out Kallmann syndrome, the lack of these features in this patient makes pathogenic variants in *ANOS1* much less likely.

Klinefelter syndrome (47,XXY) (Answer A) and pathogenic variants in the *SRY* gene (Answer D) are associated with primary hypogonadism (elevated LH and FSH concentrations, not low).

One study found pathogenic variants in 77% of 22 families with normosmic hypogonadotropic hypogonadism; pathogenic variants in *GNRHR* and *TACR3* accounted for two-thirds of identified cases, while variants in *KISS1R* accounted for only 3%. As such, it has been suggested that *GNRHR* and *TACR3* should be prioritized when screening individuals with suspected normosmic hypogonadotropic hypogonadism.

Educational Objective
Establish the etiology of male hypogonadotropic hypogonadism.

Reference(s)

Topaloğlu AK. Update on the genetics of idiopathic hypogonadotropic hypogonadism. *J Clin Res Pediatr Endocrinol.* 2017;9(Suppl 2):113-122. PMID: 29280744

Gianetti E, Tusset C, Noel SD, et al. TAC3/TACR3 mutations reveal preferential activation of gonadotropin-releasing hormone release by neurokinin B in neonatal life followed by reversal in adulthood. *J Clin Endocrinol Metab.* 2010;95(6):2857-2867. PMID: 20332248

61   ANSWER: B) Complete blood cell count

This child has had multiple fractures over a short period, and a comprehensive bone health evaluation is warranted. In addition, she has signs of anemia with pallor and tachycardia. A complete blood cell count (Answer B) revealed pancytopenia with 80% lymphocytes and 3% blast cells (immature granulocytes), leading to the diagnosis of acute lymphoblastic leukemia (ALL).

In the study by Halton et al, vertebral compression fractures were noted in 16% of children within 30 days of ALL diagnosis. Children with vertebral compression fractures were more likely to have low bone density than those without compression fractures, and they were also more likely to experience bone pain. Importantly, 45% of children with vertebral compression fractures in this study did not complain of bone pain at all. Markers of bone formation (bone-specific alkaline phosphatase and osteocalcin) are low at the time of diagnosis and bone resorption markers tend to be normal or low as well, resulting in a low bone turnover state. Trabecular bone volume and thickness have also been shown to be reduced and bone density frequently declines with treatment of leukemia because high-dosage glucocorticoids are commonly part of the chemotherapeutic regimen. Children with ALL have an increased risk for fractures during the maintenance phase of treatment. The presence of 1 vertebral fracture at diagnosis was highly associated with an increased risk for sustaining an incident vertebral fracture over the next 12 months. Given the high cure rate for pediatric ALL, these patients are more likely to have spontaneous recovery of bone density and modeling of their vertebrae without the need for bone antiresorptive therapy. However, bone health is an important parameter to monitor.

Vitamin D fortification in cow's milk is frequently 100 IU per 8 oz in the United States. This child's daily intake of 3 to 4 cups most likely provides sufficient dietary vitamin D intake, making vitamin D deficiency an unlikely cause of her skeletal fragility. Her 25-hydroxyvitamin D concentration (Answer D) is therefore likely to be normal and would not explain her fracture presentation. In addition, vitamin D deficiency (<20 ng/dL [<50 nmol/L]) is only weakly associated with increased fracture risk. Excessive intake of cow's milk can cause iron deficiency anemia, which may present with pallor and constipation in children. While complete blood cell count may be ordered for this concern, it would not show leukopenia or thrombocytopenia.

Celiac disease, screened for with tissue transglutaminase antibodies (Answer E), may be associated with low bone density and rickets, but it is not clearly associated with increased fracture risk in children.

DXA (Answer C) may be considered as part of the evaluation of a child with recurrent fractures, but it would not lead to a diagnosis, especially because vertebral compression fractures can cause falsely elevated bone density.

If bone density were low, further genetic testing may be warranted in a child with recurrent fractures; however, the key features of pallor and weight loss make osteogenesis imperfecta less likely. Therefore, *COL1A1* genetic testing (Answer A) would probably not lead to the diagnosis.

Educational Objective

Explain how fractures, including vertebral compression fractures, can be a presenting feature of leukemia.

Reference(s)

Halton J, Gaboury I, Grant R, et al; Canadian STOPP Consortium. Advanced vertebral fracture among newly diagnosed children with acute lymphoblastic leukemia: results of the Canadian Steroid-Associated Osteoporosis in the Pediatric Population (STOPP) research program. *J Bone Miner Res.* 2009;24(7):1326-1334. PMID: 19210218

Mostoufi-Moab S, Halton J. Bone morbidity in childhood leukemia: epidemiology, mechanisms, diagnosis, and treatment. *Curr Osteoporos Rep.* 2014;12(3):300-312. PMID: 24986711

Canova C, Pitter G, Zanier L, Simonato L, Michaelsson K, Ludvigsson JF. Risk of fractures in youths with celiac disease-a population-based study. *J Pediatr.* 2018;198:117-120. PMID: 29681452

Sanchez-Mostiero DO, Boussati JMA. Low back pain as an unusual presentation in a child with acute lymphoblastic leukaemia. *BMJ Case Rep.* 2022;15(3):e242843. PMID: 35246428

62 ANSWER: A) Diabetic neuropathy screening

Although the patient in this vignette is at risk for all diabetes mellitus–related complications because he has had the condition for more than 15 years, the most emergent complication to be concerned about is diabetic neuropathy (Answer A). Diabetic neuropathy can be missed without proper screening if the clinician solely depends on reported symptoms. Diabetic neuropathy is rarely described in pediatric practice, most likely because of subclinical presentation, and children may not voluntarily report diabetic neuropathy symptoms. Early diabetic neuropathy symptoms are usually related to small-fiber involvement, and the most common presentation is symmetric distal sensory polyneuropathy. Symptoms such as gait imbalance and weakness may arise with large-fiber involvement. In the literature, the incidence of diabetic neuropathy varies widely from 10% to 70% in patients with type 1 diabetes, depending on patient selection and the definitions used. On the basis of abnormal findings on nerve conduction studies, diabetic neuropathy has been estimated to occur in approximately one-half of all children with diabetes who have had the condition for 15 years or longer. However, the prevalence of diabetic neuropathy is often underestimated because it tends to be subclinical in this age group.

Although nerve conduction studies are the gold standard for diagnosis, neuropathy screening instruments are easy, accurate, and widely used options, including in children. The 2 main screening components are a questionnaire of key diabetic neuropathy symptoms and a focused neurologic examination with foot inspection, great toe vibration perception threshold, and ankle reflexes. Additional tests, such as thermal perception threshold or pinprick sensation, help to evaluate small-fiber function.

Dilated retinal examination (Answer B) is certainly essential to evaluate the entire retina and not just focus on the optic nerve and macula by nondilated manual examination or digital image capture. The patient in this vignette has been adherent to annual screening recommendations and should not be subject to earlier retinal examination unless there are specific concerns.

A 24-hour urine collection to determine the albumin-to-creatinine ratio (Answer E) is recommended for assessment of diabetic nephropathy if proteinuria is present in a random urine sample or if an abnormal albumin-to-creatinine ratio is documented on annual screening. This patient's urine screening is negative for protein and annual screening results were normal.

Performing 24-hour blood pressure monitoring (Answer D) is not indicated in this patient. Although his blood pressure and heart rate appear low, he has no symptoms and he tolerates a high level of activity (swimming) with no concerns. Postural hypotension can be a sign of autonomic dysfunction and may require screening with 24-hour ambulatory blood pressure monitoring.

A lipid profile (Answer C) should be included in his annual screening and is recommended to be repeated every 2 years if normal.

Although not listed as an answer option, psychological comorbidity with depression and anxiety is prevalent in patients with longstanding diabetes mellitus, and annual screening should be considered even if there is no indication for concern. The patient in this vignette reports being self-sufficient with diabetes care, yet he struggles to maintain a narrow blood glucose range. He is on track with educational goals and appears to have leadership qualities (serves as the captain of his swim team). However, the burden of psychological comorbidity remains, and providers should vigilantly screen before transition to college life.

Table. Screening Guidelines Adopted From American Diabetes Association Standards of Medical Care in Diabetes

Condition	Method	When to start	Follow-up frequency
Thyroid disease	Thyroid-stimulating hormone; consider antithyroglobulin and antithyroid peroxidase antibodies	Soon after diagnosis	Every 1 to 2 years if thyroid antibodies negative; more often if symptoms develop or presence of thyroid antibodies
Celiac disease	IgA tTG if total IgA normal; IgG tTG and gliadin antibodies if IgA deficient	Soon after diagnosis	Within 2 years and then at 5 years after diagnosis; sooner if symptoms develop
Hypertension	Blood pressure monitoring	At diagnosis	Every visit
Dyslipidemia	Lipid profile	Soon after diagnosis; preferably after hyperglycemia has improved and >2 years old	If LDL cholesterol <100 mg/dL, repeat at 9 to 11 years old; then, if <100 mg/dL, every 3 years
Nephropathy	Albumin-to-creatinine ratio	Puberty or >10 years old, whichever is earlier, and diabetes duration of 5 years	If normal, annually; if abnormal, repeat with confirmation in 2 of 3 samples over 6 months
Retinopathy	Dilated fundoscopy or retinal photography	Puberty or >11 years old, whichever is earlier, and diabetes duration of 3 to 5 years	If normal, every 2 years; consider less frequently (every 4 years) if hemoglobin A_{1c} <8% and eye professional agrees
Neuropathy	Foot exam with foot pulses, pinprick, 10-g monofilament sensation tests, vibration, and ankle reflexes	Puberty or >10 years old, whichever is earlier, and diabetes duration of 5 years	If normal, annually

Adapted from American Diabetes Association Professional Practice Committee; Draznin B, Aroda VR, Bakris, G. 14. Diabetes Care. 2022; 45(Suppl 1).

Educational Objective
Recommend screening for peripheral neuropathy in patients with type 1 diabetes mellitus.

Reference(s)

Ising E, Dahlin LB, Elding Larsson H. Impaired vibrotactile sense in children and adolescents with type 1 diabetes – signs of peripheral neuropathy. *PLoS One*. 2018;13(4):e0196243. PMID: 29672623

Akinci G, Savelieff MG, Gallagher G, Callaghan BC, Feldman EL. Diabetic neuropathy in children and youth: new and emerging risk factors. *Pediatr Diabetes*. 2021;22(2):132-147. PMID: 33205601

Nelson D, Mah JK, Adams C, et al. Comparison of conventional and non-invasive techniques for the early identification of diabetic neuropathy in children and adolescents with type 1 diabetes. *Pediatr Diabetes*. 2006;7(6):305-310. PMID: 17212597

American Diabetes Association Professional Practice Committee; Draznin B, Aroda VR, Bakris, G. 14. Children and adolescents: standards of medical care in diabetes-2022. *Diabetes Care*. 2022;45(Suppl 1):S208-S231. PMID: 34964865

63 ANSWER: D) Right orbit radiotherapy
Endocrine disorders frequently occur in survivors of childhood cancer, sometimes directly related to the cancer itself, but also indirectly to cancer treatment with surgery, chemotherapy, and/or radiation. By some estimates, 50% of survivors develop 1 or more endocrine problem over their lifetime. These conditions include GH deficiency, hypogonadism and pubertal disorders, and thyroid dysfunction, all of which can adversely affect childhood growth, which is the chief concern in this vignette. Since these disorders may be amenable to treatment,

and treatment is most effective if initiated early, multiple professional societies have developed consensus statements and clinical guidelines to ensure comprehensive screening for hypothalamic-pituitary complications of childhood cancer therapy.

Individuals at highest risk for GH deficiency are those with tumors directly affecting the hypothalamus and pituitary. Radiation therapy is another critical risk. In general, younger age at radiation initiation and greater cumulative radiation dose to the hypothalamus/pituitary is each associated with increased likelihood of GH deficiency and shorter time to clinical manifestation. Specifically, cranial radiation of 1800 cGy more or total body irradiation of 1200 cGy or more (fractionated) or 1000 cGy or more (single fraction) are associated with increased risk of GH deficiency. Depending on the dose and patient factors, GH deficiency can manifest between 1 and 5 years after treatment, or as late as 15 years. This timeline explains the recommendation for ongoing surveillance. In this vignette, it is important to recognize that orbital radiation (Answer D) can also lead to hypothalamic/pituitary exposure. Radiation to the flank (Answer C) would not be expected to lead to GH deficiency.

Multiagent chemotherapy (Answer B) can include agents that contribute to primary hypogonadism and thus affect pubertal growth, but this 7-year-old child is prepubertal. Chemotherapy can adversely affect growth in additional ways. In particular, treatment with cis-retinoic acid (Answer A) may lead to premature physeal closure—not GH deficiency—and may further exacerbate short stature in children who already have impaired growth from multiple other causes. Pretransplant conditioning before stem-cell transplant (Answer E) may have adverse endocrine outcomes (most notably in the absence of radiation or gonadotoxic chemotherapy). In this prepubertal child, gonadotoxic chemotherapy is less likely to affect growth.

Greater cumulative doses of radiation to the hypothalamus/pituitary are typically associated with LH/FSH or TSH deficiency (3000 cGy and 4000 cGy, respectively). Clinically, a radiation-induced decrease in growth velocity is suggested by a deviation from the pretreatment growth trajectory; for example, a decrease in height for age and sex of 1 or more standard deviations, and/or a height velocity that is less than the 25th percentile for age and sex, especially in the appropriate clinical context. Measuring growth every 6 to 12 months in children who have not yet reached skeletal maturation is appropriate as initial screening for growth impairment. Obtaining sitting height and/or arm span measurements may be valuable, especially in children who have undergone spinal radiation and thus may have disproportionate growth impairment in the axial skeleton. Provocative testing for GH deficiency and, if indicated, GH therapy, are next steps. Immunotherapy and molecularly targeted therapies can also cause GH deficiency, although in this vignette, radiation is the most clear culprit.

Educational Objective
Recommend appropriate screening for hypothalamic-pituitary complications of radiation in the context of childhood cancer treatment.

Reference(s)

Chemaitilly W, Cohen LE, Mostoufi-Moab S, et al. Endocrine late effects in childhood cancer survivors. *J Clin Oncol.* 2018;36(21):2153-2159. PMID: 29874130

Sklar CA, Antal Z, Chemaitilly W, et al. Hypothalamic-pituitary and growth disorders in survivors of childhood cancer: an Endocrine Society clinical practice guideline. *J Clin Endocrinol Metab.* 2018;103(8):2761-2784. PMID: 29982476

van Iersel L, Mulder RL, Denzer C, et al. Hypothalamic-pituitary and other endocrine surveillance among childhood cancer survivors. *Endocr Rev.* 2022;43(5):794-823. PMID: 34962573

van Kalsbeek RJ, van der Pal HJH, Kremer LCM, et al. European PanCareFollowUp Recommendations for surveillance of late effects of childhood, adolescent, and young adult cancer. *Eur J Cancer.* 2021;154:316-328. PMID: 34333209

Delgado J, Jaramillo D, Chauvin NA, et al. Evaluating growth failure with diffusion tensor imaging in pediatric survivors of high-risk neuroblastoma treated with high-dose cis-retinoic acid. *Pediatr Radiol.* 2019;49(8):1056-1065. PMID: 31055614

64 ANSWER: B) Perform pituitary-directed MRI

This patient has classic clinical features and laboratory findings of severe GH deficiency (poor growth, delayed bone age, significant disparity between current height and midparental height, low IGF-1 and IGFBP-3 concentrations). Micropenis and hypoplastic scrotum indicate hypogonadism during fetal and infantile periods. Together, these findings raise concerns for hypothalamic-pituitary dysfunction. The next step is to perform pituitary-directed MRI (Answer B) to look for congenital or acquired anatomic abnormalities. If he has a major congenital malformation (eg, ectopic posterior pituitary and pituitary hypoplasia with abnormal stalk), GH would be recommended without the need for provocative testing. Thus, ordering a GH provocative test, such as an insulin tolerance test (Answer A), is not only unnecessary now, but it also risks losing the patient to follow-up given his history. Consensus guidelines are available and are helpful for navigating the steps involved in the diagnosis and management of children with short stature and GH deficiency.

In patients with history suggestive of severe GH deficiency, GH therapy (Answer E) should not be started before brain/pituitary MRI is done to rule out potential intracranial pathology that would necessitate further investigation.

Although the patient's weight percentiles are low, his weight-for-height is appropriate; thus, referral to a nutritionist (Answer D) is not needed and would only delay the diagnosis.

This patient has growth failure and other findings, so simple reassurance (Answer C) is inappropriate.

Educational Objective
Determine when severe GH deficiency can be diagnosed without the need for GH-stimulation testing.

Reference(s)
Grimberg A, DiVall SA, Polychronakos C, et al. Guidelines for growth hormone and insulin-like growth factor-I treatment in children and adolescents: growth hormone deficiency, idiopathic short stature, and primary insulin-like growth factor-I deficiency. *Horm Res Paediatr.* 2016;86(6):361-397. PMID: 27884013

65 ANSWER: A) Continue the current levothyroxine dosage

The goals of therapy for congenital hypothyroidism are to maintain serum TSH in the age-specific reference range and free T_4 in the upper half of the age-specific reference range. After a recent levothyroxine dosage increase, this patient's TSH value is within the reference range. Although the free T_4 is mildly elevated, this alone is not an indication to reduce the levothyroxine dosage (Answer E). Overall, studies have demonstrated no adverse effects of mildly elevated free T_4 levels in children treated for congenital hypothyroidism. Therefore, current consensus guidelines recommend that if TSH is in the age-specific reference range, free T_4 concentrations above the upper normal limit can be accepted, and the levothyroxine dosage should not be reduced unless TSH is suppressed (below the lower normal limit) or clinical signs of overtreatment are present. Therefore, the most appropriate management is to continue the current levothyroxine dosage (Answer A).

Measured free T_4 concentrations may be elevated by preanalytical or analytical factors affecting the laboratory assay or can be due to drawing the blood sample within 4 hours after administration of levothyroxine. This possibility might be clarified by measuring the free T_4 by a gold-standard dialysis method (Answer C) or by ensuring that the sample was drawn at least 4 hours after the last dose of levothyroxine. However, in this case, neither of these maneuvers is necessary because demonstrating a normal free T_4 concentration would not alter clinical management.

There is no evidence that maintaining TSH in the lower part of the reference range (0.5-2.0 mIU/L) improves outcomes in congenital hypothyroidism, and consensus guidelines recommend simply maintaining TSH within the age-specific reference range. Therefore, increasing the levothyroxine dosage (Answer B) is not necessary nor advisable in light of the elevated free T_4 concentration.

Gastrointestinal absorption of levothyroxine can be impaired by co-ingestion of soy. This issue should be considered in patients in whom adequate control of hypothyroidism is difficult to establish. Switching from cow milk– to soy-based formula (Answer D) should be avoided if possible. Regardless, this patient has no evidence of abnormal levothyroxine absorption.

Educational Objective
Manage isolated mild free T_4 elevation in patients with congenital hypothyroidism.

Reference(s)
van Trotsenburg P, Stoupa A, Léger J, et al. Congenital hypothyroidism: a 2020-2021 consensus guidelines update-an ENDO-European Reference Network Initiative endorsed by the European Society for Pediatric Endocrinology and the European Society for Endocrinology. *Thyroid.* 2021;31(3):387-419. PMID: 33272083

Aleksander PE, Brückner-Spieler M, Stoehr A-M, et al. Mean high-dose l-thyroxine treatment is efficient and safe to achieve a normal IQ in young adult patients with congenital hypothyroidism. *J Clin Endocrinol Metab.* 2018;103(4):1459-1469. PMID: 29325045

66 ANSWER: C) Pseudohypoaldosteronism type 1

Pseudohypoaldosteronism (PHA) type 1 (Answer C) is a primary form of mineralocorticoid/aldosterone resistance. Affected patients often manifest symptoms early in the neonatal period or within the first month of life with salt wasting, hypotension, hyperkalemia, and metabolic acidosis despite elevated aldosterone levels. A differential diagnosis of adrenal disorders should always be considered; however, salt wasting that occurs in individuals with congenital adrenal hyperplasia (Answer A) and congenital adrenal hypoplasia (Answer B) is associated with high plasma renin activity but low aldosterone concentrations.

PHA type 2 (Answer D) (also known as Gordon hyperkalemia-hypertension syndrome) generally presents in adulthood with hypertension, which is associated with hyperkalemia, mild hyperchloremic metabolic acidosis, normal or elevated aldosterone, and low renin levels. The condition is caused by pathogenic variants in a number of genes (*WNK1*, *WNK4*, *KLHL3*, and *CUL3*). The encoded protein WNK-kinase 4, in normal circumstances, interacts with the sodium chloride co-symporter, the epithelial sodium channel, and the renal outer medullary potassium channel in an inhibitory manner to maintain normokalaemia and normotension. WNK1 has an inhibitory action on WNK4 and proteins Kelch-like 3 and Cullin 3 form a ring-like complex to ubiquitinate WNK-kinase 4. Pathogenic variants in these genes lead to excessive WNK-kinase 4 and result in PHA type 2.

Pyelonephritis (Answer E) and kidney abnormalities are other causes of transient PHA, and urine microscopy and kidney ultrasonography should always be part of the evaluation. Because this child is apyrexial, pyelonephritis is less likely.

PHA type 1 is divided into 2 forms: an autosomal dominant form sometimes referred to as renal PHA type 1 and an autosomal recessive form also known as the systemic form of PHA type 1. The autosomal dominant form is considered a milder condition. Affected patients can be asymptomatic or ill from birth. Treatment is in the form of sodium replacement, which can be reduced or completely stopped with age. Pathogenic variants in the *NR3C2* gene that encodes the mineralocorticoid receptor cause the condition. The child in this vignette had an *NR3C2* pathogenic variant. In contrast, autosomal recessive PHA type 1 is far more severe. Affected patients have salt wasting from the kidney, colon, and sweat and salivary glands. There is often severe fluid depletion, life-threatening hyperkalemia, and severe hyponatremia requiring high concentrations of sodium supplementation throughout life. Classically, the condition is associated with inappropriate urinary sodium loss and potassium retention. However, spot urinary sodium concentrations have been reported to be normal in some patients at diagnosis. Pathogenic variants in genes that encode subunits of the endothelial sodium channel (α subunit [*SCNN1A*], β subunit [*SCNN1B*], or γ subunit [*SCNN1G*]) occur in homozygous or compound heterozygous states.

Educational Objective
Diagnose pseudohypoaldosteronism type 1.

Reference(s)

Amin N, Alvi NS, Barth JH, et al. Pseudohypoaldosteronism type 1: clinical features and management in infancy. *Endocrinol Diabetes Metab Case Rep.* 2013;2013:130010. PMID: 24616761

Abraham MB, Larkins N, Choong CS, Shetty VB. Transient pseudohypoaldosteronism in infancy secondary to urinary tract infection. *J Paediatr Child Health.* 2017;53(5):458-463. PMID: 28233358

Riepe FG, Finkeldei J, de Sanctis L, et al. Elucidating the underlying molecular pathogenesis of NR3C2 mutants causing autosomal dominant pseudohypoaldosteronism type I. *J Clin Endocrinol Metab.* 2006;91(11):4552-4561. PMID: 16954160

Mabillard H, Sayer JA. The molecular genetics of Gordon syndrome. *Genes (Basel).* 2019;10(12):986. PMID: 31795491

67 ANSWER: E) Partial gonadal dysgenesis

In this vignette, the combination of undervirilization, a 46,XY karyotype, and a low AMH concentration is most consistent with partial gonadal dysgenesis (Answer E). During laparoscopy, rudimentary mullerian structures (fallopian tubes and uterus) were identified, consistent with low AMH concentrations in fetal development. 46,XY partial gonadal dysgenesis can be spontaneous, but it has also been associated with pathogenic variants in the *MAP3K1*, *WT1*, *NR5A1*, *SRY*, *DHH*, and *DMRT1* genes, among others. Establishing a more definitive diagnosis is helpful in terms of identifying gene variants that are associated with an increased risk of gonadoblastoma.

Undervirilization in an individual with a 46,XY karyotype can be caused by defects in gonadal differentiation as well as disorders of antimullerian hormone (AMH) production or action. AMH is secreted from the fetal testes beginning at the time of testicular differentiation, resulting in regression of mullerian structures. In normal males, AMH secretion continues through puberty, at which point concentrations become nearly undetectable. Low AMH production in the male fetus results in persistence of mullerian structures; however, if androgen action is not affected, normal virilization will occur. This is seen in the rare condition of persistent mullerian duct syndrome, caused by pathogenic variants in the genes encoding AMH or its receptor, and it results in persistence of the uterus and fallopian tubes with normal appearance of male external genitalia.

AMH concentrations are low in various forms of gonadal dysgenesis and generally correlate with the amount of testicular tissue present (*see figure*). In contrast, AMH concentrations are normal or high in disorders of androgen synthesis or action. As such, AMH concentrations in infancy through onset of puberty can be helpful in determining the cause of undervirilization in an individual with a 46,XY karyotype.

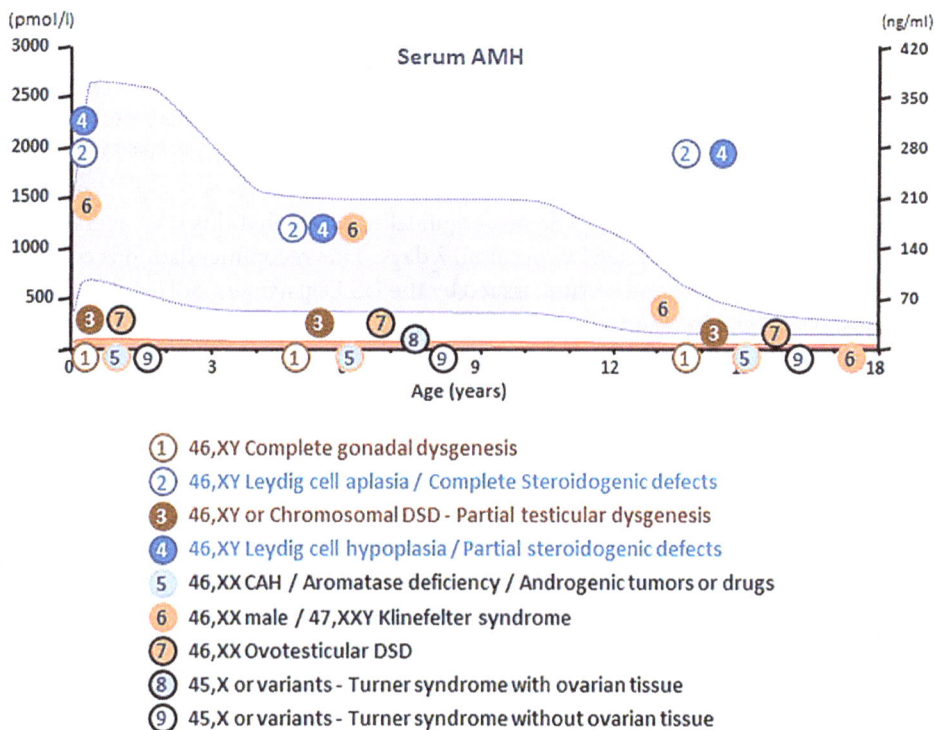

FIGURE 6 | Schematic of AMH levels in various types of disorders of sex development (DSD) in relationship to the aspect of the external genitalia and age. The shaded area represents reference levels for AMH, as obtained from ref. (22).

Adapted from Josso N & Rey RA. *Front Endocrinol* (Lausanne), 2020; 11:619. Reference intervals (shaded area) derived from Grinspon RP et al. LAREP Group. *Int J Androl*, 2011; 34(5 Pt 2).

AMH concentrations should be normal or elevated in disorders of steroidogenesis such as 5α-reductase deficiency (Answer C) and congenital adrenal hyperplasia caused by 3β-hydroxysteroid dehydrogenase deficiency (Answer A). AMH concentrations are also normal or elevated in partial androgen insensitivity syndrome (Answer D) because testicular AMH and testosterone production are intact.

46,XY ovotesticular disorders (Answer B) are extremely rare causes of disorders of sexual development and can be associated with low AMH concentrations, which generally correlate with the amount of normal testicular tissue present. However, the absence of ovarian tissue in this case makes this diagnosis less likely.

Educational Objective
Explain the role of antimullerian hormone in fetal development and the utility of its measurement when diagnosing 46,XY disorders of sexual development.

Reference(s)

Josso N, Rey RA. What does AMH tell us in pediatric disorders of sex development? *Front Endocrinol (Lausanne).* 2020;11:619. PMID: 33013698

Grinspon RP, Bedecarrás P, Ballerini MG, et al; LAREP Group. Early onset of primary hypogonadism revealed by serum anti-Müllerian hormone determination during infancy and childhood in trisomy 21. *Int J Androl.* 2011;34(5 Pt 2):e487-e498. PMID: 21831236

68 ANSWER: B) Engage in 60 minutes of moderate-to-vigorous intensity physical activity 7 days of the week

Physical activity provides multiple health benefits to children and adolescents, including improvements in cardiorespiratory fitness, muscular fitness, bone health, and cardiometabolic health. However, the 2020 World Health Organization guidelines on physical activity and sedentary behavior in children and adolescents highlight that 81% of children aged 11 to 17 years are insufficiently active across the globe. Meanwhile, excessive sedentary behavior (such as smartphone/tablet use, TV viewing, video game playing, computer use, etc) is widespread in this age group. Although the guidelines highlight that the optimal amount of physical activity that is associated with improved health outcomes cannot yet be determined with current available studies, many of the benefits are seen with an average of 60 minutes of moderate-to-vigorous intensity physical activity (MVPA) daily, so the World Health Organization currently recommends that children aged 5 to 17 years engage in at least 60 minutes of MVPA daily (420 minutes in a 7-day period). The newer guidelines state that this is an average over the week, so the physical activity does not necessarily need to occur all 7 days. This recommendation is consistent with the *Physical Activity Guidelines for Americans,* 2nd edition, issued by the US Department of Health and Human Services, which also recommends that all children and adolescents aged 6 to 17 years participate in 60 minutes or more of MVPA daily. Exercise should include aerobic activities, as well as age-appropriate muscle- and bone-strengthening exercises. The 2020 World Health Organization guidelines also recommend that children and adolescents limit the amount of time spent in sedentary pursuits, especially the amount of recreational screen time.

This child's current activity is not meeting the recommended guidelines for her age. Therefore, the most appropriate recommendation is to encourage the family to have her engage in 60 minutes of MVPA daily (Answer B).

She would need to be engaging in MVPA for an average of 60 minutes or more most days of the week before one could reassure her family that no changes in her physical activity level are recommended, regardless of her BMI (Answer E).

A child engaging in the amount of physical activity outlined in Answers A and D would also not meet current recommended guidelines.

Physical activity recommendations change by age, so younger children aged 3 to 5 years should be encouraged to be physically active throughout the day without specific time edicts (Answer C), but this would not be an appropriate recommendation for a 7-year-old child.

Educational Objective

Summarize daily physical activity recommendations for youth based on age and appreciate that most children are not meeting the proposed targets.

Reference(s)

US Department of Health and Human Services. *Physical Activity Guidelines for Americans.* 2nd edition. Washington, DC: US Department of Health and Human Services; 2018.

Styne DM, Arslanian SA, Connor EL, et al. Pediatric obesity-assessment, treatment, and prevention: an Endocrine Society clinical practice guideline. *J Clin Endocrinol Metab.* 2017;102(3):709-757. PMID: 28359099

Chaput JP, Willumsen J, Bull F, et al. 2020 WHO guidelines on physical activity and sedentary behaviour for children and adolescents aged 5-17 years: summary of the evidence. *Int J Behav Nutr Phys Act.* 2020;17(1):141.

69 ANSWER: A) Echocardiography

Tall stature in children is defined as a height that is 2 standard deviations or more above the mean for age and sex. Familial tall stature and constitutional tall stature are considered normal variants. In these situations, there is usually a family history of tall stature, and children grow at a high-normal growth velocity and have no dysmorphic features concerning for syndromic causes. Pathologic etiologies of tall stature include endocrine and nonendocrine conditions. Endocrine etiologies include gigantism/GH excess, precocious puberty (during childhood but possible short stature in adulthood if left untreated), hypogonadism or sex hormone resistance syndromes, familial glucocorticoid deficiency (type 1) and resistance, and congenital lipodystrophy syndromes. Multiple nonendocrine disorders are associated with pathologic tall stature, including exogenous obesity in young children (however, obesity-induced advancement in skeletal maturation may lead to earlier growth plate fusion and lack of tall stature in adulthood), *MC4R* pathogenic variants, Klinefelter syndrome, 47,XYY syndrome, Marfan syndrome, homocystinuria, fragile X syndrome, and cerebral gigantism (Sotos syndrome).

The patient in this vignette has a family history of tall stature (both parents are tall), but her predicted adult height is well above the midparental height. This, in addition to the presence of dysmorphic features on examination, makes familial tall stature an unlikely explanation for her growth pattern, and reassuring the family (Answer E) is incorrect.

Tall stature was identified early in life, probably well before the initial referral for evaluation at age 2 years, and it has persisted. However, her IGF-1 concentration is in the normal range and just below the mean for age with a Z-score of –0.2, making gigantism unlikely. Therefore, an oral glucose tolerance test (Answer D) to assess for GH excess is not indicated.

Estrogen has a critical role in the maturation and fusion of growth plates. Tall stature and continued growth into adulthood have been described in individuals with estrogen resistance due to loss-of-function pathogenic variants in the estrogen receptor and in individuals with aromatase deficiency, leading to a significant decrease in aromatization of androgens into estrogens. This patient has evidence of incipient thelarche, which, although slightly delayed for her age, can still be considered normal. Her delayed thelarche is unlikely to be caused by estrogen resistance due to a loss-of-function variant in the gene encoding the estrogen receptor (Answer B), as her estradiol concentration would be expected to be high.

Marfan syndrome is an autosomal dominant condition with musculoskeletal, cardiovascular, and ocular manifestations. Tall stature is one of the musculoskeletal manifestations. However, aortic root dilatation, ectopia lentis, and findings on physical examination are the cardinal features to diagnose this condition. Approximately 90% of individuals with this condition have a pathogenic variant in the *FBN1* gene that encodes fibrillin-1, a connective tissue protein. Approximately 75% of affected individuals inherit the pathogenic variant from a parent, while 25% have a de novo variant. Up to 10% of persons with a Marfan syndrome phenotype do not have an identifiable *FBN1* variant. Rare recessive *FBN1* variants leading to Marfan syndrome have also been described. Ectopia lentis is the only cardinal ocular criterion for Marfan syndrome. However, *FBN1* pathogenic variants have been identified in some patients with ectopia lentis who do not have this condition, and pathogenic variants in the *FBN1* gene alone are not enough to diagnose Marfan syndrome.

Marfan syndrome is diagnosed according to the Ghent criteria, which were revised in 2010, putting greater weight on aortic root dilatation/dissection and ectopia lentis as the cardinal clinical features, followed by genetic testing.

The Ghent criteria are based on the following aspects:

(1) Presence or absence of a family history of Marfan syndrome
(2) Imaging of the aorta for aortic diameter Z-score >2 or evidence of aortic dissection
(3) Presence of ectopia lentis
(4) Genetic testing
(5) Characteristic findings on physical examination (systemic score ≥7):
    - Wrist *and* thumb sign = 3 points; or wrist *or* thumb sign = 1 point
    - Pectus carinatum = 2 points; pectus excavatum *or* chest asymmetry = 1 point
    - Hindfoot deformity = 2 points; pes planus = 1 point
    - Pneumothorax = 2 points
    - Dural ectasia = 2 points
    - Protrusio acetabuli = 2 points
    - Reduced upper-to-lower segment ratio and increased arm span/height and no severe scoliosis) = 1 point
    - Scoliosis or thoracolumbar kyphosis = 1 point
    - Reduced elbow extension = 1 point
    - Facial features (3/5): dolichocephaly, enophthalmos, downslanting palpebral fissures, malar hypoplasia, retrognathia) = 1 point
    - Skin striae = 1 point

For individuals without a family history of Marfan syndrome, the presence of 1 of any of the following criteria is diagnostic:

- Aortic criterion (aortic diameter Z-score ≥2 or aortic root dissection) **and** ectopia lentis*
- Aortic criterion (aortic diameter Z-score ≥2 or aortic root dissection) **and** a causal *FBN1* pathogenic variant
- Aortic criterion (aortic diameter Z-score ≥2 or aortic root dissection) **and** a systemic score ≥7*
- Ectopia lentis **and** a causal *FBN1* pathogenic variant that has been identified in an individual with aortic aneurysm

For individuals with a family history (as defined by presence of the above criteria in a first- or second-degree relative), the presence of 1 of any of the following criteria is diagnostic for Marfan syndrome:

- Ectopia lentis
- Systemic score ≥7 points*
- Aortic criterion (aortic diameter Z-score ≥2 in person older than 20 years, Z-score ≥3 if younger than 20 years, or aortic root dissection)

For criteria with an asterisk (*), the diagnosis of Marfan syndrome can only be made after exclusion of vascular Ehlers-Danlos syndrome (via *COL3A1* testing), as well as Shprintzen-Goldberg syndrome and Loeys-Dietz syndrome (via an aneurysm panel comprising *TGFBR1*, *TGFBR2*, *SMAD2*, *SMAD3*, *TGFB2*, *TGFB3*, and *SKI*).

This patient has increased arm spam and decreased upper-to-lower segment ratio (1 point), 3/5 facial features (1 point), pectus carinatum (2 points), kyphosis (1 point), and protruding heels and high-arched feet (2 points). She meets the systemic score for diagnosis. The best next step is to proceed with echocardiography (Answer A).

When the patient had testing for a skeletal disorders gene panel (Answer C), a pathogenic variant in *FBN1* (c.1285C>T [p.Arg429*]) was identified. However, the clinical diagnostic criteria must be met to diagnose Marfan syndrome, even when an *FBN1* pathogenic variant is identified, as noted above.

Educational Objective
Guide the diagnostic approach for a patient with tall stature and features suggestive of Marfan syndrome.

Reference(s)

Hannema SE, Sävendahl L. The evaluation and management of tall stature. *Horm Res Paediatr.* 2016;85(5):347-352. PMID: 26845047

Loeys BL, Dietz HC, Braverman AC, et al. The revised Ghent nosology for the Marfan syndrome. *J Med Genet.* 2010;47(7):476-485. PMID: 20591885

Sakai LY, Keene DR, Renard M, De Backer J. FBN1: the disease-causing gene for Marfan syndrome and other genetic disorders. *Gene.* 2016;591(1):279-291. PMID: 27437668

Radke RM, Baumgartner H. Diagnosis and treatment of Marfan syndrome: an update. *Heart.* 2014;100(17):1382-1391. PMID: 24777611

70 ANSWER: D) Start propranolol

This patient has presumed amiodarone-induced thyrotoxicosis (AIT). Of the options given, the addition of a β-adrenergic blocker is the best next step. He is thyrotoxic and very symptomatic. While he does not have tachycardia (due to his prior cardiac procedures and current medication regimen), he has many other symptoms, including tremor, anxiety, and difficulty concentrating. Propranolol (Answer D) is one of the more lipophilic β-adrenergic blockers (as is metoprolol), and it should cross the blood brain barrier, making it a better choice to target his symptoms than more hydrophilic β-adrenergic blockers such as nadolol. The addition of a β-blocker would usually bring concern for bradycardia; however, this patient has a pacemaker and therefore β-blockade can be added safely without risk of severe bradycardia. In this patient, heart rate cannot be used as a good measure of symptom control.

Patients taking amiodarone can develop thyroid dysfunction any time they are on the drug and even several months after discontinuation due to its long half-life. Amiodarone can cause thyrotoxicosis in several ways, both related and unrelated to its iodine content.

Type 1 AIT is due to the presence of excess iodine substrate leading to overproduction of thyroid hormone (the Jod-Basedow effect). This is seen most often in persons with underlying Graves disease, persons with multinodular goiter (not common in children), or in areas with endemic low iodine levels. Thyrotropin-receptor antibodies may be positive, and ultrasonography may show increased vascularity or multiple nodules. Since excess production of thyroid hormone is the main problem, blocking thyroid hormone production with methimazole is the mainstay of treatment.

Type 2 AIT is due to the cytotoxic effect of amiodarone on the thyroid gland resulting in a destructive thyroiditis. Typically, there is no history of autoimmune thyroid disease and ultrasonography may show decreased vascularity. This thyroiditis is usually self-limited and may be brief. In patients with minimal symptoms, observation may be sufficient. However, in patients with significant symptoms, prednisone typically results in rapid improvement within a few weeks. The prednisone dosage should be slowly weaned over several months.

Based on this patient's test results, it is not clear whether he has type 1, type 2, or mixed type 1 and type 2 AIT. In this situation, it is reasonable to either start steroids alone or both steroids and methimazole and to monitor closely. Rapid improvement in thyroid laboratory test results (within 2 weeks) favors type 2 AIT and prednisone alone can be continued. However, lack of rapid response to either prednisone alone or a combination of prednisone and methimazole favors type 1 or mixed type 1 and type 2 and methimazole should be continued or added.

Neither radioactive uptake scans (Answer B) nor ^{99m}Tc pertechnetate scans (Answer C) have been shown to be useful in distinguishing type 1 from type 2 AIT. The high iodine content of amiodarone also precludes the use of radioactive iodine for ablation of a thyrotoxic gland.

Urgent subtotal thyroidectomy (Answer A) may be necessary in a patient who is critically ill and who cannot be stabilized medically. While this child is very symptomatic, he is stable and there is no indication to treat surgically without initial β-blockade followed by attempted medical management of his AIT.

Discontinuation of amiodarone (Answer E) should not be considered in this patient for several reasons:

(1) Amiodarone has a very long half-life, and its effect on the thyroid can last many months after the medication is discontinued; therefore, this step will not result in rapid improvement.
(2) Amiodarone (through inhibition of type 2 deiodinase) decreases T_3 levels. His laboratory test results show a disproportionately high free T_4 concentration compared with the total T_3 concentration. Discontinuation of amiodarone would lead to increased conversion to T_3 and could make him more thyrotoxic in the short term.
(3) This patient has a serious cardiac condition. He is doing well on his current cardiac medication regimen, and discontinuation of amiodarone could result in cardiac destabilization.

Educational Objective
Distinguish between various types of amiodarone-induced thyroid disease and recommend the best management approach.

Reference(s)
Ylli D, Wartofsky L, Burman KD. Evaluation and treatment of amiodarone-induced thyroid disorders. *J Clin Endocrinol Metab*. 2021;106(1):226-236. PMID: 33159436

Bartalena L, Bogazzi F, Chiovato L, Hubalewska-Dydejczyk A, Links TP, Vanderpump M. 2018 European Thyroid Association (ETA) guidelines for the management of amiodarone-associated thyroid dysfunction. *Eur Thyroid J*. 2018;7(2):55-66. PMID: 29594056

71 ANSWER: D) Offer GH therapy with no changes to planned MRI surveillance
Children and adolescents with brain tumors affecting the hypothalamus and pituitary frequently develop multiple pituitary hormone deficiencies, including GH deficiency. Indeed, growth impairment is a common presenting manifestation of children with craniopharyngioma, the prototypic nonmalignant hypothalamic/pituitary tumor of childhood. Treatment of children with craniopharyngioma often includes surgical resection with or without radiation therapy. Whether from the tumor itself or subsequent treatment, GH deficiency is highly prevalent, occurring in an estimated 75% of individuals. As in this case, the diagnosis of GH deficiency is often clear, with decreased height percentile (especially relative to genetic potential), decreased height velocity, low growth factors despite adequate nutrition, and delayed bone age. Thus, provocative testing (Answer E) is not necessary to establish the diagnosis, especially in this clinical scenario where the patient has short stature, decreased growth velocity, and multiple pituitary hormone deficiencies.

Endocrinologists replace some hormones affected by hypothalamic/pituitary injury (ie, vasopressin, thyroid hormone, cortisol, and sex steroids) as soon as their deficiencies are diagnosed, but GH replacement is often delayed because of theoretical concerns that the growth-promoting effects of GH could confer increased risk for tumor recurrence. Indeed, in preclinical model systems (eg, local expression of GH and associated intracellular signaling in breast cancer) and clinical examples of GH excess (eg, acromegaly), GH-axis activity and carcinogenesis demonstrate a mechanistic connection. In contrast, physiologic pituitary and/or exogenous GH are not associated with tumor formation. Consistent with these findings, observational studies of individuals with craniopharyngioma and nonmalignant intracranial tumors have not documented an association between GH treatment and increased risk of tumor recurrence. Epidemiological studies have suggested a connection between GH treatment and malignancy in individuals with cancer predisposition syndromes (eg, Noonan syndrome, Fanconi anemia, and Bloom syndrome).

A recently updated consensus statement summarizing the available evidence concurs that there is no excess risk of tumor recurrence in individuals with nonmalignant intracranial tumors who are treated with GH. In children who have completed definitive treatment for craniopharyngioma and have radiologically stable disease, GH replacement is reasonable to start as early as 3 months after treatment with a view to optimize linear growth and body composition (increased muscle and bone mass, decreased fat mass). Thus, counseling the family that GH therapy is contraindicated (Answer A) or continuing to observe for another 12 months and offering GH therapy if there is no tumor recurrence (Answer B) is incorrect. In addition to growth and body composition, observational studies also suggest that quality of life is better preserved in children with craniopharyngioma who receive GH therapy.

No change in the frequency of tumor surveillance is recommended after GH initiation, even with residual disease (thus, Answer D is correct and Answer C is incorrect). For malignant brain tumors, a waiting period of at least 12 months is advised because of the risk of tumor relapse, which is highest during the initial year after treatment.

For all patients, individualized risk-benefit assessment and discussion, along with multidisciplinary collaboration among endocrinologists, neurooncologists, and neurosurgeons, is recommended when making the decision to start GH therapy.

Educational Objective
Describe the evidence related to risks and benefits of GH therapy for survivors of nonmalignant intracranial tumors.

Reference(s)
Muller HL. The diagnosis and treatment of craniopharyngioma. *Neuroendocrinology.* 2020;110(9-10):753-766. PMID: 31678973

Boguszewski MCS, Cardoso-Demartini AA, Boguszewski CL, et al. Safety of growth hormone (GH) treatment in GH deficient children and adults treated for cancer and non-malignant intracranial tumors-a review of research and clinical practice. *Pituitary.* 2021;24(5):810-827. PMID: 34304361

Boguszewski MCS, Boguszewski CL, Chemaitilly W, et al. Safety of growth hormone replacement in survivors of cancer and intracranial and pituitary tumours: a consensus statement. *Eur J Endocrinol.* 2022;186(6):P35-P52. PMID: 35319491

Heinks K, Boekhoff S, Hoffmann A, et al. Quality of life and growth after childhood craniopharyngioma: results of the multinational trial KRANIOPHARYNGEOM 2007. *Endocrine.* 2018;59(2):364-372. PMID: 29230635

72 ANSWER: C) Electrocardiography and cardiac evaluation
This patient has autonomic nervous system dysfunction (ANSD) related to type 1 diabetes. ANSD can present with impairments in blood pressure regulation, heart rate control, and thermoregulation. The large fluctuations in blood glucose concentrations associated with type 1 diabetes tend to place these patients at particularly greater risk, even when there are no associated complications. Cardiac autonomic neuropathy is a serious and deadly component of ANSD. It is important to detect early autonomic disturbances, such as reduced heart rate variability, reduced baroreflex sensitivity, hypertension, and impending heart failure, which are all known to be dependent on functional autonomic abnormalities. The patient in this vignette is hypertensive, anxious yet bradycardic, and most likely dehydrated. Electrocardiography and echocardiography (Answer C) are necessary to assess cardiac contractility and function.

Celiac disease screening (Answer B) by measuring tissue transaminase (tTG) IgA and total IgA (tissue transglutaminase [tTG] IgG and gliadin antibodies if IgA deficient) is recommended soon after diabetes diagnosis, repeated within 2 years, and then 5 years after diagnosis. Screening should be done sooner if symptoms develop. Although the patient in this vignette should be screened for celiac disease, his symptoms are consistent with autonomic nervous system dysfunction, so such screening is not the best next step.

Highly stimulating substances, such as methamphetamines or cocaine, could induce some of the symptoms he is experiencing. This patient admits to marijuana use and vaping, but he states that he does not use other illicit drugs. A recent urine toxicology screen is negative. Thus, repeating urine toxicology screening (Answer A) is not the best next step.

His urine sample indicates mild ketosis and no proteinuria. Although urine protein screening (Answer C) is important to monitor yearly, this would not be helpful in the management of his current symptoms.

Brain MRI (Answer D) would not be helpful because there are no signs or symptoms of acute intracranial pathology.

Management of type 1 diabetes relies on an integrated regimen of diet, timely and appropriate insulin dosing, and regular exercise, all of which help improve autonomic dysfunction and prevent poor cardiac outcomes. Being aware of subtle changes in blood pressure and pulse rate is important at clinical visits. Daily physical activity should be encouraged as much as tight glycemic control.

Educational Objective
Identify autonomic dysfunction as a diabetes mellitus–related complication.

Reference(s)
Rosengård-Bärlund M, Bernardi L, Fagerudd J, et al; FinnDiane Study Group. Early autonomic dysfunction in type 1 diabetes: a reversible disorder? *Diabetologia*. 2009;52(6):1164-1172. PMID: 19340407

Weston PJ, James MA, Panerai RB, McNally PG, Potter JF, Thurston H. Evidence of defective cardiovascular regulation in insulin-dependent diabetic patients without clinical autonomic dysfunction. *Diabetes Res Clin Pract*. 1998;42(3):141-148. PMID: 9925343

McGinn R, Kenny GP. Autonomic dysfunction associated with type 1 diabetes: a role for fitness? *Clin Auton Res*. 2014;24(6):249-251. PMID: 25398261

73 ANSWER: D) *IGF1R*

The child in this vignette has short stature and a history of intrauterine growth restriction. Her body proportions are described as normal, but she has microcephaly. Additionally, her father had a similar clinical picture with intrauterine growth restriction, which seemed to partially respond to exogenous GH therapy. Her mother had no notable medical history and normal height.

Linear growth in humans is orchestrated to a great extent by the GH–IGF-1 axis. GHRH produced in the hypothalamus stimulates pituitary somatotrophs to make GH (GH/somatotropin). In turn, GH interacts with its receptor, mainly in the liver but also in peripheral tissues, to induce IGF-1 production after a series of events in the postreceptor cascade involving the JAK-STAT system. Dimerization of the GH receptor occurs after GH interacts with the extracellular domain of the receptor and is followed by association with cytoplasmic JAK2, which phosphorylates itself and phosphorylates the intracellular domain of the GH receptor. This allows recruitment of STAT5B, which homodimerizes after phosphorylation. The STAT5B homodimer then moves to the nucleus and binds to DNA to promote expression of several genes, including *IGF1* (encodes IGF-1), *IGFBP3* (encodes IGFBP-3), and *IGFALS* (encodes acid-labile subunit).

The IGF system has a pivotal role in human growth during fetal life, as well as postnatally in infancy and puberty. Intrauterine growth is largely dependent on the IGF system, which includes IGF-1 and IGF-2. It is important, however, to recognize that while IGF-1 secretion is dependent on GH postnatally, both IGF-1 and IGF-2 are secreted during intrauterine life independent of GH stimulation, except in the last few weeks before term. Insulin, placental sufficiency, and fetal nutrition are thought to be among the drivers of intrauterine IGF-1 and IGF-2 production. Consequently, prenatal GH deficiency, as seen in individuals with *GH1* gene deletions (not included in the answer options) has minimal to no effect on prenatal growth. Additionally, IGF-1 concentrations are typically low in individuals with GH deficiency, in contrast to the patient in this vignette whose IGF-1 is elevated.

Elevated IGF-1 concentrations can be seen in individuals with SSDA (short stature, Dauber-Argente type), an autosomal recessive disorder associated with loss-of-function pathogenic variants in the *PAPPA2* gene (Answer A). *PAPPA2* encodes the pregnancy-associated plasma protein-A2, or pappalysin-2, a protease that promotes IGF-1 bioavailability by cleaving it from the ternary complex it forms with the IGF-binding proteins and acid-labile subunit. Concentrations of acid-labile subunit, IGFBP-3, and IGF-1 are elevated in affected individuals; however, bioavailable IGF-1 is low. The patient in this vignette has intrauterine growth restriction, while individuals with SSDA have postnatal growth retardation that usually starts at age 6 to 8 years. The patient in this vignette most likely inherited the condition from her affected father while the mother seemed unaffected. This is consistent with a dominant mode of inheritance, while SSDA is autosomal recessive. Additional features of SSDA include mild microcephaly, small chin, thin long bones, long fingers and toes, delayed dentition, decreased enamel, and decreased dentin density.

GH insensitivity syndrome in its classic form (Laron syndrome) is associated with abnormalities of the GH receptor (Answer B), but it can also result from abnormalities in the post receptor cascade, particularly STAT5B deficiency (Answer E). Individuals with GH insensitivity syndrome have little to no impairment of prenatal growth given that the fetal IGF system (IGF-1 and IGF-2) is independent from GH stimulation as discussed above. Once again, IGF-1 levels in postnatal life are low in these individuals, contrary to what is seen in the patient presented in the vignette. Patients with GH insensitivity syndrome associated with STAT5B deficiency also have altered immune responses manifested with chronic pulmonary disease and alteration of T-cell homeostasis, features that are not characteristic of GH insensitivity syndrome due to *GHR* pathogenic variants. Interestingly, manipulated alterations of the *IGF2* gene in a mouse model cause significant reduction of intrauterine growth with no effect on postnatal growth, while *IGF1* gene abnormalities cause both intrauterine and postnatal growth failure.

Pathogenic variants in the *IGF1* gene (Answer C), which cause prenatal IGF-1 deficiency, result in both prenatal and postnatal growth failure as seen in this patient. However, IGF-1 concentrations would be low, not elevated as in this vignette. Individuals with *IGF1* pathogenic variants also present with microcephaly and intellectual disability, providing some evidence of the importance of IGF-1 for brain development.

Compound heterozygous point variants in the *IGF1R* gene (Answer D) have been described in children with intrauterine and postnatal growth failure and elevated IGF-1 concentrations, consistent with a syndrome of resistance to IGF-1, as seen in this patient. Microcephaly and normal to mildly affected neurological development can be present. No abnormalities in body proportions have been described.

Educational Objective
Explain the differential effects of GH and IGF-1 on prenatal and postnatal growth to help guide the diagnostic assessment of growth disorders.

Reference(s)
Abuzzahab MJ, Schneider A, Goddard A, et al; Intrauterine Growth Retardation (IUGR) Study Group. IGF-I receptor mutations resulting in intrauterine and postnatal growth retardation. *N Engl J Med.* 2003;349(23):2211-2222. PMID: 14657428

Gkourogianni A, Andrade AC, Jonsson BA, et al. Pre- and postnatal growth failure with microcephaly due to two novel heterozygous IGF1R mutations and response to growth hormone treatment. *Acta Paediatr.* 2020;109(10):2067-2074. PMID: 32037650

Göpel E, Rockstroh D, Pfäffle H, et al. A comprehensive cohort analysis comparing growth and GH therapy response in IGF1R mutation carriers and SGA children. *J Clin Endocrinol Metab.* 2020;105(4):dgz165. PMID: 31680140

Klammt J, Neumann D, Gevers EF, et al. Dominant-negative *STAT5B* mutations cause growth hormone insensitivity with short stature and mild immune dysregulation. *Nat Commun.* 2018;9(1):2105. PMID: 29844444

Hwa V, Fujimoto M, Zhu G, et al. Genetic causes of growth hormone insensitivity beyond GHR. *Rev Endocr Metab Disord.* 2021;22(1):43-58. PMID: 33029712

Dauber A, Munoz-Calvo MT, Barrios V, et al. Mutations in pregnancy-associated plasma protein A2 cause short stature due to low IGF-I availability. *EMBO Molec Med.* 2016;8:363-374. PMID: 26902202

74 ANSWER: C) Measure 8-AM serum cortisol and ACTH

This patient has symptoms, signs, and laboratory studies consistent with primary hypothyroidism due to autoimmune thyroiditis, which will require treatment with levothyroxine. However, there are additional abnormalities that are not explained by hypothyroidism, including nausea, weight loss, hyperkalemia, metabolic acidosis, and clinical evidence of volume depletion. These findings are suspicious for primary adrenal insufficiency, which is most often caused by autoimmune adrenalitis and should be suspected in a patient with appropriate clinical findings and/or a personal and family history of autoimmunity. Of note, hyponatremia frequently is present in patients with primary adrenal insufficiency (due to volume depletion), but it can also be observed in severe hypothyroidism due to decreased renal water excretion.

In a patient with compensated adrenal insufficiency, initiation of levothyroxine for hypothyroidism can provoke life-threatening adrenal crisis due to increased metabolic clearance of cortisol. Therefore, suspected adrenal insufficiency must be evaluated (Answer C), and treated if present, prior to initiation of levothyroxine (Answers A and B).

Despite the association, primary adrenal insufficiency is rare among children with autoimmune thyroiditis; therefore, it is not necessary to evaluate all patients with autoimmune thyroiditis for adrenal insufficiency before initiating levothyroxine. However, the possibility should be considered in any patient with autoimmune thyroiditis, and adrenal function should be evaluated if clinically indicated, prior to initiating levothyroxine.

This patient's personal and family history of autoimmunity place her at increased risk of celiac disease, which could contribute to her symptoms of nausea and weight loss. The prevalence of celiac disease in children with autoimmune thyroiditis is around 6%. Therefore, it would be reasonable to measure serum tissue transglutaminase IgA and total IgA in this patient (Answer D). However, her findings of primary adrenal insufficiency require urgent evaluation that should be performed first to avoid potentially life-threatening adrenal crisis.

Thyroid ultrasonography (Answer E) is indicated for the evaluation of known or suspected thyroid nodules and may be useful in cases of goiter (thyroid enlargement) of unknown cause. In this patient with a symmetric goiter, no palpable nodules, and positive TPO antibodies, there is no reason to suspect a thyroid nodule and the etiology of thyroid enlargement (autoimmune thyroiditis) is clear, so thyroid ultrasonography is not indicated.

Educational Objective
Evaluate and manage concurrent autoimmune hypothyroidism and primary adrenal insufficiency.

Reference(s)
Peterson RE. The influence of the thyroid on adrenal cortical function. *J Clin Invest.* 1958;37(5):736-743. PMID: 13539216

Bright GM, Blizzard RM, Kaiser DL, Clarke WL. Organ-specific autoantibodies in children with common endocrine diseases. *J Pediatr.* 1982;100(1):8-14. PMID: 7035635

Roy A, Laszkowska M, Sundström J, et al. Prevalence of celiac disease in patients with autoimmune thyroid disease: a meta-analysis. *Thyroid.* 2016;26(7):880-890. PMID: 27256300

75 ANSWER: D) Start a low-phosphate diet
Chronic hyperphosphatemia is associated with an increased risk of cardiovascular events and mortality in adult patients. While it is unclear whether these risks are increased in children, this patient's hypoparathyroidism is lifelong and thus efforts should be made to improve the calcium x phosphate product to less than $55 \text{ mg}^2/\text{dL}^2$ to reduce risk of ectopic calcifications and cardiac comorbidities. First-line treatment to reduce hyperphosphatemia in patients with hypoparathyroidism whose serum calcium levels are adequately controlled is to reduce dietary intake of phosphate (Answer D). Phosphate is plentiful in most dairy, meats, and processed foods. Thus, maintaining a low-phosphate diet can be challenging for many children, especially those who attend school and consume school lunch. Consultation with a dietician is recommended to teach families how to review ingredient lists because phosphate is not typically listed on nutrition facts labels.

If dietary interventions are not successful, phosphate binders can be added to meals to reduce the amount of phosphate absorbed from the gastrointestinal tract and increase the amount excreted in the stool. Calcium carbonate taken with meals can function as a phosphate binder, and increasing the dosage to 3 times daily (Answer A) may help reduce serum phosphate levels. However, he already has a relatively high calcium dosage for body size, a normal ionized calcium concentration, and hypercalciuria. Thus, increasing calcium carbonate is not the best next step.

Sevelamer (Answer C) is another phosphate binder. It is associated with gastrointestinal adverse effects and is therefore difficult for many children to tolerate. Given that the patient has previously tried this medication and was not able to tolerate it, this approach is unlikely to be successful.

He has an elevated urine calcium-to-creatinine ratio, which increases the risk for developing nephrocalcinosis. Higher calcitriol dosages have been associated with higher serum calcium concentrations and increased urinary calcium excretion. Urinary calcium excretion tends to be more sensitive to changes in vitamin D analogues in patients with pathogenic variants in the gene encoding the calcium-sensing receptor. While findings on kidney ultrasonography are reassuring, increasing the calcitriol dosage (Answer B) is not the best next step.

Recombinant human PTH (rhPTH) replacement therapy (Answer E) is an appealing choice, and it has been shown to reduce the need for calcium and calcitriol supplementation in small studies of pediatric patients. Two or 3 injections daily were typically needed to limit peaks and troughs of serum calcium concentrations, which can contribute to nephrocalcinosis and tetany, respectively. Continuous rhPTH infusions via pump therapy have been successful in some children but also pose additional challenges. There are limited long-term data on the safety and efficacy of rhPTH in pediatric hypoparathyroidism. Thus, this treatment is not the best next step.

Educational Objective
Explain the complications of chronic hyperphosphatemia in patients with hypoparathyroidism and recommend treatment.

Reference(s)
De Sanctis V, Soliman AT, Di Maio S, Kattamis C. The management of permanent primary hypoparathyroidism in children and adolescents: a complex task. *Pediatr Endocrinol Rev.* 2018;16(1):194-202. PMID: 30371038

Winer KK, Kelly A, Johns A, et al. Long-term parathyroid hormone 1-34 replacement therapy in children with hypoparathyroidism. *J Pediatr.* 2018;203:391-399.e1. PMID: 30470382

76   ANSWER: C) Vitamin B₁

Bariatric surgery has become increasingly acceptable as an option for youth with severe obesity and/or metabolic comorbidities. The most commonly used bariatric procedures in adolescents are Roux-en-Y gastric bypass (RYGB) and sleeve gastrectomy (SG), although the latter has become the predominant procedure. While bariatric procedures can be effective for weight reduction and reversal of metabolic comorbidities, risk for nutritional deficiencies postoperatively remains a significant concern. In a 5-year prospective cohort study of teens who underwent RYGB or SG, Xanthakos et al found that at least 2 nutritional deficiencies were detected by 5 years in 59% of patients who underwent RYGB and in 27% of patients who underwent SG, although 22.5% and 17.3% of participants, respectively, already had at least 2 deficiencies by 6 months postoperatively. In particular, there is concern that adolescents may be at heightened risk for nutritional deficiencies because of low adherence to supplementation and a longer potential lifespan with altered physiology. Thus, prompt recognition and treatment of such deficiencies is crucial to avoid complications and is the reason why lifelong micronutrient supplementation is recommended.

The patient in this vignette is exhibiting symptoms that are most consistent with vitamin B₁, or thiamine, deficiency (Answer C). Thiamine deficiency is not an uncommon complication of bariatric procedures, and recommendations are to provide prophylactic supplementation in all bariatric patients. Nausea, vomiting, and loss of appetite may be early, nonspecific signs of thiamine deficiency. If not promptly recognized and treated, thiamine deficiency can progress to Wernicke encephalopathy, which is an acute neuropsychiatric syndrome characterized by the triad of ataxia, eye movement disorders, and mental status changes. Prophylaxis of Wernicke encephalopathy following early signs and symptoms requires use of parenteral vitamin supplements because oral supplements are not absorbed in significant amounts. Data have shown that adolescent and young adult bariatric patients seem to be more protected against mental status changes, so in this patient population, attention should be paid to any sensorimotor problems that arise.

Hypoferritinemia (Answer A) and vitamin B₁₂ deficiency (Answer D) are some of the most common nutritional deficiencies reported in adolescent bariatric patients postoperatively. Both deficiencies can lead to fatigue; chronic anemia; exercise intolerance; and neurologic dysfunction such as poor concentration, restless leg syndrome, weakness, dizziness, and paresthesias.

Vitamin A deficiency (Answer B) does not seem to be a significant finding in adolescent bariatric patients after RYGB or SG procedures.

Vitamin D deficiency (Answer E) is common both preoperatively and postoperatively in adolescent and adult bariatric patients. Chronic vitamin D deficiency can impair bone health and lead to future fracture risk.

Educational Objective
Identify the most common nutritional deficiencies following bariatric surgery in adolescent patients.

Reference(s)
Xanthakos SA, Khoury JC, Inge TH, et al; Teen Longitudinal Assessment of Bariatric Surgery Consortium. Nutritional risks in adolescents after bariatric surgery. *Clin Gastroenterol Hepatol.* 2020;18(5):1070-1081.e5. PMID: 31706057

Halloun R, Weiss R. Bariatric surgery in adolescents with obesity: long-term perspectives and potential alternatives. *Horm Res Paediatr.* 2022;95(2):193-203. PMID: 34758466

Oudman E, Wijnia JW, van Dam M, Biter LU, Postma A. Preventing Wernicke encephalopathy after bariatric surgery. *Obes Surg.* 2018;28(7):2060-2068. PMID: 29693218

77 ANSWER: B) Thyroid-stimulating immunoglobulin

This infant's laboratory evaluation shows severe elevation of serum thyroid hormone, but he has no clinical findings of thyrotoxicosis. Symptoms and signs of neonatal thyrotoxicosis can include increased body temperature; decreased weight; stare; tachycardia; irritability; restlessness; or warm, moist skin. In cases of neonatal Graves disease, goiter or proptosis may be present. When the results of laboratory studies are inconsistent with the clinical presentation, preanalytical or analytical factors affecting the laboratory measurements should be considered.

This patient is being treated with biotin, which is found in some commercial supplements (often promoted for hair/nail health), but it may be used for the management of refractory neonatal seizures, of which one treatable cause is congenital biotinidase deficiency. Large doses of biotin (>5 to 10 mg daily) can confound the laboratory assessment of thyroid function due to interference with some competitive-binding assays whose design depends on the binding of biotin to the protein avidin. The direction of confounding of each analyte (falsely high or falsely low) depends on the specific assay, but in many assays, biotin causes falsely low TSH and falsely high free T_4, total and free T_3, and/or TRAb.

Since this patient is clinically euthyroid, the TSH and free T_4 abnormalities are most likely caused by biotin treatment. In this situation, false elevations most likely also would be observed in free T_3 (Answer A), total T_3 (Answer C), total T_4 (Answer D), and TRAb (Answer E). Unlike TRAb assays, which measure binding of serum antibodies to TSH receptors (often using avidin-biotin interactions), thyroid-stimulating immunoglobulin (Answer B) has traditionally been a functional assay measuring the ability of serum antibodies directly to activate TSH receptors expressed in cell systems. Such a thyroid-stimulating immunoglobulin assay is not subject to interference from biotin, and its value would be normal in this patient. Some newer assays for thyroid-stimulating immunoglobulin are binding assays rather than traditional functional assays, but to date biotin interference with thyroid-stimulating immunoglobulin assays has not been reported.

In addition to thyroid function tests, some immunoassays for other hormones (including PTH, LH, FSH, estradiol, testosterone, DHEA-S, cortisol, prolactin, and 25-hydroxyvitamin D) may use biotin and be confounded by biotin ingestion. In general, discontinuation of biotin intake for 48 to 72 hours before blood sampling is sufficient to avoid assay interference.

Educational Objective
Diagnose biotin interference in the assessment of biochemical thyrotoxicosis and distinguish laboratory thyroid assays affected by interference.

Reference(s)
Barbesino G. Misdiagnosis of Graves' disease with apparent severe hyperthyroidism in a patient taking biotin megadoses. *Thyroid.* 2016;26(6):860-863. PMID: 27043844

Li D, Radulescu A, Shrestha RT, et al. Association of biotin ingestion with performance of hormone and nonhormone assays in healthy adults. *JAMA.* 2017;318(12):1150-1160. PMID: 28973622

78 ANSWER: D) Refer to pulmonology

This patient has several classic clinical features suggestive of cystic fibrosis (recurrent pneumonia since infancy, fatty diarrhea, poor weight gain [requiring nutrition supplements], poor growth). All 50 states screen for cystic fibrosis as part of newborn screening. However, this patient had poor prenatal care and was born at home, thus delaying the diagnosis. She needs a sweat chloride test and/or genetic testing for pathogenic variants in the *CFTR* gene. Poor growth in patients with cystic fibrosis is multifactorial and is related to decreased GH release, GH resistance, growth plate abnormalities, and chondrocyte dysfunction. Confirming this patient's diagnosis and optimizing treatment for cystic fibrosis is critical to maximizing growth potential. She should be referred to pulmonology (Answer D). In persons with cystic fibrosis, short stature (<5th percentile for height) is an independent risk factor for mortality along with lung function, malnutrition, and cystic fibrosis–related diabetes. Monitoring both height and weight is critical for patients with cystic fibrosis, because height has added prognostic significance in outcomes. Higher weight-for-age at age 4 years is associated with improved pulmonary function, height, and pubertal progression.

Although some small studies have shown that GH therapy improves growth, larger studies are needed to provide clear evidence that the benefits of GH outweigh risks in patients with cystic fibrosis. Thus, GH provocative testing (Answer A) should not be performed before the underlying pathology is evaluated and treated. Newer drugs to treat cystic fibrosis using CFTR modulators (ivacaftor, lumacaftor/ivacaftor combination therapy), which target specific defects in the CFTR protein, show promising results in promoting weight gain and growth in affected children.

Most patients who have poor growth in early childhood do not catch up by adulthood. Thus, her family should not be reassured that she will most likely attain her genetic potential for height as an adult (Answer C).

She does not have any features suggestive of Turner syndrome; thus, karyotype analysis (Answer B) could further delay the diagnosis of her underlying medical condition.

In children, celiac disease could initially present with poor growth with or without any additional symptoms or signs. However, this patient has a history of recurrent hospital admissions for pneumonia, which is characteristic of celiac disease (Answer E).

Educational Objective
Suspect cystic fibrosis based on clinical presentation and identify the factors associated with morbidity and mortality in patients with poor growth.

Reference(s)

Le TN, Anabtawi A, Putman MS, Tangpricha V, Stalvey MS. Growth failure and treatment in cystic fibrosis. *J Cyst Fibros.* 2019:18(Suppl 2):S82-S87. PMID: 31679733

Thaker V, Carter B, Putman M. Recombinant growth hormone therapy for cystic fibrosis in children and young adults. *Cochrane Database Syst Rev.* 2018;8(8):CD008901. PMID: 34424546

Marks MP, Heltshe SL, Baines A, Ramsey BW, Hoffman LR, Stalvey MS. Most short children with cystic fibrosis do not catch up by adulthood. *Nutrients.* 2021;13(12):4414. PMID: 34959966

79 ANSWER: C) Perform cosyntropin-stimulation testing

The patient in this vignette has clinical signs of androgen exposure, a prepubertal LH concentration, and elevated testosterone and androstenedione suggestive of an adrenal etiology. Findings are concerning for congenital adrenal hyperplasia (CAH) due to 11β-hydroxylase deficiency, as the degree of 17-hydroxyprogesterone elevation is not sufficient to explain his presentation. Given these findings, cosyntropin-stimulation testing (Answer C) is the most likely test to identify the underlying etiology. Results are shown (*see table*).

Measurement	Baseline	Stimulated
11-Deoxycortisol	2810 ng/dL (8-235 ng/dL) (SI: 81.2 nmol/L [0.2-6.8 nmol/L])	16,000 ng/dL (SI: 462.4 nmol/L)
17-Hydroxypregnenolone	378 ng/dL (<319 ng/dL) (SI: 11.3 nmol/L [<9.6 nmol/L])	1654 ng/dL (SI: 49.8 nmol/L)
17-Hydroxyprogesterone	146 ng/dL (<208 ng/dL) (SI: 4.4 nmol/L [<6.3 nmol/L])	433 ng/dL (SI: 13.1 nmol/L)
Pregnenolone	175 ng/dL (10-156 ng/dL)	533 ng/dL

Findings of very elevated 11-deoxycortisol at baseline without a significantly elevated 17-hydroxyprogesterone concentration can be sufficient to confirm the diagnosis of CAH secondary to 11β-hydroxylase deficiency. Basal 11-deoxycortisol levels are often elevated to several thousand ng/dL in the classic form but may be normal in mild cases. Thus, cosyntropin-stimulation testing may be needed when 11β-hydroxylase deficiency is suspected. Cosyntropin-stimulated levels of 11-deoxycortisol that are 5 times the normal range confirm the diagnosis. CAH due to 11β-hydroxylase deficiency is characterized by rapid skeletal maturation, precocious puberty, and rapid somatic growth, as well as virilization in female newborns. Hypertension is mild to moderate, and it is present in approximately two-thirds of individuals with the classic form of 11β-hydroxylase deficiency. Therapeutic goals are to reduce excess androgen and mineralocorticoid precursors by use of glucocorticoid administration.

To optimize growth, hydrocortisone in 2 to 3 doses daily is the preferred treatment of 11β-hydroxylase deficiency in children. Starting glucocorticoid replacement therapy (Answer E) without confirmatory diagnostic testing would be premature. Distinguishing between CAH secondary to 11β-hydroxylase deficiency vs 21-hydroxylase deficiency is important because of the high incidence of left ventricular hypertrophy and other consequences of longstanding hypertension that can occur in up to one-third of adults with 11β-hydroxylase deficiency. Additionally, bone age advancement is much greater than in 21-hydroxylase deficiency and may necessitate different interventions.

Brain MRI (Answer B) is not indicated, as this patient has presented with peripheral precocious puberty, not central precocious puberty. Familial male-limited precocious puberty typically presents before age 4 years with signs of virilization, elevated testosterone, suppressed gonadotropins, and mild testicular enlargement but not elevated adrenal androgens or steroid precursors as seen in this vignette. Male-limited precocious puberty is caused by activating variants in the *LHCGR* gene and only manifests in males. A combination of an antiandrogen and an aromatase inhibitor (Answer D) is currently considered the most effective approach for treatment of male-limited precocious puberty, but this would not be appropriate to treat CAH due to 11β-hydroxylase deficiency.

Adrenal MRI (Answer A) would be helpful in identifying a virilizing tumor such as adrenal cortical carcinoma. Adrenal cortical tumors are very rare; the incidence is 1 to 2 per million, whereas the incidence of CAH due to 11β-hydroxylase deficiency has an incidence of 1 in 100,000 to 1 in 200,000 newborns. In children, adrenal cortical tumors are most often found in association with genetic syndromes such as Li-Fraumeni syndrome, Beckwith-Wiedemann syndrome, multiple endocrine neoplasia type 1, and Carney complex. Less than 10% of adrenal cortical tumors present with virilization alone. As such, adrenal imaging is less likely to identify the cause of this patient's presentation.

Educational Objective
Identify an uncommon form of congenital adrenal hyperplasia as a cause of peripheral precocious puberty in a boy.

Reference(s)
Khattab A, Haider S, Kumar A, et al. Clinical, genetic, and structural basis of congenital adrenal hyperplasia due to 11β-hydroxylase deficiency. *Proc Natl Acad Sci U S A.* 2017;114(10):E1933-E1940. PMID: 28228528

Haddad NG, Eugster EA. Peripheral precocious puberty including congenital adrenal hyperplasia: causes, consequences, management and outcomes. *Best Pract Res Clin Endocrinol Metab.* 2017;33(3):101273. PMID: 31027974

80 ANSWER: C) Disease recurrence after initial therapy

This child's presentation is consistent with Cushing disease; pituitary MRI showed a 7-mm adenoma, prompting surgical resection. Consensus guidelines summarize current recommendations regarding the diagnosis, management, and ongoing surveillance of individuals with Cushing disease, including children. As in this case, impaired growth velocity and accumulation of excess central adiposity is characteristic of pediatric Cushing disease. Hypercortisolism is confirmed via overnight 1-mg dexamethasone-suppression testing and midnight salivary cortisol measurement. Hypercortisolism can also be assessed via 24-hour urinary free cortisol measurement. Similar algorithms are used in both children and adults to distinguish ACTH-dependent from ACTH-independent Cushing syndrome. As in adults, surgical resection is the first-line treatment for pediatric Cushing disease.

Racial/ethnic disparities have been noted in pediatric Cushing disease. Specifically, in a study of 129 children with Cushing disease, children of self-reported non-White race had a higher summary index of disease severity at presentation, a result driven by both higher cortisol levels and larger tumor size. The extent of growth impairment in pediatric Cushing disease reflects the cumulative exposure to glucocorticoid, and non-White children also have a lower height Z-score at presentation, raising the possibility that growth impairment takes longer to prompt specialty referral. As a result of more severe disease at presentation, Cushing disease in non-White children is also more refractory to treatment, with higher rates of persistent and/or recurrent disease (thus, Answer C is correct). After diagnosis, non-White children also have less consistent long-term follow-up.

Compared with White, non-Hispanic children, Hispanic and/or African American children tend to experience delays in diagnosis; therefore, they are more likely to be diagnosed at older, not younger, ages (thus, Answer A is incorrect). Because clinical disease is more severe at diagnosis in non-White children, there appears to be less, not more, diagnostic uncertainty (thus, Answer B is incorrect). No race-specific differences have been reported in rates of genetic predisposition for Cushing disease (thus, Answer D is incorrect).

Findings regarding disparities in pediatric Cushing disease recapitulate results of other investigations, including those focused on disparities in adults with Cushing disease and in children with CNS tumors of diverse causes. In adults with Cushing disease, racial/ethnic differences in presentation and postoperative outcomes have been described and are overall similar to findings in pediatric studies. Specifically, Black individuals with Cushing disease are more likely to have hypopituitarism and larger tumors (macroadenomas) at diagnosis. Perhaps as a consequence, remission is marginally less likely in Black adults with Cushing disease as compared with remission their White counterparts. In children with brain tumors of diverse causes, as in children with Cushing disease, differences in specific tumor prevalence among subgroups (higher prevalence in White individuals in some studies) are challenging to interpret, because non-White children appear less likely to undergo prompt diagnostic evaluation. One meta-analysis noted that racial/ethnic characteristics were inconsistently reported in epidemiological studies, limiting the overall availability of summary data. Insufficient representation of children from minority backgrounds in clinical trials is also a barrier to achieving insights regarding the extent to which treatment approaches can be generalized across the diverse cohort of children affected by Cushing disease (thus, Answer E is incorrect).

Potential factors underlying disparities that have been identified across studies include structural racism, both independently and as reflected in worse socioeconomic status, decreased access to subspecialty and referral centers, language barriers, and higher background rates of obesity in non-White subgroups (which leads clinicians to less often suspect rare etiologies). Policy solutions, as well as clinician education initiatives across primary and specialty care, are needed.

Educational Objective
Describe the contribution of race/ethnicity to disparities in disease outcomes in pediatric Cushing disease.

Reference(s)
Fleseriu M, Auchus R, Bancos I, et al. Consensus on diagnosis and management of Cushing's disease: a guideline update. *Lancet Diabetes Endocrinol.* 2021;9(12):847-875. PMID: 34687601

Gkourogianni A, Sinaii N, Jackson SH, et al. Pediatric Cushing disease: disparities in disease severity and outcomes in the Hispanic and African-American populations. *Pediatr Res.* 2017;82(2):272-277. PMID: 28422946

Ioachimescu AG, Goswami N, Handa T, Pappy A, Veledar E, Oyesiku NM. Racial disparities in acromegaly and Cushing's disease: a referral center study in 241 patients. *J Endocr Soc.* 2022;6(1):bvab176. PMID: 34934883

Nieblas-Bedolla E, Christophers B, Williams JR, Power-Hays A, Jimenez N, Rodriguez A. Racial and ethnic disparities among children with primary central nervous system tumors in the US. *J Neurooncol.* 2021;152(3):451-466. PMID: 33774801

Raphael JL, Lion KC, Bearer CF. Policy solutions to recruiting and retaining minority children in research. *Pediatr Res.* 2017;82(2):180-182. PMID: 28590464

81 ANSWER: D) Use of the phone app

Adolescence is one of the peak periods for onset of type 1 diabetes mellitus. The psychosocial vulnerability of teenagers coupled with the type 1 diabetes diagnosis, especially in the setting of diabetic ketoacidosis, can cause significant emotional stress. All adolescents should learn healthy coping strategies and skills to navigate this critical period while they are emerging as young adults. Coping is defined as adolescents' efforts to regulate their emotions, cognition, and behavior, as well as their situations and contexts, in reaction to stressful events or challenging circumstances. In general, there are 2 widely accepted types of coping skills: problem-focused coping and emotion-focused coping. Problem-focused coping strategies directly address the source of stress. Such strategies use cognitive reappraisal, generating problem-solving solutions, and taking action to solve the problem. Self-discovery of a smart phone app that can be used for insulin dose calculation (Answer D) is an example of this coping strategy. This type of initiative leads to self-confidence, emotional well-being, improved quality of life, and improved metabolic outcomes. In contrast, emotion-focused coping strategies aim to reduce the negative emotional response associated with stress. Emotion-focused coping involves a wide range of strategies, including seeking emotional support, denial, venting, and withdrawing from the situation. When emotional responses such as anger or sadness are peaking and unregulated, cognitive coping strategies such as cognitive reappraisal and problem solving are needed but are difficult for many adolescents to access. Adolescents with adjustment problems are more likely to use social withdrawal, avoidance (Answer A), venting (Answer E), mental disengagement (Answer B), and wishful thinking (Answer C), which can each be useful coping strategies in certain circumstances if used temporarily. However, they are considered to have negative long-term implications.

Improving adolescents' emotional regulation, coping, and decision-making represents an essential strategy for preventing externalizing behavior and its consequences in poor health outcomes. Young persons who can effectively recognize and regulate their emotions, who are able to process and respond to personal and situational demands, and who are strategic in their coping responses have a host of tools to deal adaptively with stressors and challenges.

Educational Objective
Assess coping and resilience in adolescents with type 1 diabetes mellitus.

Reference(s)

Modecki KL, Zimmer-Gembeck MJ, Guerra N. Emotion regulation, coping, and decision making: three linked skills for preventing externalizing problems in adolescence. *Child Dev.* 2017;88(2):417-426. PMID: 28195431

Meijer SA, Sinnema G, Bijstra JO, Mellenbergh GJ, Wolters WHG. Coping styles and locus of control as predictors for psychological adjustment of adolescents with a chronic illness. *Soc Sci Med.* 2002;54(9):1453-1461. PMID: 12058860

Waugh CE, Leslie-Miller CJ, Shing EZ, Furr RM, Nightingale CL, McLean TW. Adaptive and maladaptive forms of disengagement coping in caregivers of children with chronic illnesses. *Stress Health.* 2021;37(2):213-222. PMID: 32946684

Zimmer-Gembeck MJ, Skinner EA. Review: the development of coping across childhood and adolescence: an integrative review and critique of research. *Int J Behav Dev.* 2010;35:1-17.

82 ANSWER: E) Untreated maternal hyperthyroidism

This patient has laboratory values suggestive of central hypothyroidism. In this case, his hypothyroidism is likely due to prolonged untreated maternal hyperthyroidism (Answer E). Laboratory testing should be performed to exclude hypopituitarism even though his physical examination findings are not indicative of hypopituitarism (normal phallus, no hypotension). The etiology of maternal hyperthyroidism was not known, but the most likely cause of hyperthyroidism with such an elevated free T_4 concentration in a pregnant woman is Graves disease. The presence of TRAb in the infant also supports maternal Graves disease as the cause of maternal hyperthyroidism.

Neonates of mothers with Graves disease are at significant risk of complications, both in utero and postpartum. The most well-known concern for infants born to mothers with Graves disease is the development of fetal or neonatal hyperthyroidism. Less commonly, central hypothyroidism can occur and is described in infants born to mothers with inadequate treatment of their hyperthyroidism during pregnancy. The etiology of central hypothyroidism in these infants is not clearly understood, but prolonged early exposure to high T_4 levels in utero may impair maturation of the fetal hypothalamic-pituitary-thyroid axis. Alternatively, TRAb can bind directly to the TSH receptor in the pituitary gland, resulting in suppressed TSH production. Central hypothyroidism due to maternal Graves disease is typically transient, with recovery occurring between 3 and 19 months of age. Central hypothyroidism should be treated; some specialists recommend a gradual reduction of the levothyroxine dosage as the infant's pituitary-thyroid axis recovers, while others recommend treatment until 3 years of age.

These infants remain at risk for developing neonatal Grave disease, so monitoring for emergence of hyperthyroidism is important. Central hypothyroidism can occur prior to the development of neonatal hyperthyroidism. In this infant, the TRAb levels are low; therefore, he is at very low risk of developing hyperthyroidism (TRAb levels are typically at least 2 to 4 times the upper normal limit in infants who go on to develop neonatal Graves disease).

Prematurity (Answer B) is associated with hypothyroxinemia. Transient hypothyroxinemia of prematurity is defined by low concentrations of T_4 and normal or slightly low TSH concentrations. The severity of low T_3 and TSH would not be typical for that seen in prematurity alone.

TBL1X pathogenic variants (Answer D) are associated with central hypothyroidism and hearing loss. The timing of diagnosis of central hypothyroidism is variable, but it can occur in the newborn period. In the absence of an alternative explanation, and if no additional pituitary hormone deficiencies are diagnosed, genetic evaluation for isolated central hypothyroidism should be considered.

The *PROP1* gene (Answer C) encodes a protein essential for HESX-1 repression and POUF1 expression and is essential for the development of most types of anterior pituitary cells. Pathogenic variants often present with GH deficiency as the earliest manifestation. TSH and ACTH production can be normal initially with later development of deficiencies. If there was not an alternative explanation in this case, and the patient developed additional pituitary hormone deficiencies, the possibility of a *PROP1* pathogenic variant should be considered.

FOXE1 pathogenic variants (Answer A) are associated with thyroid dysgenesis and therefore primary hypothyroidism would be expected (elevated TSH with low or normal T_4 and T_3).

Educational Objective
Identify neonatal central hypothyroidism as a complication of uncontrolled maternal Graves disease in pregnancy.

Reference(s)

van der Kaay DC, Wasserman JD, Palmert MR. Management of neonates born to mothers with Graves' disease. *Pediatrics.* 2016;137(4):e20151878. PMID: 26980880

Forghani N, Aye T. Hypothyroxinemia and prematurity. *Neoreviews.* 2008;9(2):e66-e71.

Kempers MJE, van Trotsenburg ASP, van Rijn RR, et al. Loss of integrity of thyroid morphology and function in children born to mothers with inadequately treated Graves' disease. *J Clin Endocrinol Metab.* 2007;92(8):2984-2991. PMID: 17504907

83 ANSWER: E) *PAPSS2*

Inactivating pathogenic variants in *PAPSS2* (3'-phosphoadenosine 5'-phosphosulfate synthase 2) (Answer E) have been observed in patients with premature pubarche, defined as growth of pubic hair before age 8 years. The *PAPSS2* gene encodes 1 of 2 isoforms of PAPS synthase, an enzyme involved in the synthesis of PAPS. PAPS is the sulfate donor for SULT2A1 (sulfotransferase family 2A member 1), a sulfotransferase enzyme that catalyzes the sulfonation of steroids and bile acids in the liver and adrenal glands. In the adrenal gland, SULT2A1 is the major enzyme responsible for DHEA sulfation, converting DHEA to DHEA-S. Importantly, DHEA is the principal precursor of androgen synthesis in females. The biochemical hallmark indicative of a sulfonation defect is the combination of very low or undetectable circulating DHEA-S in the presence of high DHEA (*see figure*).

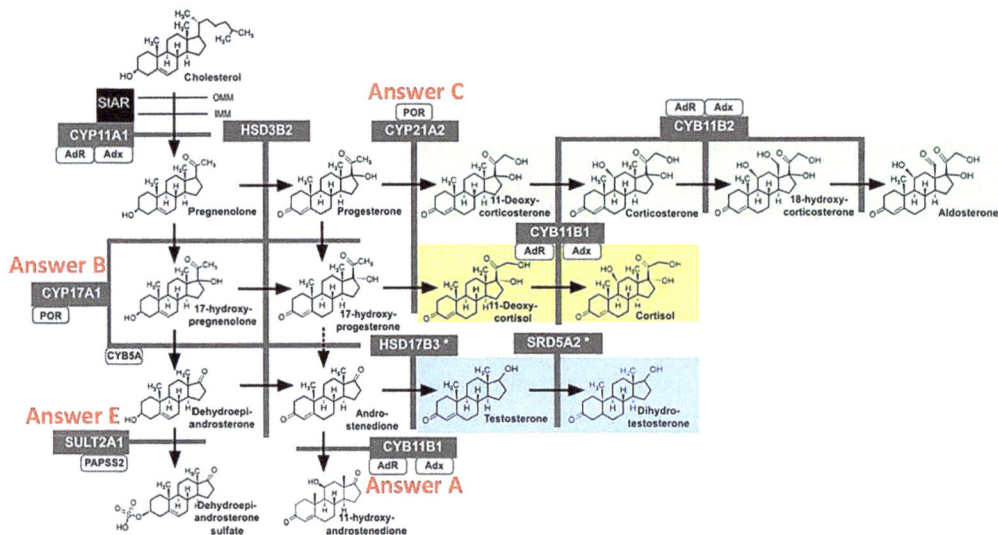

Reprinted with permission from Baranowski ES et al. *Horm Res Paediatr,* 2018; 89(5). © 2018 The Authors. Published by S. Karger AG, Basel.

Pathogenic variants in *PAPSS2* have also been documented in individuals with hyperandrogenism and polycystic ovary syndrome. Furthermore, deficiency is a cause of spondyloepimetaphyseal dysplasia (Pakistani type) and PAPSS2-related brachyolmia, in which impaired proteoglycan sulfation in chondrocytes is thought to lead to the bone phenotype. In cases of spondyloepimetaphyseal dysplasia and brachyolmia, a clear phenotype of virilization and hyperandrogenization is not always present.

Pathogenic variants in *CYP11B1* (Answer A), *CYP17A1* (Answer B), and *CYP21A2* (Answer C) all cause congenital adrenal hyperplasia, which does not have the DHEA-S/DHEA biochemical hallmark.

Pathogenic variants in *MKRN3* (Answer D) give rise to familial isolated central precocious puberty. In light of this patient's absent breast development and low gonadotropin levels, this is not a likely cause.

Educational Objective

Explain the pathophysiology of androgen excess due to PAPSS2 deficiency.

Reference(s)

Noordam Cees, Dhir V, McNelis JC, et al. Inactivating PAPSS2 mutations in a patient with premature pubarche. *N Engl J Med.* 2009;360(22):2310-2318. PMID: 19474428

Baranowski ES, Arlt W, Idkowiak J. Monogenic disorders of adrenal steroidogenesis. *Horm Res Paediatr.* 2018;89(5):292-310. PMID: 29874650

Perez-Garcia EM, Whalen P, Gurtunca N. Novel inactivating homozygous PAPSS2 mutation in two siblings with disproportionate short stature. *AACE Clin Case Rep.* 2021;8(2):89-92. PMID: 35415222

Oostdijk J, Idkowiak J, Mueller JW, et al. PAPSS2 deficiency causes androgen excess via impaired DHEA sulfation--in vitro and in vivo studies in a family harboring two novel PAPSS2 mutations. *J Clin Endocrinol Metab.* 2015;100(4):E672-E680. PMID: 25594860

Tüysüz B, Yılmaz S, Gül E, et al. Spondyloepimetaphyseal dysplasia Pakistani type: expansion of the phenotype. *Am J Med Genet A.* 2013;161A(6):1300-1308. PMID: 23633440

84 ANSWER: B) Combined oral contraceptive once daily

The presence of irregular menses, hyperandrogenism, and an elevated LH-to-FSH ratio is consistent with polycystic ovary syndrome. Endocrine Society and international consensus guidelines recommend hormonal contraceptives (Answer B) as the first-line treatment for adolescents with polycystic ovary syndrome, with the caveat that this applies if the therapeutic goal is to treat acne, hirsutism, or anovulatory symptoms. The patient in this vignette fits this description.

Polycystic ovary syndrome and nonclassic congenital adrenal hyperplasia have common features such as hirsutism and oligomenorrhea. The diagnosis of polycystic ovary syndrome necessitates ruling out other pathologic causes of hyperandrogenism. As such, laboratory testing can be helpful in distinguishing nonclassic congenital adrenal hyperplasia from polycystic ovary syndrome. Many sources suggest the use of a basal 17-hydroxyprogesterone concentration greater than 200 ng/dL (>6.06 nmol/L) as a screening cutoff for congenital adrenal hyperplasia. In the present case, an elevated testosterone level and normal adrenal androgen levels make congenital adrenal hyperplasia less likely, and oral hydrocortisone treatment (Answer C) would probably not normalize her oligomenorrhea and hyperandrogenism. Furthermore, hormonal contraceptives can improve clinical hyperandrogenism in nonclassic congenital adrenal hyperplasia without the adverse effects of long-term corticosteroid treatment.

While her prolactin concentration is mildly elevated, the degree of elevation is not significant enough to disrupt menses and would not explain the hyperandrogenemia. Thus, treatment with cabergoline (Answer A) is incorrect.

Metformin monotherapy (Answer D) is recommended if the goal is to treat a patient with polycystic ovary syndrome who also has impaired glucose tolerance or features of metabolic syndrome. The patient in this vignette has a normal BMI, normal hemoglobin A_{1c} value, and no clinical evidence of insulin resistance. In an adolescent with elevated BMI or insulin resistance, metformin alone may lower testosterone levels and improve menstrual cycle regulation, but the limited data available indicate that the benefits may not be clinically significant.

Antiandrogens (Answer E) can be beneficial in reducing hirsutism; however, evidence of efficacy in adolescents with polycystic ovary syndrome is lacking. Current guidelines recommend use of hormonal contraceptives alone for 6 months before considering the addition of antiandrogens. Furthermore, initial treatment of hirsutism with an antiandrogen necessitates the use of effective contraception due to the teratogenic potential of these medications.

There are many uncertainties and challenges in treating polycystic ovary syndrome in adolescents. Adequately powered randomized controlled trials are lacking, and there is no single intervention that treats all of the features of polycystic ovary syndrome. A recent meta-analysis showed that hormonal contraceptives or metformin alone each only minimally improved menstrual cycle regulation and hirsutism. Compared with metformin monotherapy, hormonal contraceptives increased the risk of dysglycemia, but not compared with placebo. According to recent international guidelines, addition of metformin to hormonal contraceptives is an option in adolescents with polycystic ovary syndrome who have a BMI greater than 25 kg/m². However, there are inadequate randomized controlled trials and no clear evidence that the combination of hormonal contraceptives and metformin offers benefits beyond hormonal contraceptives plus lifestyle interventions.

Educational Objective
Guide treatment of polycystic ovary syndrome in adolescents.

Reference(s)

Al Khalifah RA, Florez ID, Zoratti MJ, Dennis B, Thabane L, Bassilious E. Efficacy of treatments for polycystic ovarian syndrome management in adolescents. *J Endocr Soc.* 2020;5(1):bvaa155. PMID: 33324861

Legro RS, Arslanian SA, Ehrmann DA, et al; Endocrine Society. Diagnosis and treatment of polycystic ovary syndrome: an Endocrine Society clinical practice guideline. *J Clin Endocrinol Metab.* 2013;98(12):4565-4592. PMID: 24151290

Peña AS, Witchel SF, Hoeger KM, et al. Adolescent polycystic ovary syndrome according to the international evidence-based guideline. *BMC Med.* 2020;18(1):72. PMID: 32204714

85 ANSWER: E) Olanzapine

Antipsychotic medications are commonly used by pediatric and adolescent mental health providers for several psychiatric indications, both for labeled and off-label use. Unfortunately, negative metabolic consequences can affect up to 60% of patients and may limit long-term use. Children appear to have increased susceptibility to antipsychotic-induced weight gain, which is often rapid in nature. In addition, patients taking these agents are also at risk for other cardiometabolic abnormalities, including central obesity, insulin resistance, dyslipidemia, and systemic inflammation. Antipsychotic medications can adversely affect metabolic function through direct effects on lipids and insulin sensitivity or indirectly due to antipsychotic-induced weight gain and obesity. Antipsychotic-induced weight gain can be substantial, with average weight gain of 11 lb (5 kg) over a 12-month period. The mechanism(s) by which antipsychotic medications induce weight gain is/are poorly understood but may be related to effects on appetite and changes in energy expenditure.

Multiple studies have shown that risperidone, which is the antipsychotic medication that this child is currently taking, is associated with at least moderate weight gain, but it can be severe for some patients. In a study of 119 pediatric patients (age range 8-19 years) with schizophrenia or schizoaffective disorder treated with antipsychotic medication for 8 weeks, Taylor et al documented mean weight gain of 4.13 ± 3.79 kg for those randomly assigned to risperidone. While risperidone is associated with weight gain for many patients, olanzapine (Answer E) is associated with the most severe weight gain when comparing antipsychotic medications. Taylor et al reported mean weight gain of 7.29 ± 3.44 kg for olanzapine when compared with risperidone or molindone. Haloperidol (Answer D), which is also an antipsychotic agent, has not been found to cause more weight gain than risperidone.

Fluoxetine (Answer C) belongs to the medication class known as selective serotonin reuptake inhibitors, which in the short term may actually result in weight loss, although this effect is often not sustained in longer-term follow-up and some patients may gain weight over time.

Duloxetine (Answer B) belongs to the medication class known as serotonin and norepinephrine reuptake inhibitors. Some studies using serotonin and norepinephrine reuptake inhibitors have reported weight loss in the medication group compared with placebo, although other studies have reported no weight change or weight gain with longer-term use.

Bupropion (Answer A) is an antidepressant that has been shown to either be weight neutral or result in weight loss for some patients. Bupropion, in combination with naltrexone, has also been used in the treatment of binge-eating disorder with obesity.

Educational Objective

Explain the risks for weight gain and cardiometabolic abnormalities in youth taking antipsychotic medications.

Reference(s)

Libowitz MR, Nurmi EL. The burden of antipsychotic-induced weight gain and metabolic syndrome in children. *Front Psychiatry.* 2021;12:623681. PMID: 33776816

Taylor JH, Jakubovski E, Gabriel D, Bloch MH. Predictors and moderators of antipsychotic-related weight gain in the treatment of early-onset schizophrenia spectrum disorders study. *J Child Adolesc Psychopharmacol.* 2018;28(7):474-484. PMID: 29920116

Reekie J, Hosking SP, Prakash C, Kao KT, Juonala M, Sabin MA. The effect of antidepressants and antipsychotics on weight gain in children and adolescents. *Obes Rev.* 2015;16(7):566-580. PMID: 26016407

Grilo CM, Lydecker JA, Fineberg SK, Moreno JO, Ivezaj V, Gueorguieva R. Naltrexone-bupropion and behavior therapy, alone and combined, for binge-eating disorder: randomized double-blind placebo-controlled trial. *Am J Psychiatry.* 2022;179(12):927-937. PMID: 36285406

86

ANSWER: A) Measure serum calcium and PTH

In addition to primary congenital hypothyroidism that is mild but persistent, this patient has short stature, developmental delay, and shortened 4th/5th metacarpals. These features are suggestive of pseudohypoparathyroidism type 1a, which is caused by pathogenic inactivating variants in *GNAS*. This gene encodes the G-protein stimulatory α subunit ($G_s\alpha$), which mediates the signaling of multiple hormone receptors, including those for TSH, LH, FSH, PTH, and GHRH. Pathogenic variants in *GNAS* inherited from either parent cause a skeletal phenotype, including short stature and shortened 4th/5th metacarpals, known as Albright hereditary osteodystrophy. However, because of genetic imprinting the *GNAS* locus is expressed only from the maternal allele in some hormone-responsive tissues. Therefore, individuals who inherit a pathogenic *GNAS* variant from their mother have pseudohypoparathyroidism type 1a with hormonal deficiencies related to receptor insensitivity, including PTH resistance, primary hypothyroidism, delayed puberty, and GH deficiency. Of these, PTH resistance is most urgent to diagnose because severe hypocalcemia can result in seizures or death. Therefore, in a patient with suspected pseudohypoparathyroidism type 1a, serum calcium and PTH should be measured (Answer A). Although hypothyroidism may be present at birth, PTH resistance typically develops during childhood, and elevation of serum PTH and phosphate is often observed before hypocalcemia develops. In fact, this patient had hypocalcemia with elevated PTH.

Although GH deficiency can occur in pseudohypoparathyroidism type 1a, excluding hypocalcemia due to PTH resistance is more urgent and should be performed before considering GH-stimulation testing (Answer D) to evaluate her short stature.

SHOX deficiency (Answer C) is a genetic cause of short stature due to abnormal growth plate function. SHOX deficiency is characterized by a variety of skeletal features not present in this patient, including disproportionate shortening of the limbs (resulting in an increased upper-to-lower segment ratio or an abnormally short arm span relative to height), cubitus valgus, bowing of forearms and lower legs, and Madelung deformity of the wrist. SHOX deficiency can cause shortened fourth metacarpals but does not cause developmental delay or hormonal abnormalities.

Congenital hypothyroidism is common, detected in about 1 in 2000 infants using current newborn screening approaches; however, pseudohypoparathyroidism type 1a is a rare cause of this disorder. Congenital hypothyroidism is most often caused by thyroid dysgenesis (failure of the thyroid gland to form normally during embryogenesis), and less commonly by dyshormonogenesis (intrinsic abnormalities of thyroid hormone synthesis). Pseudohypoparathyroidism type 1a is a rare etiology of dyshormonogenesis in which impaired TSH-receptor signaling via $G_s\alpha$ leads to TSH resistance.

A clue to the diagnosis in this case is the unusual presence of congenital hypothyroidism in the patient's maternal half-sibling. Most cases of congenital hypothyroidism are caused by thyroid dysgenesis, which is almost always sporadic in occurrence: the likelihood of thyroid dysgenesis occurring in 2 siblings is less than 1%, and it is even lower in half-siblings (who share only 1 parent). Genetic causes of dyshormonogenesis include pathogenic variants in the genes encoding thyroperoxidase (*TPO*), thyroglobulin (*TG*), dual oxidase 2 (*DUOX2*) and its accessory protein (*DUOXA2*), the sodium-iodide symporter (*SLC5A5*), pendrin (*SLC26A4*), the iodine transporter SLC26A7 (*SLC26A7*), and iodotyrosine deiodinase (*IYD*). However, biallelic pathogenic variants in a single gene or heterozygous pathogenic variants in multiple genes are usually required to cause dyshormonogenesis; therefore, the co-occurrence of a genetic form of dyshormonogenesis in half-siblings is unlikely. A few genetic causes of dyshormonogenesis that may show an apparently dominant pattern of inheritance include defects of *DUOX2*, the TSH receptor (*TSHR*) or—if maternally inherited—of its downstream messenger, $G_s\alpha$ (*GNAS*). Of these, only variants in *GNAS* produce extrathyroidal manifestations as observed in this patient (pseudohypoparathyroidism type 1a).

Transplacental passage of maternal antibodies that bind to and block activation of the TSH receptor can cause congenital hypothyroidism, and this condition may recur in multiple infants born to the same mother. TSH receptor–blocking antibodies are an uncommon cause of congenital hypothyroidism (1% of cases) but should be considered in infants born to mothers who have a history of autoimmune thyroid disease or who have other children born with congenital hypothyroidism. The diagnosis can be made by measuring TRAb in the infant's serum (Answer B). However, antibody-mediated congenital hypothyroidism is transient and resolves over the first 1 to 3 months of life as maternal antibodies are cleared from the infant's circulation, so this etiology is not consistent with the patient's persistent hypothyroidism at 7 years of age.

Thyroid scintigraphy with [123]I (Answer E) can distinguish whether congenital hypothyroidism is due to thyroid dysgenesis or to dyshormonogenesis (eutopic thyroid). This distinction may be useful in infancy or early childhood to assess the likelihood of hypothyroidism being permanent: dysgenesis is permanent, whereas some cases of dyshormonogenesis are transient. In this case, hypothyroidism is already known to be permanent, and the presence of other clinical features suggests the diagnosis of pseudohypoparathyroidism type 1a, so scintigraphy is unnecessary.

Educational Objective
Identify clinical features of pseudohypoparathyroidism type 1a, a rare etiology of congenital hypothyroidism, and evaluate a patient with suspected pseudohypoparathyroidism type 1a.

Reference(s)
Brown RS, Bellisario RL, Botero D, et al. Incidence of transient congenital hypothyroidism due to maternal thyrotropin receptor-blocking antibodies in over one million babies. *J Clin Endocrinol Metab.* 1996;81(3):1147-1151. PMID: 8772590

Larrivée-Vanier S, Jean-Louis M, Magne F, et al. Whole-exome sequencing in congenital hypothyroidism due to thyroid dysgenesis. *Thyroid.* 2022;32(5):486-495. PMID: 35272499

Mantovani G, Bastepe M, Monk D, et al. Diagnosis and management of pseudohypoparathyroidism and related disorders: first international consensus statement. *Nat Rev Endocrinol.* 2018;14(8):476-500. PMID: 29959430

van Trotsenburg P, Stoupa A, Léger J, et al. Congenital hypothyroidism: a 2020-2021 consensus guidelines update-an ENDO-European Reference Network initiative endorsed by the European Society for Pediatric Endocrinology and the European Society for Endocrinology. *Thyroid.* 2021;31(3):387-419. PMID: 33272083

87 ANSWER: B) Discontinue GH and measure IGF-1 in 1 to 2 months

Patients with isolated GH deficiency, especially those whose GH peak during provocative testing is greater than 3.0 ng/mL (>3.0 µg/L), may have adequate endogenous GH production for the metabolic effects of adult life once linear growth is completed. Therefore, when there is attainment of "near-adult height," defined as a growth velocity less than 2 cm/y in the face of advanced pubertal development, measurement of IGF-1 approximately 1 to 2 months after discontinuation of therapy (Answer B) would be recommended. If low (ie, <–2 SD for age and sex), a GH provocative test should be performed to determine whether there is permanent GH deficiency. Of note, the GH cutoff at this time (5.1 ng/mL [5.1 µg/L]) is lower that the accepted cutoff peak (10.0 ng/mL [10.0 µg/L]) used to determine GH deficiency in children. Obesity causes a blunted response of GH in provocative testing and a lower cutoff should be used for the diagnosis of GH deficiency.

GH has multiple actions. One of the most important roles of GH in children and adolescents is the promotion of linear growth, mainly through the stimulation of IGF-1 production in the liver and peripherally, which, in turn, is the major promotor of chondrogenesis, but also by direct interaction with GH receptors in the growth plate. Other functions of GH include important effects on body composition (promoting lean body mass and decreasing fat mass), bone accretion, lipid metabolism, and well-being.

GH production during the growing phases of life (infancy, childhood, and puberty) is much higher than in adulthood; therefore, replacement of GH in deficient states requires significantly higher (absolute and relative to body weight) dosages in children than in adults. The use of higher GH dosages (up to 0.7 mg/kg weekly) during puberty in individuals with GH deficiency (Answer D) has been proposed by some authors to optimize linear growth by mimicking the physiologic rise of endogenous GH production during active puberty. However, the patient in this vignette had already experienced a pubertal growth spurt between 12 and 14 years of age as seen in the growth chart. Additionally, he has reached full pubertal development and is at his "near adult height" as determined by his height velocity of 1.6 cm/y. Therefore, increasing the GH dosage is incorrect.

Most children diagnosed with GH deficiency do not remain deficient as adults. Identifying those individuals with persistent GH deficiency after completion of linear growth is important because they will benefit from replacement therapy for the non–growth-related actions of this hormone.

GH deficiency can be isolated or be part of multiple pituitary hormone deficiencies. Most individuals diagnosed with isolated GH deficiency in childhood have a normal GH response to provocative testing in late adolescence or early adulthood. The exception is those whose GH provocative testing shows a very low GH peak (<3.0 ng/mL [<3.0 µg/L]). Individuals with multiple pituitary hormone deficiencies, defined as deficiency of 3 or more pituitary hormones, are significantly more likely to have GH deficiency persisting into adulthood. Persistent GH deficiency is also more likely in individuals with GH deficiency due to *genetic* causes, congenital *structural* defects of the hypothalamic-pituitary axis, and *organic* causes. Genetic etiologies of GH deficiency include abnormalities in the genes that encode transcription factors involved in pituitary gland development (eg, *POU1F1* and *PROP1*) and the gene that encodes GH (*GH1*). Individuals with genetic causes of GH deficiency frequently have affected relatives. Congenital structural abnormalities of the hypothalamic-pituitary axis can be linked to midline defects, including septo-optic dysplasia, optic nerve hypoplasia, and interrupted pituitary stalk. An ectopic posterior pituitary is not always associated with permanent GH deficiency. Organic causes of GH deficiency such as CNS tumors, most commonly suprasellar tumors such as craniopharyngiomas, and their treatment with surgical removal or radiation therapy are very likely to be associated with permanent GH deficiency.

As such, individuals with GH deficiency associated with multiple pituitary hormone deficiencies and those with genetic, structural, or organic causes do not need provocative testing to redemonstrate GH deficiency after completion of linear growth. Some propose measuring IGF-1 approximately 1 month after discontinuing GH therapy. If low (ie, <−2 SD for age and sex), no further testing is required to restart therapy at adult GH replacement dosages (Answer A), which are much lower than growth-promoting dosages.

Performing a GH-stimulation test (Answer E) while the patient is receiving GH therapy would not be recommended.

Although discontinuing GH therapy without retesting after completion of linear growth in patients with isolated GH deficiency (Answer C) is a common practice, it may eliminate the possible metabolic benefit of continued GH therapy at adult replacement dosages in individuals with GH deficiency.

Educational objective
Diagnose permanent GH deficiency in individuals with childhood-onset GH deficiency.

Reference(s)

Grimberg A, DiVall SA, Polychronakos C, et al; Drug and Therapeutics Committee and Ethics Committee of the Pediatric Endocrine Society. Guidelines for growth hormone and insulin-like growth factor-I treatment in children and adolescents: growth hormone deficiency, idiopathic short stature, and primary insulin-like growth factor-I deficiency. *Horm Res Paediatr.* 2016;86(6):361-397. PMID: 27884013

Cavarzere P, Gaudino R, Sandri M, et al. Growth hormone retesting during puberty: a cohort study. *Eur J Endocrinol.* 2020;182(6):559-567. PMID: 32337961

Secco A, di Iorgi N, Napoli F, et al. Reassessment of the growth hormone status in young adults with childhood-onset growth hormone deficiency: reappraisal of insulin tolerance testing. *J Clin Endocrinol Metab.* 2009;94(11):4195-4204. PMID: 19837937

Molitch ME, Clemmons DR, Malozowski S, Merriam GR, Vance ML; Endocrine Society. Evaluation and treatment of adult growth hormone deficiency: an Endocrine Society clinical practice guideline. *J Clin Endocrinol Metab.* 2011;96(6):1587-1609. PMID: 21602453

Mauras N, Attie KM, Reiter EO, Saenger P, Baptista J. High dose recombinant human growth hormone (GH) treatment of GH-deficient patients in puberty increases near-final height: a randomized, multicenter trial. Genentech, Inc., Cooperative Study Group. *J Clin Endocrinol Metab.* 2000;85(10):3653-3660. PMID: 11061518

88 ANSWER: B) Perform left thyroid lobectomy

This patient has a unilateral thyroid nodule with several suspicious features on ultrasonography (hypoechogenicity, irregular margins, and areas of hyperechogenicity highly suggestive of microcalcifications). The cytology is indeterminate. The 2015 American Thyroid Association guidelines for management of thyroid nodules and malignancy in children recommend lobectomy (Answer B) for a nodule with indeterminate cytology, including Bethesda IV. If surgical histology confirms malignancy, the patient should proceed with completion total thyroidectomy and central compartment neck dissection. The American Thyroid Association guidelines recommend proceeding with total thyroidectomy and potential central lymph node dissection for Bethesda VI cytology, although more recent literature suggests that some unilateral malignant nodules without lymph node metastases can be safely managed with lobectomy alone. Closely monitoring with ultrasonography (Answer E) would be inadequate.

The role of molecular pathogenic variants in cytologic samples was not formally addressed in the 2015 guidelines, as testing was not routinely used for pediatric patients at that time. Genetic testing can be helpful in determining the presurgical possibility of malignancy and can provide guidance on whether patients at high risk for malignancy should undergo total thyroidectomy as their initial surgery. Genetic testing should be used only as an adjunct to ultrasonography and cytology to aid in surgical planning. If a high-risk variant is found, total thyroidectomy can be considered as the first surgery. If a low-risk variant is found or no variant is identified, the patient's management plan should not change. The presence of lower-risk pathogenic variants or the absence of any variant should not be used to support the decision to avoid surgery.

DICER1 pathogenic variants in thyroid nodules are typically associated with papillary thyroid carcinoma with less aggressive features as opposed to more invasive disease. *DICER1* variants have also been found in benign nodules. However, as noted above, this patient's nodule had suspicious ultrasound and cytologic features and should be removed regardless of the genetic findings. Had genetic testing shown a very high-risk pathogenic variant (eg, *RET*, *BRAF*, *NTRK*), total thyroidectomy (Answers C and D) could have been considered as a first step.

Germline *DICER1* pathogenic variants are associated with a high risk of malignancy (pleuropulmonary blastoma); pulmonary cysts; thyroid gland neoplasia (multinodular goiter, adenomas, and/or thyroid cancer); ovarian tumors (Sertoli-Leydig cell tumor, gynandroblastoma, and sarcoma); and cystic nephroma. Patients with known germline *DICER1* pathogenic variants should undergo screening. Patients with a pathogenic variant in the nodule should be evaluated for the presence of a germline variant. However, the presence of a single somatic *DICER1* variant in a thyroid nodule cytology sample does not mean the patient has a germline variant that needs evaluation or follow-up (Answer A).

Proceeding with total thyroidectomy and lymph node dissection on the basis of ultrasound and cytologic features would be more extensive surgery than is necessary for a lesion that is unilateral without evidence of metastases. Although this patient had bilateral cervical lymphadenopathy, the lymph nodes were described as morphologically normal, and their presence did not increase the risk that this nodule was malignant.

Educational Objective
Explain the role of molecular genetic analysis of thyroid nodule cytology samples in surgical planning.

Reference(s)
Francis GL, Waguespack SG, Bauer AJ, et al; American Thyroid Association Guidelines Task Force. *Thyroid.* 2015;25(7):716-759. PMID: 25900731

Wasserman JD, Sabbaghian N, Fahiminiya S, et al. DICER1 mutations are frequent in adolescent-onset papillary thyroid carcinoma. *J Clin Endocrinol Metab.* 2018;103(5):2009-2015. PMID: 29474644

89 ANSWER: C) Normal BMI for age and sex; BMI has low sensitivity for detecting excess adiposity
Obesity is a global health crisis with both short- and long-term implications for adverse health outcomes. Identifying overweight/obesity in children and adolescents is important to effect change. Providers need screening tools that are cost-effective, efficient, and reliable in recognizing obesity at an early stage. While there are different methods of assessing for excess adiposity (eg, waist circumference, skinfold calipers, DXA), many of these methods are time-consuming and/or costly, which limit widespread use as screening tools. Because of ease of measurement, BMI has been widely used as a proxy for weight-related health risk because high BMI values may reflect excess adiposity. BMI is a ratio of an individual's weight to height squared (kg/m^2). It varies with age in children, so BMI in children aged 2 to 19 years is plotted on Centers for Disease Control sex-specific BMI growth charts to identify the BMI-for-age percentile, derived from a reference population. Overweight in childhood is classified as a BMI at or above the 85th percentile, but less than the 95th percentile, on the BMI-for-age growth chart. Obesity is classified as a BMI at or above the 95th percentile on the BMI-for-age growth chart. In children, the BMI cutoffs for obesity are chosen to reliably delineate a level above which a child is at higher risk for developing obesity-related comorbidities.

Obesity denotes excess body fat, whereas BMI relies on body weight, irrespective of body composition. One flaw of measuring BMI is that its calculation assumes that individuals with normal BMI have normal body fat and that increases in BMI above the normal range are proportional to increases in body fat percentage. However, BMI cannot distinguish between lean and fat mass. Additionally, recent data have highlighted that increases in adiposity over time may actually be higher than what BMI calculations indicate. Javed et al found that BMI has low sensitivity to detect excess adiposity in children and adolescents, and thus may fail to identify more than one-quarter of children (labeled as having normal weight according to BMI) with excess body fat (Answer C). While this child has a normal weight by BMI calculation, it is incorrect to state that she cannot, therefore, have excess body fat (Answer A). Javed et al also found that BMI has high, not low, specificity for detecting excess body fat (Answer E). Because her BMI is below the 85th percentile for age and sex, she does not fall into the overweight category (Answers B and D). Age also appears to be a factor in BMI interpretation. Vanderwall et al found that in children younger than 9 years, the BMI Z-score is only a weak to moderate predictor for both total fat mass and percentage of body fat. Finally, caution must be exercised when interpreting BMI across racial/ethnic groups. At similar BMI-for-age values, the amount of body fat in children and adolescents can differ by up to 5% across racial and ethnic groups. Black children have been found to have less body fat (~3%), not more, than White children with equivalent values of BMI-for-age. Further research is needed to understand whether BMI cut-points should be adjusted for children from different racial and ethnic backgrounds.

Educational Objective
Explain the benefits and limitations of using BMI in children and adolescents to detect adiposity.

Reference(s)

Vanderwall C, Clark RR, Eickhoff J, Carrel AL. BMI is a poor predictor of adiposity in young overweight and obese children. *BMC Pediatr.* 2017 2;17(1):135. PMID: 28577356

Javed A, Jumean M, Murad MH, et al. Diagnostic performance of body mass index to identify obesity as defined by body adiposity in children and adolescents: a systematic review and meta-analysis. *Pediatr Obes.* 2015;10(3):234-244. PMID: 24961794

Freedman DS, Sherry B. The validity of BMI as an indicator of body fatness and risk among children. *Pediatrics.* 2009;124(Suppl 1):S23-S34. PMID: 19720664

Centers for Disease Control and Prevention. Defining Childhood Weight Status. December 3, 2021. Available at: https://www.cdc.gov/obesity/basics/childhood-defining.html. Accessed December 2022.

90 ANSWER: C) Monitoring serum calcium every 4 to 6 months until age 2 and then every 2 years thereafter

This patient has Williams-Beuren syndrome (WBS), an autosomal dominant condition affecting 1 in 7500 individuals. Affected patients are often described as having "elfin" facies and a "cocktail personality." WBS is due to a deletion on chromosome 7 affecting the *ELN* gene, which encodes the elastin protein, an important component of connective tissue. Pathogenic variants in *ELN* explain the characteristic facial features and cardiovascular defects (supravalvular aortic stenosis is the most common defect) associated with WBS. It is not clear how deletion of this gene leads to hypercalcemia, which is thought to be secondary to increased intestinal absorption of calcium. Laboratory data are consistent with this proposed mechanism because her PTH concentration is suppressed and her vitamin D concentrations are not elevated.

While median calcium concentrations are higher in individuals with WBS than in control patients, more than 85% of affected individuals have a calcium concentration within the reference range for age. Monitoring serum calcium every 4 to 6 months for the first 2 years of life until age 2 and then every 2 years thereafter (Answer C) is the recommended approach to detect actionable hypercalcemia, although screening cannot predict future hypercalcemia episodes. Parents should be educated regarding the signs and symptoms of hypercalcemia and laboratory testing should be ordered when there are concerns. In infancy, these signs and symptoms include poor feeding, vomiting, constipation, and irritability. Children with WBS who are normocalcemic should continue to consume the recommended daily allowance of calcium for age and thus a low-calcium diet (Answer B) is not indicated. Vitamin D supplementation (Answer E) is generally avoided in early childhood and should be used with caution in older children.

Hypercalcemia occurs in approximately 15% of infants with WBS, and in most cases it can be treated with fluids and a low-calcium diet. In more severe cases, a single infusion of pamidronate effectively treats the hypercalcemia with minimal adverse effects. While there have been reports of patients requiring a second dose of pamidronate (spaced 1 week after the initial dose) to fully normalize serum calcium, there have been no reports of patients needing additional doses (Answer D) after normalization of serum calcium. While furosemide (Answer A) has historically been used to increase renal clearance of calcium in patients with hypercalcemia, it can cause dehydration, which may exacerbate hypercalcemia. Thus, it is no longer a preferred approach.

Educational Objective
Identify Williams-Beuren syndrome as a cause of infantile hypercalcemia and provide anticipatory guidance regarding the expected outcomes.

Reference(s)

Morris CA, Braddock SR; Council on Genetics. Health care supervision for children with Williams syndrome. *Pediatrics.* 2020;145(2):e20193761. PMID: 31964759

Sindhar S, Lugo M, Levin MD, et al. Hypercalcemia in patients with Williams-Beuren syndrome. *J Pediatr.* 2016;178:254-260. PMID: 27574996

Sangun O, Dundar BN, Erdogan E. Severe hypercalcemia associated with Williams syndrome successfully treated with pamidronate infusion therapy. *J Pediatr Endocrinol Metab.* 2011;24(1-2):69-70. PMID: 21528818

91 ANSWER: D) Neurofibromatosis type 1

This patient's clinical presentation and laboratory findings are consistent with central precocious puberty. Most cases of central precocious puberty in girls are idiopathic; however, the likelihood of intracranial pathology is higher with younger age at presentation. The patient in this vignette has hyperpigmented macules (café-au-lait spots) and possibly loss of visual acuity, raising concern for an optic pathway glioma associated with neurofibromatosis type 1 (Answer D). Approximately 2.4% to 5.0% of patients with neurofibromatosis type 1 develop central precocious puberty; most cases are associated with optic pathway glioma, typically located at the optic chiasm. In a comprehensive review of visual pathway gliomas in childhood, 29% of cases were associated with neurofibromatosis. While patients with optic pathway gliomas can be asymptomatic, the most common findings include vision loss, relative afferent pupillary defect, and optic atrophy on fundoscopic examination. It is also important to recognize that suprasellar lesions are a risk factor for GH deficiency in individuals with neurofibromatosis 1; thus, a pubertal growth spurt may not be seen.

Hypothalamic hamartomas (Answer B) are among the most common lesions in patients with central precocious puberty who have pathologic findings. While hypothalamic hamartomas may present with central precocious puberty only, 36% present with gelastic seizures and 25% present with both seizures and central precocious puberty. In this vignette, the absence of seizures and the presence of findings more characteristic of neurofibromatosis type 1 make hypothalamic hamartoma a less likely diagnosis.

Craniopharyngiomas (Answer A) and histiocytosis (Answer C) can also present with endocrine dysfunction but are most often associated with pituitary hormone deficiencies and very rarely present with central precocious puberty. CNS manifestations of Langerhans cell histiocytosis typically involve infiltration of the hypothalamic-pituitary region, most often causing central diabetes insipidus. This increases the risk of anterior pituitary involvement, leading to pituitary hormone deficiencies. Hypothalamic involvement results in hyperphagia and obesity; development of central precocious puberty has only been reported in 2 cases, both with anterior pituitary hormone deficiencies. As such, Langerhans cell histiocytosis is unlikely to be the cause of central precocious puberty in this vignette.

Peutz-Jeghers syndrome (Answer E) is characterized by the development of multiple polyps in the gastrointestinal tract and freckling on the lips, eyes, nostrils, fingers, and in and around the mouth. Affected girls have an increased risk of developing benign ovarian tumors that can cause peripheral precocious puberty. As the patient in this vignette has central precocious puberty, Peutz-Jeghers syndrome is unlikely.

Educational Objective
Differentiate among pathologic causes of central precocious puberty.

Reference(s)
Cantas-Orsdemir S, Garb JL, Allen HF. Prevalence of cranial MRI findings in girls with central precocious puberty: a systematic review and meta-analysis. *J Pediatr Endocrinol Metab*. 2018;31(7):701-710. PMID: 29902155

Virdis R, Sigorini M, Laiolo A, et al. Neurofibromatosis type 1 and precocious puberty. *J Pediatr Endocrinol Metab*. 2000;13(Suppl 1):841-844. PMID: 10969931

92 ANSWER: E) Pathogenic variants in the *POMC* gene

Pathogenic variants in the *POMC* gene (encoding proopiomelanocortin) (Answer E) are a rare but well-known cause of severe early-onset obesity. POMC is the precursor protein that is cleaved to ACTH and α-MSH (*see figure*). Classically, patients with homozygous variants have pale skin, red hair, and secondary adrenal insufficiency due to reduced α-MSH and ACTH, respectively. In these classic cases, one would expect low or undetectable ACTH in the presence of hypocortisolemia. However, there is increasing understanding of disease heterogeneity. For example, in persons of nonEuropean or White ancestry, variable hypopigmentation has been observed, ranging from red hair roots in a Turkish patient to absent pigmentary changes in others. Furthermore, depending on the variant's location in the gene sequence, high ACTH concentrations have also been described whereby the ACTH produced is bioinactive or has reduced function. Thus, such variants in the *POMC* gene could provide a unifying diagnosis for this child.

Figure. Processing of Proopiomelanocortin

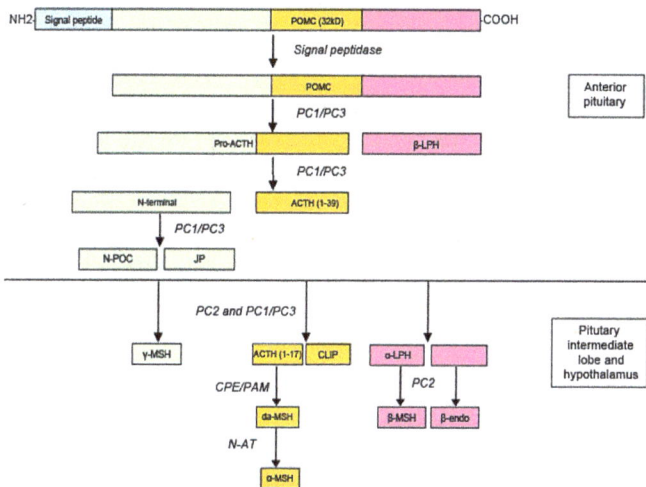

Abbreviations: POMC, proopiomelanocortin precursor protein; LPH, lipotrophin; MSH, melanococyte-stimulating hormone; CLIP, corticotropinlike intermediate peptide; JP, joining peptide; endo, endorphin; CPE, carboxypeptidase; PAM, α-amidating monooxygenase; N-AT, N-acetyltransferase.

ACTH and the various melanocyte-stimulating hormones (αβγ) are derived from the precursor protein, POMC. POMC undergoes cleavage and posttranslational modification in the pituitary, hypothalamus, and skin, by action of PC1/3 and PC2. Carboxypeptidases and aminopeptidases subsequently remove dibasic residues. Enzymes PAM and N-AT perform COOH terminal amidation and N-α-acetylation, respectively. Further modification is necessary for potency of biologically active peptides.

Deletion of the paternally inherited 15q11.2-q13 region (Answer A) and maternal uniparental disomy of chromosome 15 (Answer B) give rise to Prader-Willi syndrome, which is characterized by early initial hypotonia, feeding problems, and failure to thrive, as well as characteristic facial features, severe early-onset obesity, hyperphagia, pubertal insufficiency, intellectual disability, short stature, and distinct behaviors. In addition to these features, Prader-Willi syndrome has been associated with hypothalamic dysfunction, including central adrenal insufficiency. In one study, up to 60% of children with Prader-Willi syndrome were noted to have central adrenal insufficiency following metyrapone testing. However, others have demonstrated normal cortisol response to low- and high-dose cosyntropin-stimulation testing and insulin tolerance tests. The lack of associated features in this vignette and the patient's high ACTH concentration are not consistent with a diagnosis of Prader-Willi syndrome.

Pathogenic variants in the *BBS* genes (Bardet-Biedl syndrome genes) (Answer C) give rise to Bardet-Biedl syndrome, which encompasses a constellation of features, including truncal obesity, intellectual impairment, postaxial polydactyly, retinal degeneration, male hypogonadotropic hypogonadism, rod-cone dystrophy, complex female genitourinary malformations, kidney dysfunction, and a characteristic facial phenotype. Adrenal insufficiency is not associated with Bardet-Biedl syndrome.

Pathogenic variants in *MC4R* encoding the melanocortin 4 receptor (Answer D) are a cause of early-onset childhood obesity but are not associated with adrenal insufficiency.

Educational Objective
Develop an approach to diagnose a child with adrenal insufficiency and severe obesity.

Reference(s)

van der Velk ES, Kleinendorst L, Delhanty PJD, et al. Obesity and hyperphagia with increased defective ACTH: a novel POMC variant. *J Clin Endocrinol Metab.* 2022;107(9):e3699-e3704. PMID: 35737586

Cassidy SB, Schwartz S, Miller JL, Driscoll DJ. Prader-Willi syndrome. *Genet Med.* 2012;14(1):10-26. PMID: 22237428

Gregoric N, Groselj U, Bratina N, et al. Two cases with an early presented proopiomelanocortin deficiency—a long-term follow-up and systematic literature review. *Front Endocrinol (Lausanne).* 2021;12:689387. PMID: 34177811

Florea L, Caba L, Gorduza EV. Bardet-Biedl syndrome-multiple kaleidoscope images: insight into mechanisms of genotype-phenotype correlations. *Genes (Basel).* 2021;12(9):1353. PMID: 34573333

Meimaridou E, Hughes CR, Kowalczyk J, et al. Familial glucocorticoid deficiency: new genes and mechanisms. *Mol Cell Endocrinol.* 2013;371(1-2):195-200. PMID: 23279877

93

ANSWER: B) Reassure the family that her growth and weight gain are normal

This healthy baby had a normal prenatal course and has been appropriately achieving milestones. In the United States, the Centers for Disease Control (CDC) and the National Center for Health Statistics growth charts are based on cross-sectional data of growth from 5 national health examination surveys and 5 supplementary data sources obtained using children raised in variable conditions in the United States as a reference. The World Health

Organization (WHO) growth standard was developed using longitudinal observation of children from 6 countries, including the United States, from birth to 5 years under optimal environmental conditions. Thus, WHO standards can be applied to all children everywhere regardless of ethnicity, socioeconomic status, and type of feeding. On the CDC reference charts, the normal range is generally defined as between the 5th and 95th percentiles. On the WHO standard charts, the normal range is generally defined as between –2 SD and +2 SD Z scores, which correspond to approximately the 2nd and 98th percentiles. The standard population of children followed to generate the WHO standard charts were overall taller and thinner when compared with the children whose cross-sectional pooled data were used to create the CDC reference charts.

For children aged 0 to 2 years, the WHO standard charts are recommended for plotting height-for-age, weight-for-age, and weight-for-length to avoid misclassification, especially for those who are underweight or malnourished. On the CDC weight-for-length chart, her growth dropped to below the 5th percentile, which indicates low weight-for-length. However, when this patient's growth parameters were plotted in the WHO chart, her weight-for-length was above the 2nd percentile, which is in the healthy range (*see images*). Thus, this family should be reassured that she has normal growth and weight gain (Answer B).

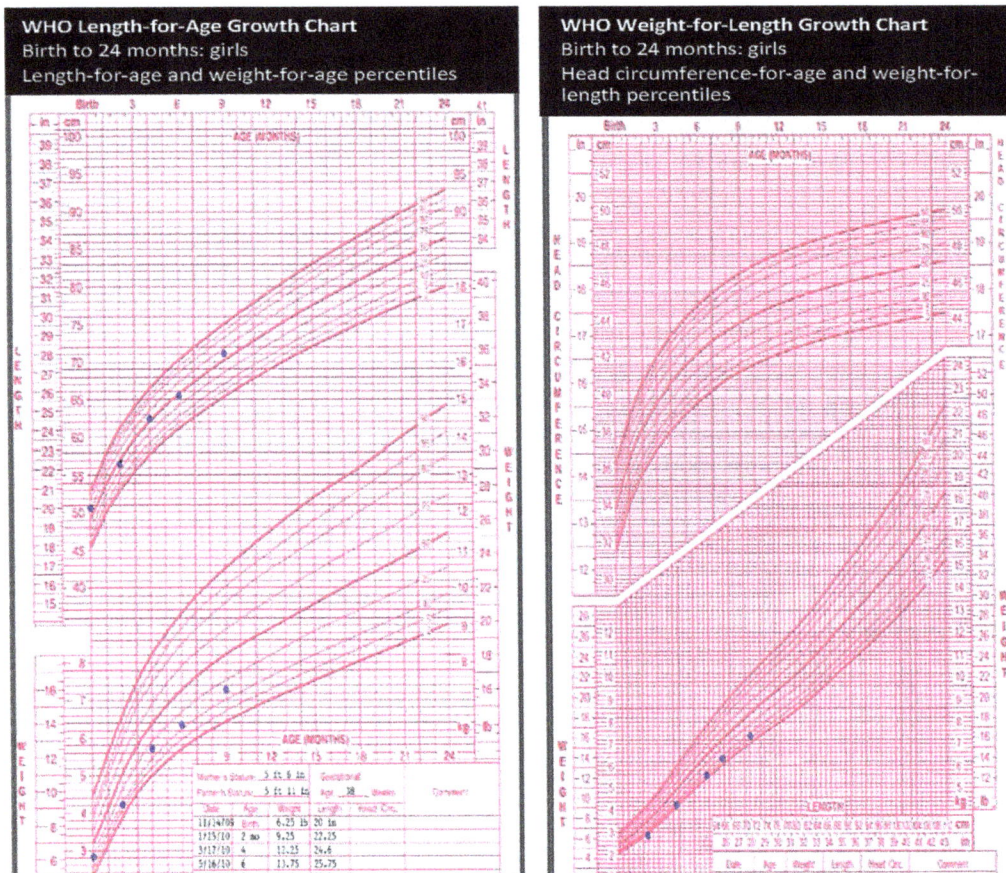

Modified from Growth Chart Training: Using the WHO Growth Charts. Centers for Disease Control and Prevention, U.S. Department of Health and Human Services. https://www.cdc.gov/nccdphp/dnpao/growthcharts/who/examples/example1.htm

Fewer children will be identified as having low weight-for-length on the WHO charts than on the CDC charts, resulting in potentially fewer children being referred for additional assessments. Even though this patient's length seems to be accelerating a bit between age 6 months and 9 months, she is most likely moving closer to her genetic potential of 66 in (167.6 cm) (approximately 75th percentile) for adult height. Thus, there is no need to check her thyroid function (Answer A).

Because her weight and length are following a normal pattern, there is no need for nutritional consultation (Answer C) or formula supplementation (Answer E).

She has no symptoms or signs suggestive of celiac disease (Answer D) such as abdominal pain, diarrhea, or poor weight gain. Celiac disease may develop any time after wheat- or gluten-containing foods are introduced into the diet, typically after 6 to 9 months of age. Infants and toddlers with celiac disease tend to have more obvious symptoms, usually gastrointestinal.

Educational Objective
Explain why the World Health Organization standard growth charts should be used when monitoring growth parameters for children aged 0 to 2 years.

Reference(s)

Mei Z, Ogden CL, Flegal KM, Grummer-Strawn LM. Comparison of the prevalence of shortness, underweight, and overweight among US children aged 0 to 59 months by using the CDC 2000 and the WHO 2006 growth charts. *J Pediatr.* 2008;153(5):622-628. PMID: 18619613

Daymont C, Hoffman N, Schaefer EW, Fiks AG. Clinician diagnoses of failure to thrive before and after switch to World Health Organization growth curves. *Acad Pediatr.* 2020;20(3):405-412. PMID: 31128383

Grummer-Strawn LM, Reinold C, Krebs NF; Centers for Disease Control and Prevention (CDC). Use of World Health Organization and CDC growth charts for children aged 0-59 months in the United States. [published correction appears in *MMWR Recomm Rep.* 2010;59(36):1184] *MMWR Recomm Rep.* 2010;10;59(RR-9):1-15. PMID: 20829749

94 ANSWER: E) Refer to medical genetics

This patient has incidentally discovered thyroid nodules. Although the nodules are not suspicious for malignancy, it is unusual for a 12-year-old child to have multiple nodules. In addition, this girl has autism, which often has an underlying genetic cause. *PTEN* pathogenic variants are commonly associated with autism, especially when an individual with autism also has macrocephaly. Whether children with autism due to *PTEN* pathogenic variants have the same risk of malignancy and thyroid disease as others with *PTEN* hamartoma syndromes, such as Cowden syndrome, is controversial. Studies on patients diagnosed with Cowden syndrome have found high rates of thyroiditis, thyroid nodules, and follicular thyroid cancer, with thyroid cancer occurring at a younger age than in the general population. However, patients in the populations studied were given a clinical diagnosis of Cowden syndrome, often due to the presence of other neoplasms (eg, colon polyps, endometrial cancer), and it is unclear if all individuals with a *PTEN* pathogenic variant have the same risks. In the absence of better data, the *PTEN* Hamartoma Tumor Syndrome Guideline Development Group has recommended screening patients with *PTEN* pathogenic variants with thyroid ultrasonography starting at age 18 years, while the National Comprehensive Cancer Network recommends annual thyroid ultrasonography starting at age 7 years. The presence of multiple thyroid nodules alone may not warrant a genetic evaluation; however, the presence of multiple nodules and other comorbidities (in this case autism) should prompt consideration of a genetic syndrome (Answer E).

The nodules described do not appear suspicious enough to warrant biopsy (Answer C). The presence of multiple nodules in and of itself should not prompt biopsy. The presence of multiple nodules in a child is unusual, and, over time, this girl will need to have multiple ultrasonography examinations. Depending on findings, FNA biopsy may be required.

Thyroidectomy (Answer D) is not warranted now. There is no evidence of malignancy, and she is able to tolerate an inexpensive, effective screening tool (ultrasonography). If an underlying genetic disorder is diagnosed, her malignancy risk may be better assessed. If the risk is very high, the family may elect to proceed with thyroidectomy through shared decision-making. At times, the psychologic burden on patients and families who require long-term close follow-up of thyroid nodules with the potential for malignant transformation is too great and they decide to proceed with thyroidectomy. If a child with severe developmental delay cannot tolerate ultrasonography or needs sedation for the procedure and is at very high risk, the family may also favor a surgical approach.

Measurement of TPO antibodies (Answer B) will not influence the further care of this child. The background echotexture is described as heterogeneous, which can be seen in Hashimoto thyroiditis, but multiple nodules are not typically present. This child is also euthyroid and the presence of TPO antibodies should not influence her care.

Interval thyroid ultrasonography is warranted, but repeated imaging in 3 months (Answer A) is too soon for there to be any discernible difference in these benign-appearing nodules. This patient will need long-term follow-up. Repeating ultrasonography more often than is necessary will unnecessarily increase health care costs and burden for this family. Follow-up ultrasonography of thyroid nodules at a 3-month interval is typically reserved for nodules that have features suspicious for malignancy if they were not biopsied or if they were biopsied and the results were indeterminate.

Educational Objective

Identify genetic syndromes in children that are associated with increased risk of follicular neoplasms of the thyroid gland.

Reference(s)

Tischkowitz M, Colas C, Pouwels S, Hoogerbrugge N, PHTS Guideline Development Group; European Reference Network GENTURIS. Cancer surveillance guideline for individuals with PTEN hamartoma tumour syndrome. *Eur J Human Genet.* 2020;28(10):1387-1393. PMID: 32533092

Bonora E, Tallini G, Romeo G. Genetic predisposition to familial nonmedullary thyroid cancer: an update of molecular findings and state-of-the-art studies. *J Oncol.* 2010;2010:385206. PMID: 20628519

95 ANSWER: D) Insulin autoantibody titers

The patient in this vignette has insulin autoimmune syndrome, most likely induced by alpha-lipoic acid. Dietary supplements containing alpha-lipoic acid can induce insulin autoimmune syndrome. In the presence of reduced nicotinamide adenine dinucleotide or reduced nicotinamide adenine dinucleotide phosphate, alpha-lipoic acid is reduced to dihydrolipoic acid, a complex that includes a sulfhydryl group. Autoimmune forms of hypoglycemia are a rare cause of low blood glucose in White populations, yet they are the third leading cause of hypoglycemia in Asian populations, especially in Japan. Other medications with a sulfhydryl group can also trigger insulin autoimmune syndrome.

Insulin autoantibody titers (Answer E) would help establish the diagnosis. Insulin autoimmune syndrome may be triggered by exposure to drugs or viruses, or it may manifest spontaneously. The *box* lists some of the medications that can trigger insulin autoimmune syndrome.

Box. Triggers of Insulin Autoimmune Syndrome

Methimazole
Propylthiouracil
Carbimazole
Alpha-lipoic acid
Glutathione
Methionine
Captopril
Hydralazine
Diltiazem
Pantoprazole

The prevalence of this condition being induced by antithyroid drugs is high in Japan and other Asian countries. The drug most frequently described as a trigger is methimazole, but there have also been case reports of propylthiouracil and carbimazole.

ABCC8 (Answer A) and *HNF1A* (Answer C) are 2 of the many genes involved in the regulation of insulin secretion from pancreatic β cells that are responsible for the underlying molecular mechanisms leading to congenital hyperinsulinemic hypoglycemia. Hyperinsulinemic hypoglycemia refers to a clinically, genetically, and morphologically heterogeneous group of disorders associated with dysregulated insulin secretion. It is the most common cause of persistent hypoketotic hypoglycemia in neonates and infants and rarely presents sporadically during the second decade of life as depicted in the vignette.

Oral glucose tolerance testing with measurement of insulin and C-peptide (Answer E) would be informative for identifying the degree of hyperinsulinism, correlating with elevated C-peptide concentrations, but it would not aid in the evaluation.

Determining alpha-lipoic acid levels with urine toxicology screening (Answer B) would also not contribute to the diagnosis.

For the differential diagnosis, one should consider most common causes of hyperinsulinemic hypoglycemia at this age, which include postprandial hyperinsulinism, dumping syndrome, insulinoma, factitious hypoglycemia, and non–islet-cell tumor hypoglycemia. To rule out insulinoma, ^{18}F-DOPA PET/CT could be considered as a next step.

The importance of testing for insulin autoantibodies in adults without diabetes who have hyperinsulinemic hypoglycemia has also been emphasized by the Endocrine Society, which includes insulin autoantibodies among the first-line tests in these patients.

Insulin autoimmune syndrome is usually self-limiting and tends to regress within 3 to 6 months after withdrawal of the triggering drug. Patients are generally advised to eat frequent, small meals that are low in carbohydrates to prevent fasting and to avoid the release of insulin associated with glucose overload of the pancreas. Uncooked cornstarch (used in patients with glycogen storage disease) can be useful for patients with insulin autoimmune syndrome to maintain stable glucose concentrations.

Educational Objective
Diagnose hypoglycemia due to insulin autoimmune syndrome secondary to alpha-lipoic acid use.

Reference(s)

Censi S, Mian C, Betterle C. Insulin autoimmune syndrome: from diagnosis to clinical management. *Ann Transl Med*. 2018;6(17):335. PMID: 30306074

Cryer PE, Axelrod L, Grossman AB, et al; Endocrine Society. Evaluation and management of adult hypoglycemic disorders: an Endocrine Society clinical practice guideline. *J Clin Endocrinol Metab*. 2009;94(3):709-728. PMID: 19088155

Furukawa N, Miyamura N, Nishida K, Motoshima H, Taketa K, Araki E. Possible relevance of alpha lipoic acid contained in a health supplement in a case of insulin autoimmune syndrome. *Diabetes Res Clin Pract*. 2007;75:366-367. PMID: 16963149

96 ANSWER: A) Autoimmune hypophysitis

Children and adults with a variety of cancers have benefited from the advent of novel targeted therapies. In particular, immune checkpoint inhibitors target tumors' ability to evade the immune system via checkpoint ligands. Antiprogrammed cell death 1 (PD-1) and anticytotoxic lymphocyte-associated protein 4 (CTLA-4) antibodies are 2 examples of immune checkpoint inhibitors. Consensus statements offer insights regarding diagnosis, grading, and overall management of toxicities related to immune checkpoint inhibitors and other immunotherapies to treat cancer. Multiple references discuss the potential of immune checkpoint inhibitors to cause autoimmune endocrine sequelae, which arise because these agents also appear to contribute to the expansion of autoreactive cell populations in specific tissues. Endocrinopathies caused by immune checkpoint inhibitors occur in up to 10% of treated individuals and can include primary hypothyroidism, thyrotoxicosis, primary adrenal insufficiency, hypophysitis (Answer A), and diabetes mellitus. Although grade IV adverse events affecting other organ systems often lead to permanent treatment discontinuation of immune checkpoint inhibitors, endocrinopathies that are well controlled by hormone replacement may not require treatment cessation. In general, immunosuppressive therapies (eg, high-dosage glucocorticoids) have not been shown to restore endocrine function.

The first pediatric phase I clinical trial of ipilimumab, an anti-CTLA-4 antibody, found that children generally present with the same range of adverse effects as adults, although effects may occur sooner, even after a single dose. In general, subsequent studies have shown similar findings. The indications and scope of treatment continue to broaden, and experience continues to accrue.

While ipilimumab therapy can cause direct toxicity in multiple organ systems (Answer B), the damage to this patient's hypothalamus/pituitary is autoimmune mediated and is thus indirect.

Pituitary apoplexy (Answer C) is typically caused by bleeding into and/or hypoperfusion of a hypothalamic/pituitary lesion. Apoplexy can cause pituitary hormone deficiencies, although the presentation is often acute. Ipilimumab is not thought to cause hypopituitarism by affecting pituitary perfusion. Also, pituitary apoplexy would tend to show characteristic imaging findings, which may vary according to the time of onset and the presence or absence of hemorrhage.

Pseudotumor cerebri syndrome (Answer D), in which symptoms such as headache and vision changes are caused by elevated pressure of cerebrospinal fluid (not related to a mechanical obstruction), can occur in association with endocrine hormone deficiencies, but it would not typically be causal.

Given the known association between immune checkpoint inhibitors and hypophysitis, this is a much more likely explanation than metastasis (Answer E).

Educational Objective
Explain the potential for immune checkpoint inhibitors to cause autoimmune hypophysitis.

Reference(s)

Ragoonanan D, Khazal SJ, Abdel-Azim H, et al. Diagnosis, grading and management of toxicities from immunotherapies in children, adolescents and young adults with cancer. *Nat Rev Clin Oncol.* 2021;18(7):435-453. PMID: 33608690

de Vries F, van Furth WR, Biermasz NR, Pereira AM. Hypophysitis: a comprehensive overview. *Presse Med.* 2021;50(4):104076. PMID: 34687912

Ihara K. Immune checkpoint inhibitor therapy for pediatric cancers: a mini review of endocrine adverse events. *Clin Pediatr Endocrinol.* 2019;28(3):59-68. PMID: 31384097

Schneider BJ, Naidoo J, Santomasso BD, et al. Management of immune-related adverse events in patients treated with immune checkpoint inhibitor therapy: ASCO guideline update. *J Clin Oncol.* 2021;39(36):4073-4126. PMID: 34724392

Merchant MS, Wright M, Baird K, et al. Phase I clinical trial of ipilimumab in pediatric patients with advanced solid tumors. *Clin Cancer Res.* 2016;22(6):1364-1370. PMID: 26534966

97 ANSWER: D) Maternal use of nasal spray

In the United States, newborn screening for 21-hydroxylase deficiency has been mandatory since 2009. The goal of screening is to identify patients with severe salt-wasting congenital adrenal hyperplasia (CAH) to prevent mortality and morbidity. In general, classic forms are readily detected, including simple virilizing CAH. Screening is based on the concentration of 17-hydroxyprogesterone, which historically was measured by radioimmunoassay and more recently by a dissociation-enhanced lanthanide fluorescence immunoassay in automated systems (DELFIA). Typically, screening laboratories set low thresholds to detect all newborns with either form of classic 21-hydroxylase deficiency (100% screening sensitivity). This means that false-positive results are relatively common. Many newborn screening programs now use a second-tier screening process using alternative methodology such as liquid chromatography–tandem mass spectrometry (LC-MS/MS) to quantify 17-hydroxyprogesterone plus measurement of additional steroids (eg, cortisol, 21-deoxycortisol, and androstenedione). Such second-tier screening is endorsed by the 2018 Endocrine Society clinical practice guidelines. Second-tier screening decreases false-positive rates by as much as 90%. However, understanding factors that can give rise to false-positive and false-negative screening results is important.

The male baby in this vignette has simple virilizing CAH that was missed on the first screen. While pregnant and breastfeeding, his mother was using nasal spray (Answer D) containing triamcinolone, which reduces 17-hydroxyprogesterone levels. Glucocorticoid is a potential factor for false-negative results, although the extent and frequency of such false-negative results are unclear.

The timing of blood sample collection for newborn screening is important. Samples are generally taken between 48 and 72 hours after birth. 17-Hydroxyprogesterone concentrations are higher in newborns right after birth and slowly decrease over a 24- to 48-hour period. Thus, sampling too early may give a false-positive result. In some cases of CAH, sampling may miss the initial rise in 17-hydroxyprogesterone. Hence, sampling after 48 hours of life is advised to avoid confounders. Later sampling on day 4 (Answer E) would not lead to a false-negative screen.

Low birth weight (<2500 g) (Answer A) and maternal preeclampsia (Answer C) are factors known to cause false-positive results because growth restriction is associated with higher 17-hydroxyprogesterone concentrations.

Typically, males have higher 17-hydroxyprogesterone concentrations than females do. Thus, male sex (Answer B) is incorrect.

Observations of these factors have resulted in laboratories adjusting the cutoff for 17-hydroxyprogesterone values based on sex, birth weight, and/or gestational age.

Educational Objective

Identify limitations of newborn screening for congenital adrenal hyperplasia.

Reference(s)

Held PK, Bird IM, Heather NL. Newborn screening for congenital adrenal hyperplasia: review of factors affecting screening accuracy. *Int J Neonatal Screen.* 2020;6(3):67. PMID: 33117906

Varness TS, Allen DB, Hoffman GL. Newborn screening for congenital adrenal hyperplasia has reduced sensitivity in girls. *J Pediatr.* 2005;147(4):493-498. PMID: 16227036

Speiser PW, Arlt W, Auchus RJ, et al. Congenital adrenal hyperplasia due to steroid 21-hydroxylase deficiency: an Endocrine Society clinical practice guideline. *J Clin Endocrinol Metab.* 2018;103(11):4043-4088. PMID: 30272171

Pearce M, DeMartino L, McMahon R, et al. Newborn screening for congenital adrenal hyperplasia in New York State. *Mol Genet Metab Rep.* 2016;7:1-7. PMID: 27331001

Houang M, Nguyen-Khoa T, Eguether T, et al. Analysis of a pitfall in congenital adrenal hyperplasia newborn screening: evidence of maternal use of corticoids detected on dried blood spot. *Endocr Connect.* 2022;11(6):e220101. PMID: 35521805

98

ANSWER: E) Stop GH therapy and urgently refer her to ophthalmology

This patient has clinical symptoms and signs suggestive of raised intracranial pressure from pseudotumor cerebri syndrome (PTCS), which is a rare but serious complication of GH therapy. GH therapy is one of the known causes of secondary PTCS. The highest risk period is within the first 2 years of starting GH therapy, although delayed presentation as late as 7 years after starting GH therapy has been documented. Using weight-based dosing for GH replacement in children with obesity may put them at risk for adverse effects such as PTCS. Patients with PTCS due to excess cerebrospinal fluid production as an adverse effect of GH therapy typically have headaches with nausea/vomiting, vision abnormalities, cranial nerve palsies (especially sixth cranial nerve palsy), and absence of anatomic abnormalities on brain imaging (CT/MRI/magnetic resonance venography). In patients who meet many of the above criteria, such as the one in this vignette, it is important to hold GH therapy while confirming the diagnosis by documenting papilledema (Answer E) and, in those who undergo lumbar puncture, elevated opening pressure and normal cerebrospinal fluid analysis. Thus, it is not appropriate to simply decrease the GH dosage and follow-up in 1 week (Answer B).

The primary goals of PTCS treatment are to prevent vision loss and to relieve symptoms of elevated intracranial pressure (eg, headache). After confirming the diagnosis of PTCS, treatment is aimed at lowering intracranial pressure and producing weight loss if patients are overweight or have obesity. Carbonic anhydrase inhibitors such as acetazolamide reduce cerebrospinal fluid production and effectively manage PTCS. The recommended starting acetazolamide dosage in children is 15 to 25 mg/kg daily divided into 2 to 3 doses (thus, Answer D is incorrect). The dosage may be gradually increased up to 100 mg/kg daily as needed (maximum 2 g daily in children and 4 g daily in adolescents). Common adverse effects include paresthesia, fatigue, metallic taste, gastrointestinal upset, and loss of appetite. Metabolic acidosis is a well-recognized adverse effect but is typically asymptomatic, well tolerated, and generally does not require treatment. If persistent, however, metabolic acidosis can result in poor growth. Surgical interventions are considered for patients with progressive vision loss due to PTCS.

This patient has a classic presentation of PTCS secondary to GH therapy. Thus, reassurance without further evaluation (Answer A) or referral to neurology for migraine headaches (Answer C) is not appropriate, as either option puts the patient at risk for vision loss due to further delay of diagnosis and treatment.

Educational Objective

Suspect pseudotumor cerebri in patients treated with GH based on the clinical presentation and recommend initial management steps.

Reference(s)

Malozowski S, Tanner LA, Wysowski DK, Fleming GA, Stadel BV. Benign intracranial hypertension in children with growth hormone deficiency treated with growth hormone. *J Pediatr*. 1995;126(6):996-999. PMID: 7776116

Martín-Begué N, Mogas E, Wolley Dod C, et al. Growth hormone treatment and papilledema: a prospective pilot study. *J Clin Res Pediatr Endocrinol*. 2021;13(2):146-151. PMID: 33006547

Sheldon CA, Paley GL, Beres SJ, McCormack SE, Liu GT. Pediatric pseudotumor cerebri syndrome: diagnosis, classification, and underlying pathophysiology. *Semin Pediatr Neurol*. 2017;24(2):110-115. PMID: 28941525

Reeves GD, Doyle DA. Growth hormone treatment and pseudotumor cerebri: coincidence or close relationship? *J Pediatr Endocrinol Metab*. 2002;15(Suppl 2):723-730. PMID: 12092686

99

ANSWER: B) Gain-of-function variant in *LRP5* (low-density lipoprotein receptor-related protein 5)

Of the more than 400 disorders described in the 2019 Nosology and Classification of Genetic Skeletal Disorders, approximately 10% are associated with osteosclerosis or high bone density. Although no strict criteria exist, it has been proposed that bone mineral density (BMD) Z-scores greater than +3.2 SD constitute high BMD. High BMD can be localized or generalized, with the former frequently due to tumors or Paget disease. Generally, conditions associated with high BMD are caused by genetic variants that lead to increased bone formation or decreased bone resorption. Many of the conditions that result in increased bone formation are associated with fracture resistance, whereas those that cause decreased bone resorption are associated with skeletal fragility.

LRP5 forms a heterozygous dimer with LRP6 on the surface of the osteoblast, leading to intracellular Wnt signaling through which β-catenin escapes phosphorylation and is able to translocate to the nucleus to activate genes associated with bone formation. The described autosomal dominant gain-of-function pathogenic variants in the *LRP5* gene (Answer B) have all occurred in the sclerostin-binding domain; thus, affected patients have unopposed bone formation leading to BMD Z-scores greater than 4.0 SD and resistance to fracture. However, given enough force, fractures can occur. Radiographic features include thickened cortices with narrowing of the medullary cavities, although not enough to affect hematopoiesis. Family studies suggest that most affected individuals are asymptomatic, although there can be macrocephaly, hypertelorism, torus palatinus (50%), and cranial nerve impingement leading to morbidity. The features presented in this vignette most closely align with a gain-of-function pathogenic variant in *LRP5*.

Sclerostin is encoded by the *SOST* gene (Answer C) and is an inhibitor of bone formation. Sclerostosis and the milder variant (Van Buchem disease) are due to genetic changes that lead to loss of function or reduced function of the *SOST* gene, respectively. Patients with sclerostosis present with cutaneous digital syndactyly (76%), tall stature, skull or mandibular thickening, oral exostoses (tori) often of the palate or mandible, cranial nerve palsies due to narrowing of the foramina (83%), bone pain, and fracture resistance. Understanding the molecular basis of this condition led to the development of an antisclerostin monoclonal antibody that is used as an anabolic agent to treat osteoporosis. The patient in this vignette is of normal stature for his age and has none of the other classic features of sclerostosis.

Loss-of-function pathogenic variants in the *CLCN7* gene (Answer D) affect the chloride channel located on the ruffled border of the osteoclast responsible for creating the acidic environment necessary for bone resorption. While severe forms (autosomal recessive osteopetrosis) often present in infancy with bone marrow failure and recurrent infections, autosomal dominant osteopetrosis is often diagnosed incidentally after evaluation for low-trauma fracture. Radiographic features of osteopetrosis include lack of differentiation between the cortex and the medullary cavity. Failure of normal bone remodeling leads to persistence of primary spongiosa (bone-within-bone), "rugger-jersey spine" due to vertebral endplate thickening, and transverse sclerotic bands within the distal femora. Fractures occur despite high bone density because of low-quality bone. Additional features include osteomyelitis, nerve compression, and dental concerns, which are not present in this vignette.

Loss-of-function pathogenic variants in the *CTSK* gene (Answer E) cause pycnodysostosis, an autosomal recessive condition characterized by short stature, skull deformities, underdeveloped facial bones, hypoplastic clavicles, short hands and feet, delayed tooth loss, delayed eruption of secondary dentition, and high BMD with increased risk for fragility fractures and delayed fracture healing. *CTSK* encodes cathepsin K, an enzyme secreted by osteoclasts and responsible degradation of bone matrix. This patient's normal stature and lack of facial dysmorphism make this answer unlikely to be the cause of his high BMD.

Excessive fluoride consumption (Answer A) is an acquired cause of generalized high BMD that may also be associated with bone and joint pain, dental discoloration, and fractures. Most multivitamins do not contain fluoride, and supplementation is only needed if the individual does not drink fluoridated water. Of note, fluoride was used historically as a treatment for osteoporosis and did lead to increased BMD, but it did not have a significant effect on fractures.

Educational Objective
Diagnose high-bone mass conditions and differentiate among those associated with skeletal fragility vs resistance to fracture.

Reference(s)
Gregson CL, Duncan EL. The genetic architecture of high bone mass. *Front Endocrinol (Lausanne)*. 2020;11:595653. PMID: 33193107

Williams BO. LRP5: from bedside to bench to bone. *Bone*. 2017;102:26-30. PMID: 28341377

100 ANSWER: D) Recommend proceeding with treatment of attention-deficit/hyperactivity disorder

This patient presents with a goiter, mild symptoms of thyrotoxicosis, and markedly elevated total T_4 and T_3. The presence of symptoms and the elevation of total T_4, free T_4, and total T_3 indicate that these findings are not caused by an abnormality of thyroid hormone binding or by laboratory artifact or assay interference; therefore, measuring free T_4 by a gold-standard dialysis method (Answer B) is not necessary. In this context, the absence of TSH suppression indicates the presence of central hyperthyroidism. The differential diagnosis includes a TSH-secreting pituitary adenoma and resistance to thyroid hormone β (RTHβ). TSH-secreting adenomas are extremely rare in children, and in this case, the diagnosis is excluded by normal findings on brain MRI. Therefore, the most likely diagnosis in this patient is RTHβ.

Thyroid hormone signaling is mediated by 2 thyroid hormone receptors (TRα and TRβ) that are encoded by distinct genes and are differentially expressed in body tissues. TRβ is highly expressed in the hypothalamus and pituitary and is the primary thyroid hormone receptor that mediates central negative feedback of thyroid hormone. RTHβ usually is caused by heterozygous loss-of-function genetic variants in the gene encoding TRβ (*THRB*). The resulting impairment in the central feedback of thyroid hormone leads to increased TSH levels and consequently elevated T_4 and T_3 levels. Because of decreased central sensitivity to thyroid hormones, TSH levels remain normal or slightly elevated despite excess circulating T_4 and T_3, leading to the common finding of goiter. The high thyroid hormone levels may cause clinical manifestations of thyrotoxicosis in tissues that express predominantly (normally functioning) TRα, such as the heart (tachycardia), gastrointestinal tract (poor weight gain, frequent stools), and nervous system (hyperactivity, attention-deficit/hyperactivity disorder). Conversely, hypothyroidism manifestations may occur from decreased thyroid hormone signaling in tissues that express TRβ, such as bone (slow growth, delayed bone age), cochlea (sensorineural hearing loss), and other areas of the brain (learning disability, developmental delay).

Because individuals with RTHβ experience hyperthyroidism in some tissues and hypothyroidism in others, there is no single treatment that will address all aspects of this disorder. Treatments that aim to normalize thyroid hormone signaling in one type of tissue are likely to exacerbate the thyroid hormone signaling abnormality in other tissues. Therefore, treatments aimed at altering thyroid hormone levels, such as levothyroxine, methimazole (Answer A), and thyroidectomy (Answer E) generally should be avoided.

Most patients with RTHβ (such as the patient in the vignette) have mild symptoms, as their elevated thyroid hormone levels largely compensate for impaired thyroid hormone sensitivity. Therefore, in most cases, no treatment is required. Patients with symptoms of attention-deficit/hyperactivity disorder—which are common—should be treated with conventional therapy for attention-deficit/hyperactivity disorder (Answer D). β-Adrenergic blockers may be used to treat symptoms of tachycardia or tremor. Large, symptomatic goiter can sometimes be treated with high-dosage liothyronine given every other day, but surgery should be avoided because goiter tends to recur.

Thyroid uptake and scan with [123]I (Answer C) may be useful in the evaluation of primary thyrotoxicosis (elevated free T_4, low TSH) to differentiate among causes due to overproduction of thyroid hormone (Graves disease or autonomous nodule), which have normal or increased uptake, from other causes in which uptake is low (thyroiditis, exogenous levothyroxine ingestion). This test is not indicated in cases of central hyperthyroidism.

Educational Objective
Diagnose resistance to thyroid hormone β and manage symptoms of this disorder.

Reference(s)
Dumitrescu AM, Refetoff S. The syndromes of reduced sensitivity to thyroid hormone. *Biochim Biophys Acta.* 2013;1830(7):3987-4003. PMID: 22986150

Pappa T, Refetoff S. Resistance to thyroid hormone beta: a focused review. *Front Endocrinol (Lausanne).* 2021;12:656551. PMID: 33868182

PEDIATRIC ENDOCRINE SELF-ASSESSMENT PROGRAM 2023-2024

Part III

This question-mapping index groups question topics according to the 7 umbrella sections of Pediatric ESAP (Adrenal, Bone, Carbohydrate and Lipid Metabolism/Obesity, Growth, Pituitary, Reproductive System, and Thyroid). Relevant **question numbers** follow each topic.